The Building Blocks of Life
A Nutrition Foundation for Healthcare Professionals

TC Callis

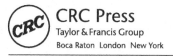

CRC Press
Taylor & Francis Group
Boca Raton London New York

CRC Press is an imprint of the
Taylor & Francis Group, an **informa** business

Designed cover image: Illustrator, Adam Speigl-James; Design Consultant: Rachael Mustoe

First edition published 2023
by CRC Press
6000 Broken Sound Parkway NW, Suite 300, Boca Raton, FL 33487-2742

and by CRC Press
4 Park Square, Milton Park, Abingdon, Oxon, OX14 4RN

CRC Press is an imprint of Taylor & Francis Group, LLC

ISBN: 978-1-032-27112-5 (hbk)
ISBN: 978-1-032-27111-8 (pbk)
ISBN: 978-1-003-29140-4 (ebk)

DOI: 10.1201/b22900

Typeset in Times
by MPS Limited, Dehradun

Dedication

For my parents who enabled me to write this.
Thank you for telling me I could be anything I wanted to be.
I wish you could have been here for this.

Contents

Acknowledgements

This book would not have been possible without the inspiration, help, and support of so many people.

Rhaya Jordan who first pointed my feet to the nutrition road.

Heather Rosa who encouraged me to ask questions, challenge assumptions, and be as curious as I could possibly be.

My dear friend Martha Halford-Fumigalli who spent time and energy finding me a publisher.

My sister-from-another-mother, Susan Johnston, whose unfailing encouragement and care over the two and a half years of writing this book has been both extraordinary and invaluable.

My beloved son, David, who never fails to make me laugh and who rolls his eyes at the merest mention of vitamin D.

And the many many friends who have been endlessly patient, understanding and forgiving when I declined invitations, bored them rigid with the intricate details of energy production, or revolted them with the inner workings of the digestive system.

Thank you all. I am blessed to have all of you in my life.

Author

For nearly two decades TC worked backstage in London's West End theatres and in the film and TV industry. But in 1999, looking for a new challenge she embarked on a Batchelor of Science degree course in Nutritional Therapy at the University of Westminster. Three years of rigorous scientific study firmly cemented her passion for nutrition and her belief in a thorough and questioning approach to evidence.

Graduating with a 2:1 BSc Hons in 2002, TC went on to work for the UK Food Standards Agency, the government department charged with ensuring food safety and standards across the United Kingdom of Great Britain and Northern Ireland. In eight years of working for the government, TC came to realise the vital importance of an evidence-based regulatory framework to ensure food safety. However, she also noted with some concern that the UK government's nutrition policy was not always as robustly up-to-date as it could be. Realising that lobbying for change to national nutrition policy would be easier outside of government, TC moved into industry.

From 2010 to 2020 she worked for the Proprietary Association of Great Britain (PAGB), a trade association representing the manufacturers of over-the-counter medicines, consumer-facing medical devices and food supplements. During her time there, TC raised the profile of vitamin D at the national level; initiated and drove a collaborative project where the wider food supplements industry and government worked together to gain a health claim on folic acid reducing the risk of neural tube defects; commissioned multiple peer review papers and academic reports on the state of nutrition in the UK; wrote Nutrition Fact Sheets for the independent charity the Self Care Forum; successfully lobbied government at EU and national level to allow the use of the word "antioxidant" in the advertising and marketing of foods, and co-ordinated nine trade associations with varying agendas in responding to UK government consultations on the use of single-use plastics and recycling.

At the beginning of 2020, TC left the industry to start working on a book. With this book, TC hopes to redress some of the imbalances in nutrition awareness that UK government policy has imposed, as well as increase understanding of nutrition amongst primary care practitioners.

Introduction

This book is not intended to be a textbook or primer. It does not set out each body system in relation to nutrition. Instead, it looks at how and why nutrition supports life and health, with a particular focus on micronutrients. And it will, hopefully, encourage readers to pursue further learning around nutrition, in greater detail, and in a more tailored and structured way, further down the line.

You cannot get more fundamental than nutrition. It underpins the structure and function of every cell in our bodies. It impacts our physical and mental health long before conception and informs every aspect of our health until the moment of our death. There is increasing evidence that feast or famine, deficiency or excess in the diets of our grandparents shows up in our genetic coding, which in turn influences our health throughout our lives.[1,2]

We can do nothing to amend the diets of our ancestors. But there is a lot we can do for ourselves because good nutrition is essential to good health, and to good health outcomes. In the current climate of overstretched health services and funding cuts, we all need to take more responsibility for our own health and well-being, in what we eat and in understanding how what we eat informs that health and well-being.

Just as nutrition underpins and informs our health, our diets and our relationship with food are deep rooted in our inner core. What we eat, why we make the choices we do in relation to food, where and even when we eat are all associated with our sense of self and self-value, and our relationships with others. Food is so much more than simply eating. It is pleasure, it is socialising, it is consoling, it is love. It is our response to stress and equally our response to happiness. Our relationship with food begins early in life and our eating patterns, likes and dislikes seem to be set between the ages of three and eight.[3,4] Amending those patterns can be one of the most difficult of all behavioural changes because of the complex psychosocial implications such change can have.[5,6]

Despite its central importance to health, very little nutrition has been included in the training of most mainstream healthcare practitioners (HCPs) in the UK. Awareness of self-care and social prescribing is growing among HCPs[7,8] but, apart from concerns around obesity and diabetes, nutrition is rarely viewed as relevant in mainstream medicine, in either policy or messaging. Yet nutrition can be used to modify, improve, reverse and prevent a remarkable range of health issues, all of which have the potential to significantly reduce costs to our over-burdened NHS in the long term. Of course, nutrition is not the answer to all our ills, but it supports our physical and mental health in all sorts of ways that we are beginning to understand in far greater depth than ever before.

This book is intended to provide HCPs, who all too often simply don't have the time to go and find out for themselves, some basic principles and information on nutrition. And it will hopefully stimulate an interest in the subject to inspire readers to go and look at areas of nutrition that this book does not cover.

Because every nutrient has multiple functions which affect multiple systems, there are some issues and key nutrients which are "cross-cutting". Vitamin D and obesity have specific chapters in this book, as well as repeated mentions in other chapters. Both have been high on the nutrition agenda for some time; public health and mainstream medicine are now starting to catch up on these hot topics.

The subject of supplementation is also repeatedly raised throughout the book. The UK diet is dire. Nearly 60% of the calories consumed here derive from ultra-processed foods, which are calorie-dense but nutrient-poor.[9] Government data shows intake of many vitamins and minerals falls far below that which is needed to maintain health.[10] And intake of fruits and vegetables is at an all-time low.[11] Almost everyone needs a boost of a wide range of nutrients, and the easiest way to do that is to take food supplements.

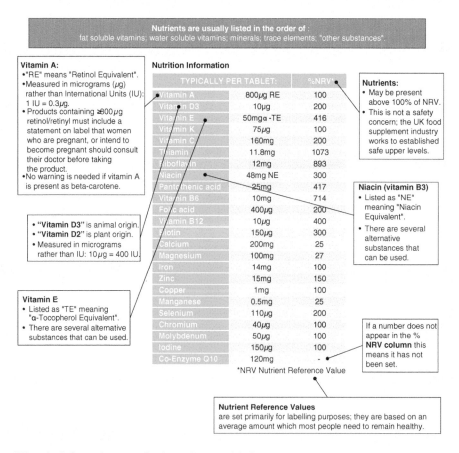

Nutrients are usually listed in the order of :
fat soluble vitamins; water soluble vitamins; minerals; trace elements; "other substances".

Vitamin A:
• "RE" means "Retinol Equivalent".
• Measured in micrograms (μg) rather than International Units (IU): 1 IU = 0.3μg.
• Products containing ≥800μg retinol/retinyl must include a statement on label that women who are pregnant, or intend to become pregnant should consult their doctor before taking the product.
• No warning is needed if vitamin A is present as beta-carotene.

• "**Vitamin D3**" is animal origin.
• "**Vitamin D2**" is plant origin.
• Measured in micrograms rather than IU: 10μg = 400 IU.

Vitamin E
• Listed as "TE" meaning "α-Tocopherol Equivalent".
• There are several alternative substances that can be used.

Nutrition Information

TYPICALLY PER TABLET:		%NRV*
Vitamin A	800μg RE	100
Vitamin D3	10μg	200
Vitamin E	50mgα -TE	416
Vitamin K	75μg	100
Vitamin C	160mg	200
Thiamin	11.8mg	1073
Riboflavin	12mg	893
Niacin	48mg NE	300
Pantothenic acid	25mg	417
Vitamin B6	10mg	714
Folic acid	400μg	200
Vitamin B12	10μg	400
Biotin	150μg	300
Calcium	200mg	25
Magnesium	100mg	27
Iron	14mg	100
Zinc	15mg	150
Copper	1mg	100
Manganese	0.5mg	25
Selenium	110μg	200
Chromium	40μg	100
Molybdenum	50μg	100
Iodine	150μg	100
Co-Enzyme Q10	120mg	-

*NRV Nutrient Reference Value

Nutrients:
• May be present above 100% of NRV.
• This is not a safety concern; the UK food supplement industry works to established safe upper levels.

Niacin (vitamin B3)
• Listed as "NE" meaning "Niacin Equivalent".
• There are several alternative substances that can be used.

If a number does not appear in the % **NRV column** this means it has not been set.

Nutrient Reference Values
are set primarily for labelling purposes; they are based on an average amount which most people need to remain healthy.

What the information on a food supplements label means.

Food supplements don't need to be expensive. They are widely available from health food stores, pharmacies, discount stores, and supermarkets. No specific products or brands are recommended anywhere in this book. From a nutrition perspective, the generic ones are generally as good as the branded ones and are certainly cheaper!

If you want to recommend that a patient takes a food supplement, advise them to read the label. The important bit is the nutrition information table on the back of the packet or tub. This lists the nutrients and how much of each is contained in the product.

Some chapters contain summary tables for quick reference, others do not because they are not appropriate. There are also nutrient "cheat sheets" at the back of the book, which consist of single-page quick reference guides to each vitamin and mineral, as well as a number of other substances such as omega-3 fatty acids. To reduce repetition, food sources for micronutrients are primarily noted in the cheat sheets.

Each chapter can be read in isolation. But reading the book from cover to cover provides a deep dive into some aspects of nutrition. It's a good place to start to build a foundation in understanding the complexities and scope of just how what we eat, when we eat, and overall nutrition impacts health and well-being, for us and for future generations.

REFERENCES

1 Brygren, L.O., Muller, P., Brodin D., Kaati, G., Gustafsson, J.A., & Kral J.G. (2017). Paternal grandparental exposure to crop failure or surfeit during a childhood slow growth period and epigenetic marks on third generation's growth, glucoregulatory and stress genes. *bioRxiv.* doi: https://doi.org/10.1101/215467

2 Kaati, G., Bygren, L.O., Pembrey, M., & Sjöström, M. (2007). Transgenerational response to nutrition, early life circumstances and longevity. *European Journal of Human Genetics: EJHG, 15*(7), 784–790. https://doi.org/10.1038/sj.ejhg.5201832

3 Mallan, K.M., Fildes, A., Magarey, A.M., & Daniels, L.A. (2016). The relationship between number of fruits, vegetables, and noncore foods tried at age 14 months and food preferences, Dietary Intake Patterns, Fussy Eating Behavior, and Weight Status at Age 3.7 Years. *Journal of the Academy of Nutrition and Dietetics, 116*(4), 630–637. https://doi.org/10.1016/j.jand.2015.06.006

4 De Cosmi, V., Scaglioni, S., & Agostoni, C. (2017). Early taste experiences and later food choices. *Nutrients, 9*(2), 107. https://doi.org/10.3390/nu9020107

5 Kelly, M.P., & Barker, M. (2016). Why is changing health-related behaviour so difficult? *Public Health* Volume 136, 109–116. https://doi.org/10.1016/j.puhe.2016.03.030

6 Higgs, S., & Thomas, J. (2016). Social influences on eating. *Current Opinion in Behavioural Sciences*, (9), 1–6. https://doi.org/10.1016/j.cobeha.2015.10.005

7 Smith, P. (2021). Self care should be central to the future of healthcare. *Guidelines in Practice,* https://www.guidelinesinpractice.co.uk/public-health/self-care-should-be-central-to-the-future-of-healthcare/456188.article

8 Bickerdike, L., Booth, A., Wilson, P.M., Farley, K., & Wright, K. (2017). Social prescribing: Less rhetoric and more reality. A systematic review of the evidence. *BMJ Open, 7*(4), e013384. https://doi.org/10.1136/bmjopen-2016-013384

9 Rauber, F., Louzada, M., Martinez Steele, E., Rezende, L., Millett, C., Monteiro, C.A., & Levy, R.B. (2019). Ultra-processed foods and excessive free sugar intake in the UK: A nationally representative cross-sectional study. *BMJ Open*, 9(10), e027546. https://doi.org/10.1136/bmjopen-2018-027546

10 Derbyshire, E. (2019). UK dietary changes over the last two decades: A focus on vitamin & mineral intakes. *Journal of Vitamins and Minerals,* 2, 104. doi:10.29011/JVM-104.100004

11 The Food Foundation (2021). Veg Facts 2021. https://foodfoundation.org.uk/sites/default/files/2021-09/Peas-Please-Veg-Facts-2021.pdf

1 Nutrition Basics

THE BASICS

You may believe you know the basics already, but the purpose of this book is to stimulate interest and raise awareness about aspects of nutrition that may be surprising.

- Nutrients are substances that provide nourishment to the body.
- They are needed for growth and development as well as for ongoing support and maintenance of health.
- Nutrients are classified as essential if they must be obtained from the diet and cannot be synthesised in sufficient quantities by the body.
- An insufficient intake of nutrients from the diet can lead to poor health and disease.
- Nutrients are split into two groups, macronutrients, and micronutrients.

MACRO- AND MICRONUTRIENTS ARE SPLIT UP INTO SMALLER AND MORE COMPLEX GROUPS

Some nutrients are synthesised within the body, for example some of the B vitamins and vitamin K are synthesised in small amounts by gut bacteria. But we cannot make enough of them in our bodies to ensure a sufficient supply to support health and therefore they are considered essential.

MACRONUTRIENTS

Macronutrients are things we need in relatively large amounts. Fats, proteins, carbohydrates, fibre, and water are all macronutrients. Some of the macronutrients provide calories which the body uses to create energy, and some provide building materials for structures and chemicals. Some support the colonies of microorganisms that inhabit our gut, while others provide lubrication to our systems and organs.

Most public health messaging targeting diet, health, and nutrition in the UK focuses on macronutrients because some of these nutrients are associated with obesity.

FATS

The fats and oils found in animal and plant foods are an essential part of the diet. They are a concentrated source of energy; they are components of cell

DOI: 10.1201/b22900-2

structures, the brain, and the nervous system; they enable us to absorb fat-soluble vitamins and they are used to produce hormones, neurotransmitters, and immune cells.[1]

Despite decades of demonisation by public health bodies, increasing evidence is showing that fats are not "the enemy" when it comes to health.[2] It is the nature and quality of the fat that is the real issue. There are multiple different types of fat, some, like the omega-3 fatty acids, are extremely beneficial, while others, like trans fats, can be extremely harmful to health. What may come as news to some readers is that saturated fats are being rehabilitated, with many nutrition researchers and scientists calling for a significant re-evaluation of their position in the diet.[3]

PROTEINS

Proteins are made up of amino acids, organic compounds which are a mixture of carbon, hydrogen, oxygen, and nitrogen; some also contain phosphorus and sulphur. Amino acids are the building blocks for our bodies; they are essential in tissue growth and repair and for the synthesis of proteins, structural components, hormones, and neurotransmitters.

We need 20 different amino acids, however only nine amino acids are classified as essential and must be obtained from the diet. A healthy body can synthesise the other eleven from amino acids in the proteins that we consume.[4] A food that contains all nine essential amino acids is called a complete protein. This can be an issue for vegetarians and vegans as, although there are many protein-containing plant foods, very few contain all nine essential amino acids. Therefore, vegetarians and vegans need to combine a range of different protein-containing foods to obtain sufficient levels of essential amino acids.[5]

CARBOHYDRATES

Carbohydrates are found in grains, legumes, fruits, vegetables, milk products, nuts and seeds, as well as sugary processed foods and sweets. They are classified as simple carbohydrates (sometimes known as simple sugars) and complex carbohydrates, which include starch and fibre.

Simple carbohydrates are the most basic form. They are made up of a single unit of sugar (monosaccharide) or two units of sugar (disaccharides). They are found in fruit, honey, and milk, as well as in refined sugar. When simple carbohydrates are ingested, they are rapidly broken down into glucose, the primary fuel for energy production.[6]

Complex carbohydrates are made up of three or more sugars, bonded together into complex chemical structures. They are found in fruit, vegetables, whole grains, pulses, nuts and seeds. It takes our digestion much longer to break down complex carbohydrates and these are often called "slow release."[7]

Digestion and metabolism break simple sugars and starches down into the most basic sugar molecule, glucose, for use in energy generation.

FIBRE

Fibre is a type of complex carbohydrate. It is so important that, even though we cannot digest it, it is now categorised as a macronutrient in its own right. Multiple different types of fibre have been identified. Four that are of key importance are soluble fibre, insoluble fibre, resistant starch and fermentable saccharides (sometimes called FODMAPs (Fermentable Olig-, Di-, Mono-saccharides And Polyols).[8]

Soluble fibre absorbs water during digestion, slowing the passage of digested food through the bowel and softening faecal matter. Insoluble fibre adds bulk to stools but essentially passes straight through us, unchanged. Resistant starch and FODMAPs are the types of fibre which fuel and support the microbiome, the colonies of trillions of microorganisms that inhabit our gut.[9]

Evidence is growing that appropriate levels and types of fibre are essential for our health. Intakes of 25 g/day can have a significant beneficial impact but average fibre intake for adults in the UK is currently only around 19.7 g/d.[10]

WATER

Even though water provides no calories, it is a macronutrient. We need it in large amounts because many of the metabolic processes in our bodies occur in water. However, we cannot produce enough through metabolism, or gain enough through food consumption alone.

The UK Eatwell Guide states that we should drink "6–8 glasses" of liquid (which includes water, lower fat milk, sugar-free drinks, and tea and coffee).[11] However, there is no guidance on what size those glasses should be. Should they be pint glasses or tumblers? Perhaps a small wine glass or a goblet? A bone china teacup or a large mug? Although there is no widespread international consensus on how much we should drink, recent work indicates that we should probably consume a total (from food and drink) of 1.8 L of water a day.[12]

The inclusion of "lower fat milk" and "sugar-free drinks" in the guidance is equally concerning. There is increasing evidence that dairy fat contains substances that are highly beneficial, particularly to cardiovascular and metabolic health.[13,14] At the same time, evidence that artificial sweeteners stimulate a pro-inflammatory environment and have a negative impact on the gut microbiome is also building.[15]

MICRONUTRIENTS

Micronutrients are nutrients which we need in small, or even miniscule amounts. Vitamins, minerals, trace elements, essential fatty acids (the omega-3 fats), and phytonutrients – chemicals contained within plants – are all micronutrients. The World Health Organisation refers to micronutrients as "magic wands" because they enable the body to drive metabolism, produce enzymes and hormones, and synthesise other substances like immune cells, which are all essential for growth, development, and overall health.[16]

Many of the micronutrients are discussed in detail at appropriate points throughout this book. In addition, nutrient "cheat sheets" have been included in the final section where vitamins, minerals, omega-3 fatty acids, and several phytonu-trients each have a quick reference single page noting recommended intakes, whether they are nutrients of concern (i.e. if intakes in the UK are below what they should be), their functions, risks from both insufficiency and excess, dietary sources, and other relevant or interesting information.

VITAMINS

Vitamins are organic compounds essential to life which are required in small amounts. They drive the processes of metabolism and work as co-enzymes which bind to enzymes to support their functions. They function as antioxidants; they are essential for the working of the immune and nervous systems; and are needed for growth and development.[17] There are 13 vitamins currently classified as essential and they are sub-divided into fat soluble (vitamins A, D, E and K) and water soluble (the B vitamin complex (eight substances) and vitamin C).

MINERALS

Minerals are inorganic compounds which are essential for life. They provide materials for body structures, not just bones and teeth, but also proteins and cell walls. They ensure proper fluid balance and are essential in nerve transmissions and muscle function. They work with vitamins in energy metabolism and are needed in the formation of red blood cells, hormones, and neurotransmitters. They are essential in foetal development, and overall growth and development. They regulate blood pressure and are vital to the function of the immune system.[17] There are 17 essential minerals which are sub-divided into two groups; minerals and trace elements.

OMEGA-3 FATTY ACIDS

Omega-3 fatty acids are polyunsaturated fatty acids (PUFAs) that are classified as essential fatty acids (EFAs) because they must be derived from the diet. There are three omega-3 fats which are particularly relevant to human health and wellbeing; alpha-linolenic acid (ALA); eicosapentaenoic acid (EPA); and docosahexaenoic acid (DHA). They are key structural components in cell membranes, and are particularly high in retinal, brain, and sperm cells. They are used to make signalling molecules that modulate a wide range of functions including stimulating and/or inhibiting inflammation, the regulation of immune cells, the manufacture and regulation of hormones, and the regulation of the cardiovascular system.[1]

PHYTONUTRIENTS

Phytonutrients are naturally occurring compounds in plant foods; fruit, vegetables, legumes (peas, beans and lentils), and whole grains. There is a huge range of these chemicals, and they can have significant beneficial effects. They are often brightly coloured, act as antioxidants and support specific organs and functions. For example lycopene, found in red and orange coloured fruit and vegetables is known to have a favourable effect on the cardiovascular system whilst lutein and zeaxanthin, found in marigold petals, are known to be protective of the eyes, helping reduce the risk of certain ocular diseases.[18,19] Even though we cannot manufacture these compounds in our bodies, phytonutrients are not considered to be "essential", but they play an important role in supporting health and wellbeing.

DEFICIENCY OR INSUFFICIENCY

Insufficiency is not as overt as outright deficiency. Intakes may be suboptimal, but not necessarily low enough to cause deficiency disease. However, both deficiency and insufficiency of any of the micronutrients can cause disease, or disfunction within the systems or metabolic processes that the nutrients work within.

Sufficiency on the other hand is not necessarily optimal. Sufficiency of micronutrients supports overall physical and mental health and wellbeing but does not necessarily improve things. Optimal intake can improve infant, child and maternal health, strengthen the immune system and reduce the risk of non-communicable diseases.

NUTRIENT INTAKES – TERMINOLOGY

There are a lot of different measurements for nutrients and the plethora of acronyms can get rather confusing at times.

Nutrition intake requirements are sometimes known as Dietary Reference Values (DRVs). In the UK these are set at population levels and are split by age and gender. There are four different types:

- Estimated Average Requirements (EARs) are used to estimate energy requirements.
- Reference Nutrient Intakes (RNIs) are used for vitamins and minerals and are supposedly the amount needed to ensure that the needs of 97.5% of the population are met.
- Lower Reference Nutrient Intakes (LRNIs) are set for vitamins and minerals; intakes below LRNI mean that deficiency is likely to occur.
- Safe Intakes (SIs) are used where there is insufficient data to set an EAR, a RNI or a LRNI.

Most people are aware of the EAR for calories (although it is unlikely that many people will know the term EARs in this context); for women the current calorie intake recommendation is set at 2,000 and for men it is 2,500.[20]

RNIs for nine vitamins and 11 minerals were set by the Committee on Medical Aspects of Food and Nutrition Policy (COMA) in 1991.[21] They are split by age, ranging from 0–3 months to 50+ and gender. Despite significant advances in nutrition science, most RNIs have not been re-evaluated since they were set back in 1991.

The only vitamin to have been re-evaluated since 1991 is vitamin D. Public health concerns around chronic and widespread vitamin D deficiency led Public Health England to ask the Scientific Advisory Committee on Nutrition (SACN) to re-examine intake recommendations for this nutrient. Their report, published in 2016, recommended a doubling of the previous RNI and advised widespread supplementation of vitamin D across all UK populations.[22]

In addition, measurements called Nutrient Reference Values (NRVs) are set for all vitamins and minerals that are classified as essential. These are set under labelling legislation at EU level and take into account population intake requirements.[23] However, the spread of dietary habits across the EU is so varied that it is almost impossible to ensure that a single number will cover all needs and therefore NRVs are primarily used for labelling purposes. It is not yet known whether, following the exit of the UK from the European Union, these will continue to be incorporated into UK food law or whether, along with other food standards, the UK government decides to get rid of them.

Safe Upper Levels (SULs) for vitamins and minerals in the UK were established in a report, published in 2003 by the Expert Group on Vitamins and Minerals (EVM).[24] This evaluated data that was current at that time for 14 vitamins (including β-carotene, which is a form of vitamin A) and 22 minerals. The report sought to establish safe upper intake levels for total dietary intake, as well as for additional supplementation. In some cases, guideline levels were set because insufficient data existed. Some of the minerals have not been established as essential but they occur in our diets, for example the trace elements germanium and vanadium. These minerals have not been included in this book as there is no evidence that they are essential to health.

NATIONAL DIET AND NUTRITION SURVEY

The UK government measures food intakes through the National Diet and Nutrition Survey (NDNS), a rolling programme of dietary surveys which has been gathering data for nearly two decades.[25] The UK also maintains a database, McCance and Widdowson's Composition of Foods Integrated Dataset which lists data on the nutrient content of many common UK foods.[26] The data gathered by the NDNS enables nutrient intakes to be evaluated, using information from McCance and Widdowson, across UK populations and against RNIs.

NDNS data shows worrying trends in both excess and insufficiency across a wide range of nutrients, all of which have the potential to have long term negative health impacts. Many of these concerns will be discussed in later chapters. However, McCance and Widdowson does not collect data on all nutrients discussed in this book, particularly some of the minerals, and therefore NDNS data cannot reflect intakes for these substances.

GOVERNMENT GUIDELINES

The UK government has set out what we should be eating in the Eatwell Guide.[11] There are concerns that the Guide is not entirely evidence based and that the food and drink industry, rather than independent experts, played a significant part in its development.[27]

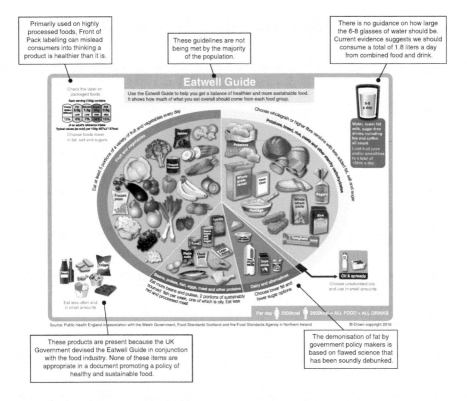

Primarily used on highly processed foods, Front of Pack labelling can mislead consumers into thinking a product is healthier than it is.

These guidelines are not being met by the majority of the population.

There is no guidance on how large the 6-8 glasses of water should be. Current evidence suggests we should consume a total of 1.8 liters a day from combined food and drink.

These products are present because the UK Government devised the Eatwell Guide in conjunction with the food industry. None of these items are appropriate in a document promoting a policy of healthy and sustainable food.

The demonisation of fat by government policy makers is based on flawed science that has been soundly debunked.

Is the Eatwell Guide up to the job?

Equally there are concerns that UK dietary guidelines are not being met by the population.[28] It seems almost nobody adheres to the recommendations made by the Guide.[29] There are probably several reasons for this. The high cost of complying is certainly a factor, and all too often public health messaging does not consider issues like social and economic factors, mental health issues, or geographic constraints.[30,31] In addition, the UK Government public health communication is lacklustre at the best of times, and this communication has proved to be particularly poor in the area of diet and nutrition over the last two decades.[32]

Based on the evidence set out in this book, it does seem that the Guide was put together without any consideration of the government's own NDNS data, or an understanding of how and why people eat in the way that they do.

THERE IS NOTHING SIMPLE ABOUT NUTRITION

When thinking about nutrition multiple factors need to be taken into account. Age, gender, socioeconomic status, level of education, marital and parental status, any religious affiliations, cultural background and the likes and or dislikes of an individual all need to be considered. And that is just the top layer. Add in the extraordinary complexities of the digestive system and the amazing microbiome that we are learning more about each day. Then pile on the nutritional biochemistry that keeps us alive and (hopefully) healthy.

Clearly all this cannot be squeezed into a single book. It can't all be squeezed into a three-year degree. But what a book (and a degree) can do is stimulate an interest in the subject and inspire a reader to go and find out more.

REFERENCES

1 Erasmus, U. (1993). Fats that heal fats that kill. Burnaby BC Canada: *Alive Books*.

2 Temple, N.J. (2018). Fat, sugar, whole grains and heart disease: 50 years of confusion. *Nutrients, 10*(1), 39. https://doi.org/10.3390/nu10010039

3 Astrup, A., Magkos, F., Bier, D.M., Brenna, J.T., de Oliveira Otto, M.C., Hill, J.O., King, J.C., Mente, A., Ordovas, J.M., Volek, J.S., Yusuf, S., & Krauss, R.M. (2020). Saturated fats and health: A reassessment and proposal for food-based recommendations: JACC state-of-the-art review. *Journal of the American College of Cardiology, 76*(7), 844–857. https://doi.org/10.1016/j.jacc.2020.05.077

4 Lopez, M.J., Mohiuddin, S.S. (2021). Biochemistry, essential amino acids. In: StatPearls [Internet]. Treasure Island (FL): StatPearls Publishing. Available from: https://www.ncbi.nlm.nih.gov/books/NBK557845/

5 Gorissen, S., Crombag, J., Senden, J., Waterval, W., Bierau, J., Verdijk, L.B., & van Loon, L. (2018). Protein content and amino acid composition of commercially available plant-based protein isolates. *Amino Acids, 50*(12), 1685–1695. https://doi.org/10.1007/s00726-018-2640-5

6 Holesh, J.E., Aslam, S., Martin, A. (2021). Physiology, carbohydrates. In: StatPearls [Internet]. Treasure Island (FL): StatPearls Publishing. Available from: https://www.ncbi.nlm.nih.gov/books/NBK459280/

7 Vinoy, S., Laville, M., & Feskens, E.J. (2016). Slow-release carbohydrates: Growing evidence on metabolic responses and public health interest. Summary of the symposium held at the 12th European Nutrition Conference (FENS 2015). *Food & Nutrition Research, 60*, 31662. https://doi.org/10.3402/fnr.v60.31662

8 Barber, T.M., Kabisch, S., Pfeiffer, A., & Weickert, M.O. (2020). The health benefits of dietary fibre. *Nutrients, 12*(10), 3209. https://doi.org/10.3390/nu12103209

9 Hijová, E., Bertková, I., & Štofilová, J. (2019). Dietary fibre as prebiotics in nutrition. *Central European Journal of Public Health, 27*(3), 251–255. https://doi.org/10.21101/cejph.a5313

10 Public Health England and the Food Standards Agency (2020). *National Diet and Nutrition Survey Rolling programme Years 9 to 11 (2016/2017 to 2018/2019)*. https://assets.publishing.service.gov.uk/government/uploads/system/uploads/attachment_data/file/943114/NDNS_UK_Y9–11_report.pdf

11 Public Health England. (2016). *The Eatwell Guide (updated 2018)*. https://www.gov.uk/government/publications/the-eatwell-guide

12 Armstrong, L.E., & Johnson, E.C. (2018). Water intake, water balance, and the elusive daily water requirement. *Nutrients, 10*(12), 1928. https://doi.org/10.3390/nu10121928

13 Bruno, R.S., Pokala, A., Torres-Gonzalez, M., & Blesso, C.N. (2021). Cardiometabolic health benefits of dairy-milk polar lipids. *Nutrition Reviews, 79*(Suppl 2), 16–35. https://doi.org/10.1093/nutrit/nuab085

14 Hirahatake, K.M., Astrup, A., Hill, J.O., Slavin, J.L., Allison, D.B., & Maki, K.C. (2020). Potential cardiometabolic health benefits of full-fat dairy: The evidence base. *Advances in Nutrition, 11*(3), 533–547. https://doi.org/10.1093/advances/nmz132

15 Basson, A.R., Rodriguez-Palacios, A., & Cominelli, F. (2021). Artificial sweeteners: History and new concepts on inflammation. *Frontiers in Nutrition, 8*, 746247. https://doi.org/10.3389/fnut.2021.746247

16 World Health Organisation *Nutrition: Micronutrients.* http://www.who.int/nutrition/topics/micronutrients/en/

17 Eastwoo M. (2003). *Principles of human nutrition (2nd ed.).* Wiley-Blackwell: Hoboken, New Jersey.

18 Mozos, I., Stoian, D., Caraba, A., Malainer, C., Horbańczuk, J.O., & Atanasov, A.G. (2018). Lycopene and Vascular Health. *Frontiers in Pharmacology, 9*, 521. https://doi.org/10.3389/fphar.2018.00521

19 Koushan, K., Rusovici, R., Li, W., Ferguson, L.R., & Chalam, K.V. (2013). The role of lutein in eye-related disease. *Nutrients, 5*(5), 1823–1839. https://doi.org/10.3390/nu5051823

20 Scientific Advisory Committee on Nutrition (2011). *Dietary Reference Values for Energy.* https://www.gov.uk/government/publications/sacn-dietary-reference-values-for-energy

21 Department of Health (1991). *Dietary Reference Values: A Guide.* https://assets.publishing.service.gov.uk/government/uploads/system/uploads/attachment_data/file/743790/Dietary_Reference_Values_-_A_Guide__1991_.pdf

22 Scientific Advisory Committee on Nutrition (SACN) *Recommendations on vitamin D.* https://assets.publishing.service.gov.uk/government/uploads/system/uploads/attachment_data/file/537616/SACN_Vitamin_D_and_Health_report.pdf

23 EUR-Lex (2018) *Consolidated version: Regulation 1169/2011 on the provision of food information to consumers.* http://eur-lex.europa.eu/legal-content/EN/TXT/PDF/?uri=CELEX:32011R1169&from=en

24 Expert Group on Vitamins and Mineral. (2003). *Safe upper levels of vitamins and minerals.* https://cot.food.gov.uk/sites/default/files/vitmin2003.pdf

25 Public Health England. (2021). National diet and nutrition survey. https://www.gov.uk/government/collections/national-diet-and-nutrition-survey

26 Public Health England. (2021). McCance and Widdowson's composition of foods integrated dataset (CoFID). https://www.gov.uk/government/publications/composition-of-foods-integrated-dataset-cofid

27 Harcombe, Z. (2017). Designed by the food industry for wealth, not health: The 'Eatwell Guide'. *British Journal of Sports Medicine, 51*(24), 1730–1731. https://doi.org/10.1136/bjsports-2016–096297

28 Prentice, S. (2020). Supporting adherence to the UK's Eatwell Guide in the general public. *Independent Nurse.* https://www.independentnurse.co.uk/clinical-article/supporting-adherence-to-the-uks-eatwell-guide-in-the-general-public/229140/

29 Scheelbeek, P., Green, R., Papier, K., Knuppel, A., Alae-Carew, C., Balkwill, A., Key, T.J., Beral, V., & Dangour, A.D. (2020). Health impacts and environmental footprints of diets that meet the Eatwell Guide recommendations: Analyses of multiple UK studies. *BMJ Open, 10*(8), e037554. https://doi.org/10.1136/bmjopen-2020–037554

30 Jones, N., Tong, T., & Monsivais, P. (2018). Meeting UK dietary recommendations is associated with higher estimated consumer food costs: An analysis using the National Diet and Nutrition Survey and consumer expenditure data, 2008–2012. *Public Health Nutrition, 21*(5), 948–956. https://doi.org/10.1017/S1368980017003275

31 Moseley, K.L. (2021). From Beveridge Britain to Birds Eye Britain: Shaping knowledge about 'healthy eating' in the mid-to-late twentieth-century. *Contemporary British History*, 35, 4, 515–544. doi: 10.1080/13619462.2021.1915141

32 Mozaffarian, D., Angell, S.Y., Lang, T., & Rivera, J.A. (2018). Role of government policy in nutrition-barriers to and opportunities for healthier eating. *BMJ, 361*, k2426. https://doi.org/10.1136/bmj.k2426

2 Malnutrition

WHAT IS MALNUTRITION?

DEFINITIONS

The National Institute for Health and Care Excellence (NICE) defines malnutrition as an individual having a body mass index (BMI) below 18.5 kg/m^2, suffering unintentional weight loss of more than 10% in the last 3–6 months, or having a BMI of less than 20 kg/m^2 and unintentional weight loss of greater than 5% within the last 3–6 months.[1]

This is very simplistic, yet also unnecessarily complex. It evaluates malnutrition within the narrow parameters of BMI and macronutrient intake without any consideration of either muscle mass or micronutrient intake.

The NHS defines malnutrition as a serious condition that occurs when a person's diet does not contain the right amount of nutrients.[2] Despite sounding more basic than the NICE version, this definition covers more ground and does not specifically include or exclude either macro or micronutrients.

The World Health Organisation defines malnutrition as "deficiencies, excesses, or imbalances in a person's intake of energy and/or nutrients".[3] This is perhaps the truest definition; it is easy to understand and allows for complex implications. Because malnutrition can include excess intakes of nutrients as well as shortfalls.

Since the early 1980s, malnutrition in the form of obesity has been growing in UK populations.[4] The burden of malnutrition, where under and/or over nutrition results in obesity and/or micronutrient deficiencies has, until fairly recently, more commonly been linked with developing countries. But it is becoming increasingly prevalent in the UK.[5]

PREVALENCE OF MALNUTRITION IN THE UK

The most recent available UK government figures show malnutrition was an underlying cause in 74 deaths and a contributory factor in 343 deaths in NHS hospitals in England and Wales in 2017 (the most up-to-date figures available when writing this book).[6] These numbers are the highest they have been for a decade. If death certificates, which include deaths outside hospitals for 2017 are considered, the numbers are even higher; malnutrition is noted as the underlying cause of 90 deaths whilst 391 note malnutrition as a contributory factor.[7]

Although worrying, these figures are the extreme end of macronutrient malnutrition, where age, disease, and complex social factors mesh, reducing overall food intake to dangerous levels. But provisional figures from NHS digital for hospital admissions for scurvy, rickets and malnutrition 2017–2018 show malnutrition is not confined to the elderly.[8] Although those aged 60+ do constitute the majority, there are disturbing numbers among those younger than 60 with diagnosed malnutrition, particularly for the specific micronutrient deficiency diseases of scurvy and rickets.

The issue of malnutrition in the UK has gained some press attention and has even been debated in Parliament.[9,10] On 5 November 2019 in the House of Lords, the Parliamentary Under Secretary of State for the Department of Health and Social Care, Baroness Blackwood of North Oxford (Conservative), stated that "malnutrition is a common clinical health problem …" adding that "the government intend reviewing hospital food policy". But malnutrition does not usually develop in hospital, it occurs in the community, which may then lead to hospitalisation. And it is extremely concerning to think that despite government Ministers believing that malnutrition is a "common clinical health problem", no policy to tackle the issue has been developed.

In 2019, the cost of NHS diagnosed malnutrition cost over £19 billion of the annual health and social care budget.[11]

THE DIFFERENCE BETWEEN MACRONUTRIENT AND MICRONUTRIENT MALNUTRITION

Despite the rise in macronutrient malnutrition, individuals not getting enough proteins, fats and carbohydrates remains, thankfully, relatively rare in the UK. Although, with the increase in poverty, food and fuel insecurity, and food bank use, those numbers will continue to rise.[12] However, macronutrient malnutrition can be either a lack of intake or excess intake and it is important to recognise that obesity, as an imbalance in intake, is also malnutrition. The issues of obesity, including some of the causes behind it, are discussed in detail in Chapter 4.

Micronutrient malnutrition on the other hand relates almost exclusively to insufficient intake. It is barely acknowledged by policy makers in the UK, yet the issue is rising. It may not manifest as outright deficiency disease, but it is just as valid when considering malnutrition because of the impact insufficiency or deficiency has on health and wellbeing.

Micronutrients of Concern in the UK

Vitamins	Minerals	Other Substances
Vitamin A	Calcium	Choline
Vitamin B2	Iron	Omega-3 fatty acids
Folic acid	Iodine	Co-enzyme Q10
Vitamin B12	Magnesium	
Vitamin C	Potassium	
Vitamin D	Selenium	
	Zinc	

UNDERNUTRITION IS PART OF MALNUTRITION

The quality of the average UK diet has declined significantly over the last 20 years.[13] Nearly two decades after the launch of the public health "five-a-day" campaign 77% of adults are eating less than the recommended quantity of vegetables, and a third of children under 10 are eating less than one portion of vegetables per day.[14] The poor quality and lack of balance in the UK diet has implications, both for intakes of micronutrients, and for the health of the nation as a whole.

Analysis of UK dietary data shows a large percentage of the population have intakes for a range of nutrients which fall below the Lower Reference Nutrient Intake (LRNI), the level at which deficiency is likely to occur.

Cohorts Where Intake of Specific Nutrients Fall Below the LRNI, Putting Them at Risk of Deficiency[13]

Teenagers (total)
- 38% fail to achieve LRNI for selenium
- 32% fail to achieve LRNI for iron
- 22% fail to achieve LRNI for zinc
- 21% fail to achieve LRNI for vitamin A
- 20% fail to achieve LRNI for iodine

Teenage girls
- 54% fail to achieve LRNI for iron
- 27% fail to achieve LRNI for iodine
- 26% fail to achieve LRNI for riboflavin (vitamin B2)
- 24% fail to achieve LRNI for vitamin A
- 22% fail to achieve LRNI for calcium
- 15% fail to achieve LRNI for folate

Women 18–64
- 45% fail to achieve LRNI for selenium
- 27% fail to achieve LRNI for iodine
- 27% fail to achieve LRNI for iron
- 16% of women of childbearing age fail to achieve LRNI for folate

65+ years
- 52% fail to achieve LRNI for selenium
- 19% fail to achieve LRNI for potassium
- 16% fail to achieve LRNI for magnesium

Vitamin D

No LRNI has been set for vitamin D. The current RNI is set at 10 µg yet the average UK intake for vitamin D is only 2.7 µg per day.[13] As discussed in Chapter 6, on vitamin D, the current RNI is far too low to maintain health and wellbeing. In addition, the plasma level of vitamin D that the government claims as sufficient is viewed as extreme deficiency by the rest of the world. Therefore, the figures below are unlikely to accurately reflect the real situation of deficiency in the UK.

Prevalence of Severe Vitamin D Deficiency in the UK[15]

Total population
- The following UK cohorts are severely deficient:
  - 57.2% of South Asian descent
  - 38.5% of African descent (including Afro Caribbean)
  - 33.1% of East Asian descent
  - 17.5% of white European descent

OMEGA-3 FATTY ACIDS

No recommended intake levels have ever been set for the omega-3 fatty acids in the UK.

Government advice is to consume at least two portions of fish per week, one of which should be oily.[16] Oily fish is one of the richest sources of two key omega-3 fatty acids, eicosapentaenoic acid (EPA) and docosahexaenoic acid (DHA). A portion is defined as 140 g.

140 g of salmon, the most commonly consumed oily fish in the UK, provides approximately 1,117 mg of combined EPA and DHA.[17]

Average Oily Fish Intake in the UK and Approximate Omega-3 Intake Calculated from McCance and Widdowson[17]

Age	Oily Fish Intake/Week[13]	Approximate Omega-3 Intake/Week
4–18	14 g	112 mg
19–64	54 g	431 mg

WHAT ARE THE HEALTH IMPLICATIONS OF THESE NUTRIENT SHORTFALLS?

VITAMIN A

Vitamin A is essential to the health and function of the eyes, particularly the retina. It regulates over 500 genes involved in cell proliferation and differentiation. It maintains the integrity of skin and mucosal cells which form the body's first line of defence against infection. It regulates the synthesis and function of many of the cells of the immune system. It is needed in the creation of red blood cells and helps to increase levels of haemoglobin.[18]

Low levels of vitamin A can cause night blindness and xerophthalmia and increase the risk and severity of infections, particularly respiratory infections.[19] It is needed for iron absorption and low levels can exacerbate or even trigger iron deficiency anaemia.[20] And although excess vitamin A in pregnancy is associated with teratogenic effects, insufficient vitamin A creates just as much risk of malformation in the foetal development of skin, heart, lungs, kidneys, eyes, and limbs.[21]

Vitamin A intakes in the UK have fallen by 21% over the last two decades.[13]

VITAMIN D

Virtually every cell in the body has vitamin D receptors, although science is still working out what many of them do. Vitamin D deficiency leads to rickets, osteomalacia, and secondary hyperparathyroidism, causing muscle and bone pain and increasing the risk of bone breakage and osteoporosis.[22]

Vitamin D enhances immunity and modulates inflammation.[23] Deficiency, or even insufficiency, has been linked to the development of many disease conditions including some cancers, type II diabetes, multiple sclerosis, cardiovascular disease, respiratory diseases (including tuberculosis), and inflammatory diseases such as Lupus, Crohn's disease, and eczema.[24,25]

Vitamin D levels in the UK are alarmingly low with around 40% of the UK population having serum levels indicating severe deficiency.[26]

RIBOFLAVIN (VITAMIN B2)

Riboflavin is essential in the formation of the co-enzyme flavin adenine dinucleotide (FAD) which is used in energy metabolism, and within several antioxidant systems which protect cell membranes from oxidative damage. It forms part of flavoenzymes that are needed for the metabolism of iron and other B vitamins.[27,28] It also works with vitamins B6, B12, and folic acid in the biochemical pathway that changes the amino acid methionine into the amino acid cysteine.[29] If there is insufficient of any of these nutrients, the pathway does not work effectively, and homocysteine, a key marker in predicting cardiovascular disease, is created instead.[30]

Riboflavin's range of functions means that low levels have wide-reaching impacts: increased tiredness and fatigue; increased risk of deficiency of iron, folate, and other B vitamins; increased risk of cardiovascular events; and increased oxidation, which in turn increases the risk of some cancers and some neurological disorders.[31]

Intakes of riboflavin have fallen by 11% over the last two decades.[13]

FOLATE (FOLIC ACID)

Folate is key to the healthy formation of the foetal neural tube in the first 12 weeks of pregnancy.[32] It is also essential in the synthesis of DNA and RNA, the production of new cells and the maintenance of existing cells.[19]

Low levels of folate slows the creation and repair of cells and, where cells have a rapid turnover, for example, bone marrow and red blood cells, this can have negative impacts, such as megaloblastic anaemia.[33] Folate's role in homocysteine metabolism means that chronic low levels of folate (as well as riboflavin, B6, and B12), increase the risk of cardiovascular disease.[34]

90% of women of childbearing age in the UK have red blood cell folate levels below the level that protects against neural tube defects.[13]

CALCIUM

Calcium insufficiency during the first two decades of life results in low bone mass and bone mineral density when they should be at their peak. This increases the risk of osteoporosis in later life.[35]

Calcium's functions go much further than structure and strength. It is an intercellular messenger that mediates the contraction of skeletal, cardiac, and smooth muscle, including blood vessels.[19] It is essential in insulin secretion.[36] It facilitates the movement of substances across cellular membranes,[37] And it is needed for the transmission of nerve impulses, effective coagulation, and the release of neurotransmitters.[38]

Chronic calcium insufficiency is about far more than osteoporosis. It increases the risk of several cancers, inflammatory bowel disease, metabolic syndrome and both types of diabetes, high blood pressure, and cardiovascular disease.[39] At a more immediate level, low blood levels of calcium cause muscle cramps and joint pain.[40]

The number of teenagers, women, and older people in the UK who are at risk of calcium deficiency has nearly doubled in the last two decades.[13]

MAGNESIUM

Magnesium is required for the synthesis and function of hundreds of enzymes that are involved in energy metabolism, regulate protein synthesis (including DNA and RNA), enable the active transport of potassium, calcium, and other minerals across cell membranes, facilitate muscle and nerve functions and cell signalling, regulate blood pressure, and support blood glucose control.[41,42] Its role in protein synthesis means it is also essential in the structure of bone, teeth, cell membranes, and mitochondria.[43] And it is key to maintaining our intercellular homeostatic balance of sodium, calcium, and potassium.[44]

Subclinical deficiency is one of the leading causes of chronic diseases, including cardiovascular disease and increased blood pressure, metabolic syndrome and type II diabetes, weakened bone and muscular weakness, neurological issues including migraines and increased risk of stroke, and increased chronic low-grade inflammation.[45]

Hardly anyone in the UK has an intake of magnesium that meets the RNI, and nearly 13% of adults have intakes below the LRNI.[46] However, intakes are not sufficiently low to qualify as outright deficiency, instead much of the UK is suffering from chronic subclinical deficiency or insufficiency.

The trouble is, most healthcare practitioners are unaware of the wide-ranging implications of magnesium insufficiency and so levels of magnesium are rarely checked. Anyone experiencing any of the health issues noted above should have their magnesium levels checked; current thinking is that individuals with serum magnesium levels below 0.9 mmol/L should be advised to take supplemental magnesium.[47]

IRON

There are four proteins that transport oxygen, haemoglobin, myoglobin, neuroglobin, and cytoglobin, and they are all dependent on iron.[48] It is needed in energy metabolism, and in immune function, particularly the proliferation and maturation of immune cells.[19,49] And it is essential in cognition, both in the development of foetus and child, and in lifelong cognitive function.[50]

The body has no specific iron excretion mechanism, therefore deficiency is likely to be the result of either blood loss, malabsorption, or insufficient intake. Iron deficiency anaemia is the most common consequence of low iron levels and it is linked with reduced circulating oxygen, increased tiredness and fatigue and reduced immune function.[51] Iron deficiency in pregnancy has a negative impact on foetal brain development and lifelong cognition.[52]

Over 40% of women, including teenage girls (but less than 2% of men), in the UK have iron intakes that put them at risk of deficiency.[46]

IODINE

Iodine is a key component of the thyroid hormones thyroxine (T4) and triiodothyronine (T3), which are central to the regulation of reproduction, growth, development, and metabolism.[19] And new evidence is emerging of the importance of iodine in the regulation of the function of some immune cells.[53]

Iodine is particularly important during pregnancy and lactation because thyroid hormones are essential in the growth and development of the brain. Low iodine intakes in pregnancy have a negative impact on foetal neurodevelopment which can reduce cognitive ability throughout life.[54]

Most women in the UK fall below recommended intakes for iodine, and 27% of women and teenage girls have intakes below the LRNI.[46] This puts any children these women may have at risk of a lifetime of cognitive disability. The UK recommended intakes for iodine are amongst the lowest in the developed world and there is no guidance for increased intake for pregnant and breastfeeding women.[55]

SELENIUM

Selenium is essential in several antioxidant systems.[56] Glutathione peroxidase neutralises free radicals, is a cofactor of other antioxidant enzymes, regenerates vitamins C and E, helps to regulate cell proliferation and protects the mitochondria, where energy production takes place.[57] Thioredoxin reductase protects against oxidation and supports cell differentiation and growth.[58] Iodothyronine deiodinase is an antioxidant which also regulates thyroid function, converting T4 to the biologically active T3.[59] Selenium is also involved in the regulation and modulation of immunity and inflammation and is essential in sperm production and health.[60,61]

Because of selenium's range of functions, insufficiency can have extensive negative impacts. Low levels of selenium are linked with reduced immune function, an increased risk of neurological dysfunction, an increased risk of developing gastrointestinal, lung, and prostate cancers, an increased rate of cognitive decline in older people and an increased risk of developing cataracts.[62,63,64,65] Selenium insufficiency is also associated with impaired thyroid function and reduced fertility in both sexes.[66]

UK government data shows low intakes for selenium in all cohorts. Over 50% of women and nearly 26% of men have intakes that fall below the LRNI, putting a significant proportion of the population at risk of severe deficiency.[46]

ZINC

Zinc is a component of over 300 enzymes that are involved in cell communication, proliferation and differentiation, the regulation of inflammatory responses and the function of the immune system.[67] Zinc is needed for the metabolism of fats, proteins and carbohydrates, the absorption and utilisation of vitamin A, and the synthesis of insulin.[68,69] It is essential in RNA and DNA synthesis, in maintaining the structure and integrity of all cell membranes, in wound healing, and in the senses of taste and smell.[70,71] And it is central to fertility for both genders, as well as in foetal and neonatal development.[72,73]

Because zinc works in so many different areas, multiple symptoms are associated with zinc deficiency. Loss of appetite, loss of sense of taste and smell, poor wound healing and skin lesions, weight loss, hair loss, fatigue, reduced fertility, increased maternal morbidity, reduced growth and reduced immunity are all signs of zinc deficiency.[74,75]

The body does not store zinc reserves and, although only around 7% of the UK population have zinc intakes below the LRNI, most of the UK population have zinc intakes that fall below the RNI.[46] This chronic low-grade insufficiency will inevitably have an impact on the health and wellbeing of the nation as a whole.

OMEGA-3

Omega-3 (and omega-6) fatty acids are components of the phospholipids in cell membranes, where they facilitate fluidity, flexibility, and permeability.[76] They are used to synthesise eicosanoids, signalling molecules used in the regulation of the vascular, renal, gastrointestinal, and reproductive systems.[77] Eicosanoids can be either pro or anti-inflammatory; omega-6 are more pro-inflammatory whilst omega-3 are more anti-inflammatory. Omega-3 fats are also essential in foetal development, particularly of the brain and retina, and they are vital to the continued healthy function of these tissues throughout life.[78]

Low levels of omega-3 create pro-inflammatory conditions and can negatively impact our health and wellbeing, from skin health to mental health.[79,80] Low intakes of omega-3 increase the risk of developing cardiovascular disease and neurodegenerative diseases such as Alzheimer's and Parkinson's.[81,82] Even the ever-sceptical Cochrane Database acknowledges that insufficient omega-3 creates poor outcomes in pregnancy for both infant and mother.[83]

Of the three main omega-3 fatty acids, the most useful for humans are EPA and DHA. ALA needs to be converted into EPA and DHA before it can be used, and unfortunately, the conversion process is inefficient in humans.[84]

The primary source of EPA and DHA is oily fish, however, intakes in the UK have been low for a long time and intakes among children, teenagers, young adults and women are particularly low.[85] As a consequence, omega-3 intakes are a real cause for concern.

REAL LIFE

We live in interesting times. The quality of the average UK diet is falling whilst obesity and food insecurity are increasing. In 2017, the UK was second in a European ranking for adult obesity and food insecurity and sixth in the same ranking for childhood obesity and food insecurity.[86] A record 2.5 million emergency three-day food parcels were distributed by the Trussell Trust from April 2020 to March 2021, a 33% increase on the previous year.[87] Low income is a key reason for people seeking emergency food parcels and there is a clear link between poverty and poor health outcomes.[88] However, poverty is not the only factor in the deficits within the UK diet.

There is a lack of knowledge and understanding of nutrition, food, and how to cook in the UK.[89] Teaching cooking in schools began to decline in the 1980s, and 10% of UK adults have never learned to cook.[90] This lack of knowledge is probably one of the drivers for the increased consumption of a type of food known as "ultra-processed".

Ultra-processed foods are made in factories from industrial ingredients, most of which would not be used in homemade foods. They are usually high in calories and low in micronutrients. And it is often these types of foods being distributed by food banks because they do not require refrigeration or much in the way of cooking facilities.

More than half of the calories in the average UK diet derive from ultra-processed foods.[91] Over half of all food purchased within the UK is ultra-processed.[92] This is a serious public health issue; for every percentage point increase in household availability of ultra-processed foods, there is an accompanying increase of 0.25% in the prevalence of obesity, and high consumption of ultra-processed foods increases all-cause mortality risk by 62%.[93,92]

OTHER ISSUES

As if all of this were not enough to take in, our food supply depends on the health (or lack of it) of our soil. And the health of our soil depends on its mineral content, its microbiome, the mycorrhizal (fungal) networks, and probably other factors that we have yet to determine. It is only recently that the value of the microbial and fungal communities in our soil have been acknowledged, and acceptance of the underground mycorrhizal "wood wide web" connecting plant life is still ongoing. What we are finding out is that our farming practices over the last seven or eight decades have had a negative impact on many elements of soil health.[94]

We farm intensively, which removes minerals from the soil, most of which we do not replace. Most fertilizers contain nitrogen, phosphate, potassium, and sulphur, only four of the 17 minerals that are considered to be essential to human health.[95]

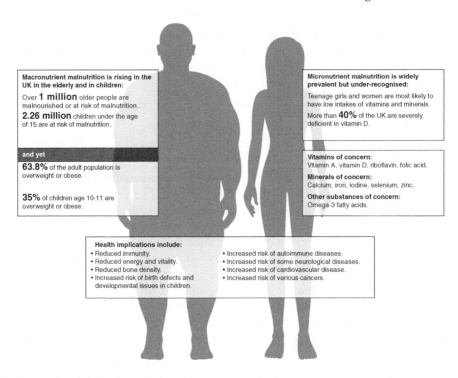

Macronutrient malnutrition is rising in the
UK in the elderly and in children:

Over **1 million** older people are
malnourished or at risk of malnutrition.

2.26 million children under the age
of 15 are at risk of malnutrition.

and yet

63.8% of the adult population is
overweight or obese.

35% of children age 10-11 are
overweight or obese.

Micronutrient malnutrition is widely
prevalent but under-recognised:

Teenage girls and women are most likely to
have low intakes of vitamins and minerals.

More than **40%** of the UK are severely
deficient in vitamin D.

Vitamins of concern:
Vitamin A, vitamin D, riboflavin, folic acid.

Minerals of concern:
Calcium, iron, iodine, selenium, zinc.

Other substances of concern:
Omega-3 fatty acids.

Health implications include:
• Reduced immunity.
• Reduced energy and vitality.
• Reduced bone density.
• Increased risk of birth defects and
  developmental issues in children.

• Increased risk of autoimmune diseases.
• Increased risk of some neurological diseases.
• Increased risk of cardiovascular disease.
• Increased risk of various cancers.

The dichotomy of malnutrition.

This impacts the mineral content of the food we grow and of the animals that eat the vegetation. McCance and Widdowson's composition of foods integrated dataset is an analysis of foods, grown in the UK. The first edition was published in 1940 and there have been seven updated editions since. An evaluation of the data from 1940 to 2019 found that some of the mineral content of fruit and vegetables has fallen significantly:[96]

- Iron content has fallen by 50%
- Copper content has fallen by 49%
- Magnesium content has fallen by 10%

CONFUSING PUBLIC HEALTH MESSAGES

Unfortunately, much of the UK diet is neither varied nor balanced. However, no one has yet come up with a clear definition of what "varied", "balanced" or even "moderation" means in relation to diet, and so it can be difficult to tell where a diet sits on the spectrum.[97] The various government departments in charge of public health messaging linked to diet and nutrition have had nearly 20 years to get the 5-a-day message embedded into public consciousness. They failed. Whilst people recognise the message, there is little understanding of what it means.[98] Commonly asked questions include the following:

- What exactly constitutes fruit and vegetables?
  - Any plant food that has not been processed including all green and coloured fruit and vegetables, nuts, seeds, and pulses. NOT potatoes – but sweet potatoes are OK.
- Does it have to be fresh?
  - No, frozen, tinned, or dried are also fine.
- What is a portion size?
  - Around 80 g fresh, tinned, or frozen, for dried foods, 30 g.
- Why does eating five apples a day not "count"?
  - Five of the same thing is not variety.
- Why is eating a range of fruit and vegetable every day important?
  - We need all the different nutritional elements in our diet that a range of fruit and vegetables brings. This includes all of the different vitamins and minerals, carbohydrates, proteins, and different fats and fibres.

A lack of knowledge is probably a factor in the extremely poor intake of fruit and vegetables across much of the population. Only 31% of adults and 8% of teenagers actually eat five portions of fruit and vegetables a day.[14] A fifth of the vegetable intake of children and teenagers comes from ultra-processed food like baked beans and pizza.[14]

None of the above is helped by the fact that there are 16 different government departments making food policy in England.[99] Added to which there are at least three more from the devolved administrations of Scotland, Wales, and Northern Ireland. None of these departments are particularly good at internal communications, let alone inter-departmental communications. And for many, the idea of communicating with either industry or the general public is absolute anathema.

SOLUTIONS?

There are some partial solutions to the issues outlined above. Some of them are quite simple, some less so. Some of them are cheap, again, some less so. But there are no 100% simple, achievable solutions; as with most things in life, there has to be a multifactorial approach.

EDUCATION

The teaching of cooking in schools declined from the 1980s onwards. It was finally lost to the national curriculum in 1993.[100] The subjects of cooking and nutrition were reintroduced to the curriculum in 2013, but decreases in lesson length, funding, and teaching resource means it has had little impact.[101] And the generations passing through school from 1993 to 2013 missed out on learning vital life skills. Those children became adults and had children of their own, but too many had no knowledge to pass on.[102]

There are long-term benefits to educating children in food, nutrition, and cooking. But in the here and now it does not address the issue of millions of adults who, if faced with raw ingredients, would have difficulties in producing a meal.

A public health programme designed to teach adults to cook would be a good place to start, if only the government were willing.

SOCIAL PRESCRIBING

Social prescribing enables healthcare professionals (HCPs) to refer patients to a range of local non-clinical services to improve their health and wellbeing. It has been discussed for many years, but the idea has only really gained ground in the last decade or so. As a relatively recent entry onto the main stage of healthcare, there is little robust evidence of its effectiveness, either in being cost-effective, or in its positive impact on the lives of patients.[103] But that is changing, and a social prescribing network was set up in 2018 to facilitate links between healthcare professionals, providers and users of social prescribing.[104,105]

Many HCPs may see social prescribing as more appropriate for vulnerable individuals. But poor diet makes everyone vulnerable to physical and mental ill health. Improving knowledge and understanding of food and cooking create positive outcomes for health and wellbeing through improved diet and nutrition.[106,107]

CLEAR MESSAGES

Creating clear messaging is something that needs to be done at government level. Nutrition policy in relation to public health once sat with the Department of Health. Then it shifted to the Food Standards Agency. Then it shifted back to the Department of Health and Social Care. Then it moved to Public Health England and from there, to the UK Health Security Agency. It looks as if it is currently squashed into the Office for Health Improvements and Disparities, but given the current shifting political grounds in the UK, that may well change.

Educating the younger generation will, hopefully, shift the country's eating patterns back to something more generally healthy. But this is a long-term solution that does not address the immediate challenges. Social prescribing could have the potential to substantially increase an understanding of and uptake of the 5-a-day messaging. But finding effective and appropriate projects to refer patients to may be challenging.

A QUICK FIX?

The nutrition policy makers in the UK government are not fans of the food supplements industry. Their view is that everyone should be able to get everything they need from a varied and balanced diet (although they do make a few very limited exceptions). But a large proportion of the UK population not only do not eat a varied and balanced diet, they may not even know what one is.

Start thinking about nutrition. Have a conversation about how patients are eating. Not just from a calories in-calories out viewpoint, but from the perspective of micronutrients. Given the significant and worrying micronutrient shortfalls that much of the UK population is suffering from, suggesting that everyone should take a multivitamin and mineral supplement is probably a good idea. If they can afford it, adding in an omega-3 fish oil or algal oil supplement could be beneficial too. And everyone, regardless of diet, needs to be taking a 25 μg vitamin D supplement every day from the beginning of September to the beginning of May.

Because boosting nutrient intake is the best kind of self-care, it protects health and wellbeing in the long term.

REFERENCES

1 NICE (2017). Nutrition support for adults: Oral nutrition support, enteral tube feeding and parenteral nutrition. https://www.nice.org.uk/guidance/cg32/chapter/guidance

2 NHS (2020). Overview: Malnutrition. https://www.nhs.uk/conditions/malnutrition/

3 WHO (2021). Malnutrition. https://www.who.int/news-room/fact-sheets/detail/malnutrition

4 Davey R.C. (2004). The obesity epidemic: Too much food for thought? *British Journal of Sports Medicine*, *38*(3), 360–363. https://doi.org/10.1136/bjsm.2003.007443

5 Lucas, E., Galán-Martín, Á., Pozo, C., Guo, M., & Guillén-Gosálbez, G. (2021). Global environmental and nutritional assessment of national food supply patterns: Insights from a data envelopment analysis approach. *The Science of the Total Environment*, *755*(Pt 1), 142826. https://doi.org/10.1016/j.scitotenv.2020.142826

6 ONS (2018). Deaths where malnutrition was the underlying cause of death or was mentioned anywhere on the death certificate, persons, NHS hospitals in England and Wales, 2001 to 2017. https://www.ons.gov.uk/peoplepopulationandcommunity/birthsdeathsandmarriages/deaths/adhocs/009064deathswheremalnutritionwastheunderlyingcauseofdeathorwasmentionedanywhereonthedeathcertificatepersonsnhshospitalsinenglandandwales2001to2017

7 Glickman, M. (2018). Deaths involving malnutrition have been on the rise. NHS neglect is not to blame. *Office for National Statistics.* https://blog.ons.gov.uk/2018/02/14/deaths-involving-malnutrition-have-been-on-the-rise-but-nhs-neglect-is-not-to-blame/

8 NHS Digital (2018). Hospital admissions for scurvy, rickets and malnutrition. https://digital.nhs.uk/data-and-information/find-data-and-publications/supplementary-information/2018-supplementary-information-files/hospital-admissions-for-scurvy-rickets-and-malnutrition

9 Nelson, N. (2019). Malnutrition cases treated by the NHS have almost trebled under Tory government. *The Mirror.* https://www.mirror.co.uk/news/uk-news/malnutrition-cases-treated-nhs-almost-18955553

10 Lords Chamber Debate (2019). Health and social care: Malnutrition. *Hansard.* https://hansard.parliament.uk/Lords/2019-11-05/debates/41E4B3AF-A735-4FD0-B37D-908568A7D374/HealthAndSocialCareMalnutrition

11 Cheung, T. (2019). Malnutrition – An epidemic. *NHS Shrewsbury and Telford Hospital Trust.* https://www.sath.nhs.uk/staff-blog/malnutrition-an-epidemic/

12 Bramley, G., Treanor, M., Sosenko, F., Littlewood, M., (2021). State of hunger: Building the evidence on poverty, destitution, and food insecurity in the UK. *The Trussell Trust.* https://www.trusselltrust.org/wp-content/uploads/sites/2/2021/05/State-of-Hunger-2021-Report-Final.pdf

13 Derbyshire, E. (2019). UK Dietary Changes Over the Last Two Decades: A focus on vitamin & mineral intakes. *Journal of Vitamins and Minerals*, *2*, 104. https://www.gavinpublishers.com/articles/research-article/Journal-of-Vitamins-Minerals/uk-dietary-changes-over-the-last-two-decades-a-focus-on-vitamin-mineral-intakes

14 Tobi R., Wheeler A., Gurung I., Sutherland J., (2021). Veg Facts 2021. *The Food Foundation.* https://foodfoundation.org.uk/sites/default/files/2021-09/Peas-Please-Veg-Facts-2021.pdf

15 Sutherland, J.P., Zhou, A., Leach, M.J., & Hyppönen, E. (2021). Differences and determinants of vitamin D deficiency among UK biobank participants: A cross-ethnic and socioeconomic study. *Clinical Nutrition, 40*(5), 3436–3447. https://doi.org/10.1016/j.clnu.2020.11.019

16 NHS Eat Well (2018). Fish and shellfish. https://www.nhs.uk/live-well/eat-well/fish-and-shellfish-nutrition/

17 Public Health England (2021). McCance & Widdowson Composition of Foods Integrated Dataset (CoFID). https://www.gov.uk/government/publications/composition-of-foods-integrated-dataset-cofid

18 Linus Pauling Institute (2015). Vitamin A. *Micronutrient Information Center, Oregon State University.* https://lpi.oregonstate.edu/mic/vitamins/vitamin-A

19 Eastwood, M. (2003). Principles of Human Nutrition (2nd ed.). Hoboken, New Jersey: Wiley-Blackwell.

20 Michelazzo, F.B., Oliveira, J.M., Stefanello, J., Luzia, L.A., & Rondó, P.H. (2013). The influence of vitamin A supplementation on iron status. *Nutrients, 5*(11), 4399–4413. https://doi.org/10.3390/nu5114399

21 Bastos, Maia, S., Rolland Souza, A.S., Costa Caminha, M.F., Lins da Silva, S., Callou Cruz, R., Carvalho Dos Santos, C., & Batista Filho, M. (2019). Vitamin A and pregnancy: A narrative review. *Nutrients, 11*(3), 681. https://doi.org/10.3390/nu11030681

22 Linus Pauling Institute (2017). Vitamin D. *Micronutrient Information Center, Oregon State University* https://lpi.oregonstate.edu/mic/vitamins/vitamin-D

23 Yin, K., & Agrawal, D.K. (2014). Vitamin D and inflammatory diseases. *Journal of Inflammation Research, 7,* 69–87. https://doi.org/10.2147/JIR.S63898

24 Martens, P.J., Gysemans, C., Verstuyf, A., & Mathieu, A.C. (2020). Vitamin D's effect on immune function. *Nutrients, 12*(5), 1248. https://doi.org/10.3390/nu12051248

25 Holick, M.F., & Chen, T.C. (2008). Vitamin D deficiency: A worldwide problem with health consequences. *The American Journal of Clinical Nutrition, 87*(4), 1080S–6 S. https://doi.org/10.1093/ajcn/87.4.1080S

26 Calame, W., Street, L., & Hulshof, T. (2020). Vitamin D serum levels in the UK Population, including a mathematical approach to evaluate the impact of vitamin d fortified ready-to-eat breakfast cereals: Application of the NDNS Database. *Nutrients, 12*(6), 1868. https://doi.org/10.3390/nu12061868

27 Mosegaard, S., Dipace, G., Bross, P., Carlsen, J., Gregersen, N., & Olsen, R. (2020). Riboflavin deficiency-implications for general human health and inborn errors of metabolism. *International Journal of Molecular Sciences, 21*(11), 3847. https://doi.org/10.3390/ijms21113847

28 Powers, H.J., Hill, M.H., Mushtaq, S., Dainty, J.R., Majsak-Newman, G., & Williams, E.A. (2011). Correcting a marginal riboflavin deficiency improves hematologic status in young women in the United Kingdom (RIBOFEM). *The American Journal of Clinical Nutrition, 93*(6), 1274–1284. https://doi.org/10.3945/ajcn.110.008409

29 Blom, H.J., & Smulders, Y. (2011). Overview of homocysteine and folate metabolism. With special references to cardiovascular disease and neural tube defects. *Journal of Inherited Metabolic Disease, 34*(1), 75–81. https://doi.org/10.1007/s10545-010-9177-4

30 Ponti, G., Ruini, C., & Tomasi, A. (2020). Homocysteine as a potential predictor of cardiovascular risk in patients with COVID-19. *Medical Hypotheses, 143,* 109859. https://doi.org/10.1016/j.mehy.2020.109859

31 Saedisomeolia, A., & Ashoori, M. (2018). Riboflavin in human health: A review of current evidences. *Advances in Food and Nutrition Research, 83,* 57–81. https://doi.org/10.1016/bs.afnr.2017.11.002

32 Imbard, A., Benoist, J.F., & Blom, H.J. (2013). Neural tube defects, folic acid and methylation. *International Journal of Environmental Research and Public Health*, *10*(9), 4352–4389. https://doi.org/10.3390/ijerph10094352

33 Linus Pauling Institute (2014). Folate. *Micronutrient Information Center; Oregon State University*. https://lpi.oregonstate.edu/mic/vitamins/folate

34 Ma, Y., Peng, D., Liu, C., Huang, C., & Luo, J. (2017). Serum high concentrations of homocysteine and low levels of folic acid and vitamin B_{12} are significantly correlated with the categories of coronary artery diseases. *BMC Cardiovascular Disorders*, *17*(1), 37. https://doi.org/10.1186/s12872-017-0475-8

35 National Institute of Health (2020). Fact sheet for health professionals: Calcium. *Office of Dietary Supplements*. https://ods.od.nih.gov/factsheets/Calcium-HealthProfessional/

36 Klec, C., Ziomek, G., Pichler, M., Malli, R., & Graier, W.F. (2019). Calcium signaling in ß-cell physiology and pathology: A revisit. *International Journal of Molecular Sciences*, *20*(24), 6110. https://doi.org/10.3390/ijms20246110

37 Cooper D, & Dimri M. (2021) Biochemistry, calcium channels. In: StatPearls [Internet]. Treasure Island (FL): StatPearls Publishing. Available from: https://www.ncbi.nlm.nih.gov/books/NBK562198/

38 Linus Pauling Institute (2017). Calcium. *Micronutrient Information Center; Oregon State University*. https://lpi.oregonstate.edu/mic/minerals/calcium

39 Peterlik, M., & Cross, H. (2009). Vitamin D and calcium insufficiency-related chronic diseases: Molecular and cellular pathophysiology. *European Journal of Clinical Nutrition* **63,** 1377–1386. https://doi.org/10.1038/ejcn.2009.105

40 Mason, P. (2007). Dietary Supplements, Third Edition; *Pharmaceutical Press:* London.

41 Linus Pauling Institute (2019). Magnesium. *Micronutrient Information Center, Oregon State University*. https://lpi.oregonstate.edu/mic/minerals/magnesium

42 National Institutes of Health (2022). Fact Sheet for Health Professionals: Magnesium. *Office of Dietary Supplements*. https://ods.od.nih.gov/factsheets/Magnesium-Health Professional/

43 Jahnen-Dechent, W., & Ketteler, M. (2012). Magnesium basics. *Clinical Kidney Journal*, *5*(Suppl 1), i3–i14. https://doi.org/10.1093/ndtplus/sfr163

44 Vormann, J. (2003). Magnesium: Nutrition and metabolism. *Molecular Aspects of Medicine*, *24*(1–3), 27–37. https://doi.org/10.1016/s0098–2997(02)00089-4

45 Ismail, A., Ismail, Y., & Ismail, A.A. (2018). Chronic magnesium deficiency and human disease; time for reappraisal? *QJM: An International Journal of Medicine*, *111*(11), 759–763. https://doi.org/10.1093/qjmed/hcx186

46 Derbyshire, E. (2018). Micronutrient intakes of British adults across mid-life: A secondary analysis of the UK National Diet and Nutrition Survey. *Frontiers in Nutrition*, *5*, 55. https://doi.org/10.3389/fnut.2018.00055

47 DiNicolantonio, J.J., O'Keefe, J.H., & Wilson, W. (2018). Subclinical magnesium deficiency: A principal driver of cardiovascular disease and a public health crisis. *Open Heart*, *5*(1), e000668. https://doi.org/10.1136/openhrt-2017-000668

48 Tosqui, P., & Colombo, M.F. (2011). Neuroglobin and cytoglobin: Two new members of globin family. *Revista Brasileira de Hematologia e Hemoterapia*, *33*(4), 307–311. https://doi.org/10.5581/1516–8484.20110082

49 Nairz, M., & Weiss, G. (2020). Iron in infection and immunity. *Molecular Aspects of Medicine*, *75*, 100864. https://doi.org/10.1016/j.mam.2020.100864

50 Ferreira, A., Neves, P., & Gozzelino, R. (2019). Multilevel impacts of iron in the brain: The cross talk between neurophysiological mechanisms, cognition, and social behavior. *Pharmaceuticals*, *12*(3), 126. https://doi.org/10.3390/ph12030126

51 Linus Pauling Institute (2016). Iron. *Micronutrient Information Center; Oregon State University* https://lpi.oregonstate.edu/mic/minerals/iron#function

52 Dev, S., & Babitt, J.L. (2017). Overview of iron metabolism in health and disease. *Hemodialysis International. International Symposium on Home Hemodialysis, 21 Suppl 1*(Suppl 1), S6–S20. https://doi.org/10.1111/hdi.12542

53 Bilal, M.Y., Dambaeva, S., Kwak-Kim, J., Gilman-Sachs, A., & Beaman, K.D. (2017). A role for iodide and thyroglobulin in modulating the function of human immune cells. *Frontiers in Immunology, 8*, 1573. https://doi.org/10.3389/fimmu.2017.01573

54 Patience, S. (2018). Iodine deficiency: Britain's hidden nutrition crisis. *Independent Nurse.* http://www.independentnurse.co.uk/clinical-article/iodine-deficiency-britains-hidden-nutrition-crisis/174833/

55 Woodside, J.V., & Mullan, K.R. (2021). Iodine status in UK-An accidental public health triumph gone sour. *Clinical Endocrinology, 94*(4), 692–699. https://doi.org/10.1111/cen.14368

56 Zoidis, E., Seremelis, I., Kontopoulos, N., & Danezis, G.P. (2018). Selenium-dependent antioxidant enzymes: Actions and properties of selenoproteins. *Antioxidants, 7*(5), 66. https://doi.org/10.3390/antiox7050066

57 Pizzorno, J. (2014). Glutathione!. *Integrative Medicine (Encinitas, Calif.), 13*(1), 8–12. https://www.ncbi.nlm.nih.gov/pmc/articles/PMC4684116/

58 Mustacich, D., & Powis, G. (2000). Thioredoxin reductase. *The Biochemical Journal, 346 Pt 1*(Pt 1), 1–8. https://www.ncbi.nlm.nih.gov/pmc/articles/PMC1220815/

59 St Germain, D.L., Galton, V.A., & Hernandez, A. (2009). Minireview: Defining the roles of the iodothyronine deiodinases: Current concepts and challenges. *Endocrinology, 150*(3), 1097–1107. https://doi.org/10.1210/en.2008–1588

60 Huang, Z., Rose, A. H., & Hoffmann, P.R. (2012). The role of selenium in inflammation and immunity: From molecular mechanisms to therapeutic opportunities. *Antioxidants & Redox Signaling, 16*(7), 705–743. https://doi.org/10.1089/ars.2011.4145

61 Moslemi, M. K., & Tavanbakhsh, S. (2011). Selenium-vitamin E supplementation in infertile men: Effects on semen parameters and pregnancy rate. *International Journal of General Medicine, 4*, 99–104. https://doi.org/10.2147/IJGM.S16275

62 Kieliszek, M. (2019). Selenium-fascinating microelement, properties and sources in food. *Molecules, 24*(7), 1298. https://doi.org/10.3390/molecules24071298

63 Kieliszek, M., Lipinski, B., & Błażejak, S. (2017). Application of sodium selenite in the prevention and treatment of cancers. *Cells, 6*(4), 39. https://doi.org/10.3390/cells6040039

64 Steinbrenner, H., & Sies, H. (2013). Selenium homeostasis and antioxidant seleno-proteins in brain: Implications for disorders in the central nervous system. *Archives of Biochemistry and Biophysics, 536*(2), 152–157. https://doi.org/10.1016/j.abb.2013.02.021

65 Post, M., Lubiński, W., Lubiński, J., Krzystolik, K., Baszuk, P., Muszyńska, M., & Marciniak, W. (2018). Serum selenium levels are associated with age-related cataract. *Annals of Agricultural and Environmental Medicine: AAEM, 25*(3), 443–448. https://doi.org/10.26444/aaem/90886

66 Mojadadi, A., Au, A., Salah, W., Witting, P., & Ahmad, G. (2021). Role for selenium in metabolic homeostasis and human reproduction. *Nutrients, 13*(9), 3256. https://doi.org/10.3390/nu13093256

67 Sanna, A., Firinu, D., Zavattari, P., & Valera, P. (2018). Zinc status and autoimmunity: A systematic review and meta-analysis. *Nutrients, 10*(1), 68. https://doi.org/10.3390/nu10010068

68 Khorsandi, H., Nikpayam, O., Yousefi, R., Parandoosh, M., Hosseinzadeh, N., Saidpour, A., & Ghorbani, A. (2019). Zinc supplementation improves body weight management, inflammatory biomarkers and insulin resistance in individuals with obesity: A randomized, placebo-controlled, double-blind trial. *Diabetology & Metabolic Syndrome, 11*, 101. https://doi.org/10.1186/s13098-019-0497-8

69 Christian, P., & West, K.P., Jr (1998). Interactions between zinc and vitamin A: An update. *The American Journal of Clinical Nutrition*, *68*(2 Suppl), 435S–441 S. https://doi.org/10.1093/ajcn/68.2.435 S

70 Lin, P.H., Sermersheim, M., Li, H., Lee, P., Steinberg, S.M., & Ma, J. (2017). Zinc in wound healing modulation. *Nutrients*, *10*(1), 16. https://doi.org/10.3390/nu10010016

71 Joachimiak, M.P. (2021). Zinc against COVID-19? Symptom surveillance and deficiency risk groups. *PLoS Neglected Tropical Diseases*, *15*(1), e0008895. https://doi.org/10.1371/journal.pntd.0008895

72 Wilson, R.L., Grieger, J.A., Bianco-Miotto, T., & Roberts, C.T. (2016). Association between maternal zinc status, dietary zinc intake and pregnancy complications: A systematic review. *Nutrients*, *8*(10), 641. https://doi.org/10.3390/nu8100641

73 Allouche-Fitoussi, D., & Breitbart, H. (2020). The role of zinc in male fertility. *International Journal of Molecular Sciences*, *21*(20), 7796. https://doi.org/10.3390/ijms21207796

74 Saritha, M., Gupta, D., Chandrashekar, L., Thappa, D.M., & Rajesh, N.G. (2012). Acquired zinc deficiency in an adult female. *Indian Journal of Dermatology*, *57*(6), 492–494. https://doi.org/10.4103/0019-5154.103073

75 Prasad A.S. (2013). Discovery of human zinc deficiency: Its impact on human health and disease. *Advances in Nutrition*, *4*(2), 176–190. https://doi.org/10.3945/an.112.003210

76 Surette M.E. (2008). The science behind dietary omega-3 fatty acids. *Canadian Medical Association Journal*, *178*(2), 177–180. https://doi.org/10.1503/cmaj.071356

77 Calder P.C. (2020). Eicosanoids. *Essays in Biochemistry*, *64*(3), 423–441. https://doi.org/10.1042/EBC20190083

78 Swanson, D., Block, R., & Mousa, S.A. (2012). Omega-3 fatty acids EPA and DHA: Health benefits throughout life. *Advances in Nutrition*, *3*(1), 1–7. https://doi.org/10.3945/an.111.000893

79 Sawada, Y., Saito-Sasaki, N., & Nakamura, M. (2021). Omega 3 fatty acid and skin diseases. *Frontiers in Immunology*, *11*, 623052. https://doi.org/10.3389/fimmu.2020.623052

80 DiNicolantonio, J.J., & O'Keefe, J.H. (2020). The importance of marine omega-3s for brain development and the prevention and treatment of behavior, mood, and other brain disorders. *Nutrients*, *12*(8), 2333. https://doi.org/10.3390/nu12082333

81 Mason, R.P., Libby, P., & Bhatt, D.L. (2020). Emerging mechanisms of cardiovascular protection for the omega-3 fatty acid eicosapentaenoic acid. *Arteriosclerosis, Thrombosis, and Vascular Biology*, *40*(5), 1135–1147. https://doi.org/10.1161/ATVBAHA.119.313286

82 Avallone, R., Vitale, G., & Bertolotti, M. (2019). Omega-3 fatty acids and neurodegenerative diseases: New evidence in clinical trials. *International Journal of Molecular Sciences*, *20*(17), 4256. https://doi.org/10.3390/ijms20174256

83 Middleton, P., Gomersall, J.C., Gould, J.F., Shepherd, E., Olsen, S.F., & Makrides, M. (2018). Omega-3 fatty acid addition during pregnancy. *The Cochrane Database of Systematic Reviews*, *11*(11), CD003402. https://doi.org/10.1002/14651858.CD003402.pub3

84 M.B., & Mensink, R.P. (2006). Conversion of alpha-linolenic acid in humans is influenced by the absolute amounts of alpha-linolenic acid and linoleic acid in the diet and not by their ratio. *The American Journal of Clinical Nutrition*, *84*(1), 44–53. https://doi.org/10.1093/ajcn/84.1.44

85 Derbyshire. E. (2019). Oily fish and omega-3s across the life stages: A focus on intakes and future directions. *Frontiers in Nutrition*, *6*, 165. https://doi.org/10.3389/fnut.2019.00165

86 The Food Foundation (2017). UK and global malnutrition: The new normal. https://foodfoundation.org.uk/wp-content/uploads/2017/07/1-Briefing-Malnutrition_v4.pdf

87 The Trussell Trust (2021). End of Year Stats. https://www.trusselltrust.org/news-and-blog/latest-stats/end-year-stats/

88 Joseph Rowntree Foundation (2018). UK Poverty 2018. https://www.jrf.org.uk/report/uk-poverty-2018

89 Jamie Oliver Food Foundation (2017). A report on the food education learning landscape. http://www.akofoundation.org/wp-content/uploads/2017/11/2_0_fell-report-final.pdf

90 Caraher, M. (2012). Cooking in crisis: Lessons from the UK. https://core.ac.uk/download/pdf/301300908.pdf

91 Rauber F., da Costa Louzada M.L., Steele E.M., Millett C., Monteiro C.A., Levy R.B. (2018). Ultra-processed food consumption and chronic non-communicable disease -related dietary nutrient profile in the UK (2008–2014). *Nutrients,* 10(5), 587. doi: 10.3390/nu10050587

92 Monteiro, C., Moubarac, J., Levy, R., Canella, D., Louzada, M., & Cannon, G. (2018). Household availability of ultra-processed foods and obesity in nineteen European countries. *Public Health Nutrition, 21*(1), 18–26. doi:10.1017/S136898001 7001379

93 Rico-Campà, A., Martínez-González, M.A, Alvarez-Alvarez, I., Mendonça, R.dD, de la Fuente-Arrillaga, C., & Gómez-Donoso C. (2019). Association between consumption of ultra-processed foods and all cause mortality: SUN prospective cohort study. *BMJ,* 365, l1949. https://doi.org/10.1136/bmj.l1949

94 Begum, T. (2021). Soil degradation: The problems and how to fix them. *Natural History Museum.* https://www.nhm.ac.uk/discover/soil-degradation.html

95 Agricultural Industries Consortium (2020). AIC Fertiliser Statistics Report 2020. https://www.agindustries.org.uk/resource/aic-fertiliser-statistics-report-2020.html

96 Mayer, A.B., Trenchard, L., & Rayns, F. (2021). Historical changes in the mineral content of fruit and vegetables in the UK from 1940 to 2019: A concern for human nutrition and agriculture. *International Journal of Food Sciences and Nutrition,* 1–13. Advance online publication. https://doi.org/10.1080/09637486.2021.1981831

97 Moseley, K.L. (2021). From Beveridge Britain to Birds Eye Britain: Shaping knowledge about "healthy eating" in the mid-to-late twentieth-century. *Contemporary British History.* https://doi.org/10.1080/13619462.2021.1915141

98 Appleton, K.M., Krumplevska K., Smith E., Rooney C., MCKinley M.C., & Woodside J.V. (2018). Low fruit and vegetable consumption is associated with low knowledge of the details of the 5-a-day fruit and vegetable message in the UK: Findings from two cross-sectional questionnaire studies. *Journal of Human Nutrition and Dietetics* 31(1), 121–130. https://doi.org/10.1111/jhn.12487

99 Parsons, K., Sharpe R., & Hawkes C. (2020). Who makes food policy in England? A map of government actors and activities. *Food Research Collaboration.* https://foodresearch.org.uk/publications/who-makes-food-policy-in-england-map-government-actors/

100 Caraher, Martin, & Dixon, Paul & Lang, Tim & Carr-Hill, Roy. (1999). The state of cooking in England: The relationship of cooking skills to food choice. *British Food Journal.* 101. 590–609. https://doi.org/10.1108/00070709910288289

101 AKO Foundation (2017). A report on the food education learning landscape. https://www.schoolfoodmatters.org/sites/default/files/%ef%80%a1%ef%80%a1FELL%20REPORT%20FINAL.pdf#overlay-context=news/food-education-learning-landscape-report

102 Vaughan, A., (2016). Failure to teach cooking at school 'contributing to £12bn a year food waste". *The Guardian.* https://www.theguardian.com/environment/2016/jul/13/failure-teach-cooking-at-school-contributing-food-waste

103 Bickerdike, L., Booth, A., Wilson, P.M., Farley, K., & Wright, K. (2017). Social prescribing: Less rhetoric and more reality. A systematic review of the evidence. *BMJ Open*, *7*(4), e013384. https://doi.org/10.1136/bmjopen-2016–013384

104 Vidovic, D., Reinhardt, G.Y., & Hammerton, C. (2021). Can social prescribing foster individual and community well-being? A systematic review of the evidence. *International Journal of Environmental Research and Public Health*, *18*(10), 5276. https://doi.org/10.3390/ijerph18105276

105 The Social Prescribing Network (2018). https://www.socialprescribingnetwork.com/

106 Farmer. N., Touchton-Leonard. K., & Ross A. (2018). Psychosocial benefits of cooking interventions: A systematic review. *Health Educations and Behaviour*, 45(2), 167–180. 10.1177/1090198117736352

107 Sampson, A., & Poole S.C. (2017). Shoreditch Trust. An independent evaluation of Food for Life cook and eat course. https://www.shoreditchtrust.org.uk/assets/Uploads/Food-For-Life-Report-May-2017.pdf

3 Digestion

Entire books could be written about every subject noted here. So, the structures and organs of the gastrointestinal (GI) system will not be discussed in detail. And, unless relevant, food sources and concerns around nutrient intake levels in the UK will not be raised. The intention is to highlight some of the more complex or surprising aspects of digestion and absorption, and the immunity, mental health, and overall health and wellbeing that the digestive system impacts on.

Whilst the heart and the brain are central to who we are, the digestive system is the core of what we are. Without it, nothing functions. The GI system is far more than the sum of its parts; the processes of digestion and absorption, and the inhabitants of the GI tract all do far more than "simply" digest and absorb. The digestive system protects us as a central part of the immune system. It influences our thinking, producing more neurotransmitters than the brain. And it supports some of the most complex ecosystems we know about, colonies of hundreds of trillions of microorganisms, collectively known as the microbiome.

DIGESTION AND ABSORPTION

Saliva isn't just about lubrication; it has multiple vital functions.

Saliva contains hundreds of chemicals, enzymes and proteins, many of which restrict or prevent microbial and fungal growth.[1] It also contains gel forming components which help to trap pathogens.[2] The combined action of these elements are some of our first line of defence against infections at one of the key entry points to the body.[3]

Saliva also contains some digestive enzymes which start the chemical process of digestion and trigger activity further down the GI tract.

The smell of food, and the action of chewing stimulates the release of salivary amylase.[4] Although food is only in the mouth for a few seconds, salivary amylase starts breaking down starch immediately. This usually stops once food hits the acidic environment of the stomach, although if the enzyme happens to be trapped inside a large ball of food it continues to work for as long as it is protected from acid.[5] But salivary amylase also has another function. As soon as it is released, it stimulates the pancreas to release insulin, preparing for glucose management once sugars from digested food have been absorbed. This "early warning system" supports overall glucose tolerance.[6]

Lingual lipase starts to break up (hydrolyse) fats in the mouth. Yet the digestion of fats is not really what this enzyme is about.[7] The breaking up of fat in the mouth again stimulates the pancreas, this time to start producing pancreatic lipase which prepares fats for absorption further down the GI tract.[8] Interestingly, this only happens when food requires substantial chewing. Food which needs little or no

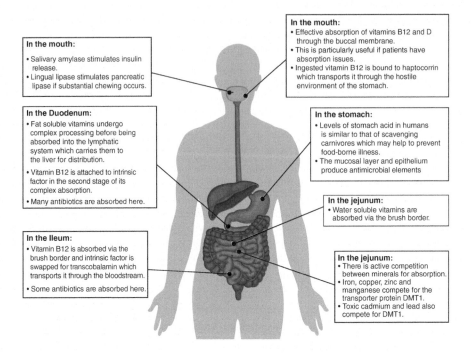

In the mouth:
• Effective absorption of vitamins B12 and D through the buccal membrane.
• This is particularly useful if patients have absorption issues.
• Ingested vitamin B12 is bound to haptocorrin which transports it through the hostile environment of the stomach.

In the mouth:
• Salivary amylase stimulates insulin release.
• Lingual lipase stimulates pancreatic lipase if substantial chewing occurs.

In the Duodenum:
• Fat soluble vitamins undergo complex processing before being absorbed into the lymphatic system which carries them to the liver for distribution.
• Vitamin B12 is attached to intrinsic factor in the second stage of its complex absorption.
• Many antibiotics are absorbed here.

In the stomach:
• Levels of stomach acid in humans is similar to that of scavenging carnivores which may help to prevent food-borne illness.
• The mucosal layer and epithelium produce antimicrobial elements

In the jejunum:
• Water soluble vitamins are absorbed via the brush border.

In the Ileum:
• Vitamin B12 is absorbed via the brush border and intrinsic factor is swapped for transcobalamin which transports it through the bloodstream.
• Some antibiotics are absorbed here.

In the jejunum:
• There is active competition between minerals for absorption.
• Iron, copper, zinc and manganese compete for the transporter protein DMT1.
• Toxic cadmium and lead also compete for DMT1.

Digestion and absorption.

chewing, for example ultra-processed food (foods containing highly manipulated ingredients created in factories) does not seem to trigger the same fat detection/enzyme release response.[7]

Some absorption of two key nutrients also takes place in the mouth.

Vitamins B12 and D both diffuse through the buccal membrane into the dense network of capillaries lining the mouth under the tongue and inside the cheeks.[9,10]

A study using toothpaste fortified with vitamin B12 found that sufficient vitamin B12 was absorbed in this way to correct deficiency.[9] Another study found that spraying a 50 μg (microgram) dose of B12 under the tongue of vegetarians and vegans every day reversed mild deficiency.[11] And a randomised trial evaluating vitamin D absorption from gel capsules and two different mouth sprays found that serum levels of vitamin D improved significantly in all groups.[12]

Oral absorption is important for both vitamins B12 and D. Intakes of both are low in the UK, and both have complex absorption routes which can easily be disrupted. It may be advisable to recommend oral sprays for these two nutrients for any patients who may have GI conditions that increase the risk of malabsorption.

In order to allow absorption, the gut needs to be permeable, but that permeability has to be highly selective. The lining of the gut is made up a single layer of epithelial cells which sit snuggly packed against each other, forming tight junctions. If something goes wrong with those tight junctions, then intestinal permeability can be increased, letting through things like imperfectly digested proteins, that really should not be entering the blood stream.[13] This is sometimes called "leaky gut".

Most nutrients are absorbed in the small intestine. The inside of the small intestine is covered in tiny finger-like projections called villi and microvilli, also known as the "brush border". The brush border massively increases the available surface area for absorption and nutrients must pass through it to be absorbed into the blood. Many micronutrients have substance specific transporters which carry them across.

Fat Soluble Vitamins

Vitamins A, D, E and K are all fat soluble, therefore they cannot be absorbed unless they are consumed in a meal which also contains some fat.

All fats are broken up by lipase enzymes, then emulsified through the churning action of the stomach and gut. The action of bile salts and pancreatic juice continues emulsification once fats enter the duodenum.[14] Emulsified fats are broken into even smaller particles called micelles. These are coated in bile salts and cholesterol to form microscopic units called chylomicrons which are absorbed into the lymphatic system.[15] Chylomicrons travel through the body and are deposited, with lymph, into the venous circulation near the heart.[16] From there they travel in the blood to the liver, at which point the various types of fat begin to follow different routes.

The fat-soluble vitamins all take different pathways, all of which are complex. Vitamin A is a good example because it is available in two different forms, retinyl (from animal foods) and β-carotene (from vegetable foods). When retinyl is consumed, it is converted to retinol whilst it is still inside the micelles. It is further transformed in the liver, into retinal or retinoic acid, depending on the function for which is it intended.[17] Vitamin A consumed in the form of β-carotene takes a different journey. It is not metabolised within micelles and is only converted into retinol in the liver if the body's vitamin A status is low.[18]

The health, or disease, of the GI tract will of course affect how well any nutrient is absorbed. However, there are several additional factors which can reduce the bioavailability (how easily a substance is absorbed and utilised) of the fat-soluble vitamins.[19]

A low fat, high fibre diet reduces fat absorption, diminishing the bioavailability of fat-soluble vitamins.[20,21] Taking fat-soluble vitamin supplements with black coffee and a breakfast of high fibre cereal and low-fat milk means they will not be absorbed, instead becoming what sceptics often accuse food supplements of being – expensive excreta.

Older people have less efficient digestive processes and age-related malabsorption is a serious issue.[22] Production of bile acids, essential in the metabolisation and absorption of fats, also tend to fall with age.[23] As a result, it is not uncommon to find low levels of fat-soluble vitamins in those over the age of 65.[24]

Individuals who are overweight or obese tend to have lower levels of circulating fat-soluble vitamins. This is likely to be because these substances are taken out of circulation and stored in body fat deposits, rather than being used for the biochemical processes they are needed for.[25,26]

Pharmaceuticals can also have a negative impact on the absorption of fat-soluble vitamins because they reduce the overall absorption of fats. The anti-obesity medicine Orlistat inhibits the production of the enzymes that break down dietary fat for absorption.[27] Statins reduce cholesterol synthesis, but cholesterol is essential in the absorption and utilisation of all fats, and reduced cholesterol can therefore lead to reduced fat absorption.[28] Bile sequestrant medications such as cholestyramine can also reduce fat absorption because bile is needed to break up and emulsify fats prior to absorption.

WATER SOLUBLE VITAMINS

Most water-soluble vitamins are absorbed in the small intestine, where substance specific carriers transport them through the brush border and into capillary blood.[29] But, in nutrition there are always exceptions, and the exception in the absorption of water-soluble vitamins is vitamin B12.

B12 is found in animal foods and food supplements. Although some is manufactured by microorganisms in the gut microbiome, it is not enough to ensure health in humans. B12 is very fragile and it protects itself by hooking onto proteins.[30] In food, it binds to animal proteins, but it must be separated from these before it can be absorbed.

In the mouth, B12, complete with the proteins it was attached to in food, is bound to a protein in saliva called haptocorrin which protects it in the hostile acidic environment of the stomach. In the stomach, gastric acid and enzymes split off the proteins it was bound to in its original food matrix, but leave it still attached to haptocorrin.[30]

The B12-haptocorrin complex travels from the stomach into the duodenum where pancreatic protease enzymes split off the haptocorrin. But the vitamin still needs protecting and so it binds itself to intrinsic factor, a protein that is produced by the parietal cells of the stomach. The B12-intrinsic factor complex moves down into the ileum where it is absorbed through the brush border. Here, intrinsic factor is swapped for yet another protein, transcobalamin. It is transcobalamin that transports B12 through the bloodstream and holds it in storage in the liver.[30]

Around 50% of our vitamin B12 is stored in the liver and it can take several years for these stores to run down. This can happen if we don't consume enough, for example in vegetarianism or veganism.[31] Stores can be depleted if there are absorption issues that impact the health of the gut, like coeliac or Crohn's disease. And as we age, intrinsic factor production falls which is why low vitamin B12 levels are often seen in the elderly. In addition, some medications, (metformin, proton pump inhibitors and H2 antagonists) can reduce the production of intrinsic factor.[32]

MINERALS

There are 17 minerals currently considered essential to human health. Most are absorbed in the small intestine, although some absorption of electrolyte minerals dissolved in water happens in the colon.[33] Mineral absorption can be either passive or active and some minerals take both routes.

Passive absorption happens when a mineral is dissolved in water (ionised) and that water is absorbed. It also happens if the concentration of an ionised mineral, that is not bound to any large molecule or protein, is greater than the concentration of the same mineral in extracellular fluids within the interstitial space.[34]

Active absorption is also known as transcellular absorption. This requires substance specific transport proteins to bind to a mineral, carry it through the cells of the brush border and push it out the other side, into extracellular fluids and blood. Many of these transport proteins are dependent on specific nutrients. For example, calcium is transported by proteins which are regulated by vitamin D while phosphate absorption is enabled by a transporter that needs both vitamin D and sodium.[35,36]

Iron is one of the few minerals that is only absorbed through active transport. Iron is highly toxic and levels in the body must be tightly regulated, but our only mechanism for iron excretion are blood loss (hardly a viable evolutionary trait) and minor losses through the breakdown of red blood cells and the sloughing of mucosal cells.[37] Therefore, iron levels in the body are regulated by absorptive control, storage in peripheral tissues like skin and mucous which are discarded rapidly, and specialist cells of the liver which act as the central iron store for the body.[38]

Dietary iron is found in two forms; haem iron (HI) in foods from animals, and non-haem iron (NHI) in both plant and animal foods.

Most iron in the diet is NHI which is insoluble and cannot be absorbed. Acids like vitamin C (ascorbic acid) and stomach acid change NHI into an absorbable form.[37] Some substances, including phytates (found in grains and seeds), oxalates (found in leafy greens and legumes), tannins (found in tea, coffee, wine and chocolate) and polyphenols (widely found in brightly coloured fruit and vegetables, nuts, chocolate, tea and coffee and many other plant-based foods) can actively block the absorption of NHI. These chemicals form strong bonds with iron, creating compounds called chelates, which cannot be absorbed.[39]

If NHI is converted to an absorbable form and manages to avoid being bound to any of the above-mentioned chemicals, it can be absorbed. It is carried into brush border cells by DMT1, a substance specific transporter.[40] Inside the brush border NHI is picked up by a protein called ferroportin which transports it through the cells. It is then passed to another protein called transferrin which carries NHI in the blood through the body.[39] Any NHI that is not needed by the body is stored in cells within the brush border. If it is not absorbed, NHI is discarded with these cells which are sloughed off at the end of their life cycle.[33]

HI makes up only 10–15% of dietary iron consumed in a standard omnivorous diet but accounts for more than 40% of total iron absorbed.[41] The mechanisms of absorption for haem iron are not yet fully understood, but it seems that HI is much more easily absorbed than NHI.

Some minerals make use of the same transporter proteins and this can impact on their absorption. DMT1 transports iron, copper, zinc and manganese, as well as the toxic metals cadmium and lead.[42] Iron deficiency stimulates increased production of DMT1 which then increases the uptake of manganese, cadmium and lead.[43] The balancing act can work the other way too, as long-term excess intakes of zinc and copper can reduce iron absorption.[42]

IMMUNITY

The complexities affecting the digestion of food and absorption of nutrients are perfectly choreographed by our digestive system and it is important to have some understanding of how it all works. But the digestive system is not simply a muscular tube full of chemicals running from mouth to anus. Everything we ingest passes through it, exposing it to more threats than any other part of the body. Therefore, some of its most important work is as a first line of defence, a complex barrier system that protects against pathogens we may consume.

A key element of GI immunity is the mucosal immune system which extends throughout the GI tract. The mouth, as the first point of entry, is heavily supplied with mucosal-associated lymphoid tissue (MALT). It makes up the tonsils and salivary glands, producing T cells, B cells and antibodies for release into the mouth and throat.[44] MALT also produces interleukins, chemicals that regulate immune and inflammatory responses. Interleukins in the mouth have key roles in maintaining the integrity of the mucosal barrier and the balance of the oral microbiome.[45]

The stomach also has its own immune system.[46] Stomach acid dissolves chemical bonds in food molecules, particularly proteins, and ionises minerals like calcium, magnesium, iron and zinc, dissolving them in gastric juice. The acid also helps to destroy food borne pathogens.[47] Scavenging animals that eat carrion, which has a high risk of microbial contamination, have extremely acidic stomachs. Herbivores have much lower levels of stomach acid, probably because their diet has a far lower risk of contamination. Omnivores, such as bears and pigs, fall somewhere in the middle of the two. But humans, generally classified as omnivores, have levels of stomach acid similar to that of scavengers, perhaps as a remnant of our deep evolutionary past.[48]

Proton pump inhibitors (PPIs) and H_2 antagonist medications, as well as age and chronic stress, all reduce stomach acid production. Reduced stomach acid may increase susceptibility to food-borne illness.[49] It can also change the make-up of the microbial colonies in the stomach.

Until the discovery of Helicobacter Pylori in 1982 it was thought that the high acidity of the stomach kept it sterile.[50] However, recent research has found that the stomach hosts its own unique microbiome. It is not yet clear what role that microbiome plays in human health and disease.[51] But evidence indicates a relationship between the gastric microbiome and the development of gastric cancer, although more research is needed to determine if that relationship is positive or negative.[52]

The epithelium lining the stomach produces antimicrobial peptides, which actively suppress certain pathogens.[53] It also produces mucus, which lines the stomach in two layers. The outer layer contains microorganisms, many of which are different from those found in the mouth and the gut.[54] The inner layer of mucus is densely packed with immune cells, reducing the chance of pathogens reaching the stomach lining.[55]

As digested food exits the stomach, it enters an environment that is a battleground between the microorganisms that exist naturally in our gut and any invading pathogens.

Like a long road with multiple names, what was called MALT in the mouth and stomach is known as gut-associated lymphoid tissue or GALT in the intestines. GALT is the largest grouping of lymphoid tissue in the body, and it produces a huge amount of our immune cells.[56] It constantly samples gut contents and can tell the difference between pathogens and the normal microbiome.[57] And when pathogens are detected, GALT actively delivers them to immune cells in the epithelium.[58]

The mucosal barrier in the gut is incredibly complex. It must be semipermeable to allow passage to nutrients for absorption whilst at the same time, providing a physical barrier to protect against pathogenic microorganisms.[59] Its depth and make-up varies, depending on where it is, but this protective layer does not always prevent successful invasion.[60] It is an ongoing arms race, as pathogens evolve novel methods of movement to burrow through it, and enzymes that can dissolve it.[61]

From a systemic perspective, one of the most important functions of the immune system of the gut is the education of our immune cells. The complexity of the gut microbiota provides a perfect training ground. Encounters with microorganisms within the gut stimulates the production of regulatory T cells, which direct immune cells to be tolerant to "self", whilst responding to foreign antigens.[62]

THE MICROBIOME

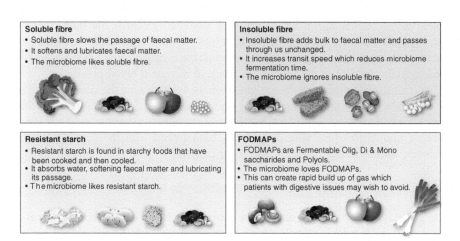

Soluble fibre
- Soluble fibre slows the passage of faecal matter.
- It softens and lubricates faecal matter.
- The microbiome likes soluble fibre.

Insoluble fibre
- Insoluble fibre adds bulk to faecal matter and passes through us unchanged.
- It increases transit speed which reduces microbiome fermentation time.
- The microbiome ignores insoluble fibre.

Resistant starch
- Resistant starch is found in starchy foods that have been cooked and then cooled.
- It absorbs water, softening faecal matter and lubricating its passage.
- The microbiome likes resistant starch.

FODMAPs
- FODMAPs are Fermentable Olig, Di & Mono saccharides and Polyols.
- The microbiome loves FODMAPs.
- This can create rapid build up of gas which patients with digestive issues may wish to avoid.

How the microbiome responds to different types of fibre.

The microbiome is as unique and individual as our fingerprints or DNA and is made up of bacteria, viruses, yeasts, fungi, protozoa and even parasites.[63] Its inhabitants are a mixture of probiotics (the good guys), pathogens (the bad guys) and commensals (are they just hanging around?). There are microbiomes on our skin, in our mouth, in our ears, in our lungs and in our gut. Every nook and cranny of every body is home to a vast range of microorganisms, and they all communicate with each other.[64]

. Probiotics are defined as live microorganisms which adhere to epithelial linings wherever they happen to take up residence in or around the body, and which provide a health benefit to the host.[65]

Commensals used to be viewed as organisms that were naturally present in and on our bodies and could, under the right conditions, turn to the dark side and become pathogens. But the Human Microbiome Project has found that commensals are far more likely to work with the good guys in regulating our metabolism and immune system and maintaining a balance which helps to defend against colonisation by pathogens.[66]

Each different environment in and on our bodies is home to a unique mix of microorganisms, although there is overlap with many microorganisms being found in several areas.

THE MICROBIOME IN THE MOUTH

The mouth is the second-most diverse microbial community in the body, hosting over 700 species of microorganisms.[67] Current evidence suggests that the greater the diversity within the oral microbiome, the healthier the mouth.[68] And like all microbiomes, there are good guys and there are bad guys.

Some particularly "good guys" are nitrate-reducing oral bacteria which act on nitrates (chemicals found in some food), chemically reducing them to nitrites which are then further reduced to nitric oxide (NO) during digestive processes. NO is a potent antimicrobial agent and a powerful vasodilator which the body uses to help regulate blood pressure.[69,70] But sometimes our actions can shift the balance of bacteria. Using disinfecting mouthwashes stops the creation of NO in the mouth.[71] And reduction of NO in the mouth can result in increased blood pressure.[72]

An unbalanced oral microbiome has been associated with the development of Alzheimer's disease and systemic lupus erythematosus.[73,74] And oral bacteria that create issues in the mouth can have a negative impact elsewhere in the body. Oral bacteria known to cause gum disease has been linked with the development of diabetes, cardiovascular diseases, and some cancers.[75,76,77]

THE MICROBIOME IN THE GUT

The gut plays host to an extraordinarily complex and dynamic microbiome. It is a community of hundreds of trillions of microorganisms which gets started before birth, and how we are born (either vaginal birth or caesarean section), can influence our microbiome throughout our lives.[78,79] The symbiotic relationship between us and our microbiome has been going on for a long time. Recent research has found that tens of thousands of years ago, some of our distant ancestors were carrying around some of the exact same species of microbes in their guts![80]

Diversity is key to the success of the microbiome; loss of diversity can result in pathogens increasing and commensals turning bad. This in turn can negatively impact on the immune system, can increase inflammation, and can reduce the integrity of the tight junctions in the gut wall and the overall health of the gut.[81] But over the last century the human microbiome has been getting smaller. And it has been happening so fast that we have not had time to find out what it is that we have been losing.[82]

Some of the probiotic inhabitants of our gut synthesise nutrients. Perhaps the best-known example of this is vitamin B12. This nutrient cannot be made directly by either plants or animals, instead it is manufactured by bacteria.[83] The microbiome also synthesises some other vitamins: B1; folate; biotin; B2; B5; and vitamin K. This production supplies some of the nutritional needs of the cells lining the gut.[84] But gut bacteria alone cannot provide enough of any of these nutrients to fully meet our needs and therefore it is imperative that we obtain them from our diet.

As with all microbiomes, some of the inhabitants of the gut are probiotic, some are pathogens, but the majority are commensals, which can be swayed, depending on the gut environment. Unfortunately, the balance between these three can easily be tipped away from the beneficial and towards the pathogenic. This is known as dysbiosis and it can be brought about by a number of factors, many of which are within our own control.

A diet low in fibre but high in sugar and ultra-processed foods can create a gut environment that favours pathogens more than probiotics.[85] Ultra-processed food, which comes up repeatedly in this book, is defined as:

"industrial formulations with many ingredients which include substances not commonly used in food preparations, and additives intended to imitate sensory qualities of unprocessed or minimally processed foods, used to disguise undesirable qualities of the final product".[86]

Currently ultra-processed food provides around 57% of total energy intake in the average UK diet.[87]

Antibiotics can have a negative impact on the microbiome, dramatically reducing both diversity and overall numbers. Even a short course can have a long-term effect on the microbial communities that inhabit the GI tract.[88] However, the negative impact of antibiotics may depend on where they are absorbed. Topically applied or intravenous antibiotics have a relatively low impact on the colonies of microorganisms in the gut. Most oral antibiotics are absorbed in the duodenum and ileum and some are more easily absorbed than others. If antibiotics are easily absorbed, higher up in the gut, then less reaches the colon where much of the microbiome resides.[89]

The gut microbiome is also extremely sensitive to stress because stress triggers changes to steroid hormone production which can have a negative impact on bacterial colonies in the gut.[90] This may be why stress is such a significant strut in the umbrella of inflammatory bowel disease (IBD).[91] Interestingly, we may be able to modify our response to stress by adding specific types of bacteria into the gut through consumption of some probiotic supplements.[92]

There are links between dysbiosis and a range of chronic diseases, particularly those associated with inflammation. These include metabolic disorders like obesity and diabetes; high blood pressure; auto-immune disorders like rheumatoid arthritis, psoriasis and atopic allergic responses; and even colorectal cancers.[93,94,95,96,97]

Even slightly reduced microbial diversity in the gut has been linked with inflammation and disease markers for both acute and chronic disease.[98,99] Obesity, diet, lifestyle and levels of physical activity all impact on the overall diversity of the microbiome.[100] A varied diet, regular exercise and a healthy body weight are all associated with a greater diversity of microorganisms in the gut.

FIBRE

Our gut microbiome is clearly important – so how can we support it? On the surface the answer is simply "lots of fibre". But there is fibre, and then there is fibre.

The UK recommendation for daily fibre intake for adults is 30 grams per day. But only 9% of adults meet that recommendation, average fibre intake for most adults in the UK is only around 19.7 grams a day.[101]

Fibre has a range of benefits, many of which go far beyond keeping the contents of our gut moving. Intakes of fibre above 25 grams per day improve both insulin sensitivity and overall metabolic health, provide a beneficial influence on inflammation within the gut and across the wider body, and reduce the risk of cardiovascular disease and colorectal cancer.[102,103] How much of this is down to the fibre itself, and how much is down to the microbiome has not yet been fully explored.

What we do know is that the probiotic organisms in our gut love dietary fibre. The human gut did not evolve to break fibre down effectively, but the microbiome is all about breaking fibre down, largely by fermentation.[104] There are lots of different types of fibre and all are important for our health.

Soluble fibre absorbs water and turns into gel during digestion. The gel slows down the processes which digest proteins, fats and carbohydrates. This means a slower and more prolonged release of nutrients for absorption. The gel also softens and lubricates faecal matter, making it pass through the gut more easily. Sources of soluble fibre include fruit, vegetables, oat bran, barley, flax seed, psyllium and pulses (beans, peas and lentils). The microbiome quite likes soluble fibre.[104]

Insoluble fibre does not absorb much water, instead it adds bulk to stools which gives the gut something to push against in peristaltic motion (the muscular contractions that move the contents of the digestive system along from mouth to anus). Sources of insoluble fibre include wheat bran, the skins of fruit and vegetables, nuts, seeds, and whole grains. The microbiome mostly ignores insoluble fibre and so it generally passes through us largely unchanged.[105]

Resistant starch is, (as the name suggests), not digested. Although it is not strictly fibre, it acts quite a lot like soluble fibre. It is found in whole grains, seeds and pulses, and is formed when some starchy foods like potatoes, rice and pasta are cooked. The level of resistant starch increases if these foods are cooked and then cooled before consumption. Reheating the foods does not reduce the level of resistant starch and, because we cannot digest it, it does not provide any calories, so potatoes which have been cooked and cooled have a lower calorific value than the equivalent amount of freshly cooked potatoes (same goes for pasta, rice, beans etc). The microbiome really likes resistant starch.[106]

And then there are Fermentable Olig-, Di-, Mono-saccharides And Polyols, or FODMAPs, that, like resistant starch, are a kind of carbohydrate. The inhabitants of the microbiome absolutely love FODMAPs and rapidly ferment them. The effect of that fermentation can be swiftly felt as it produces a large amount of gas very quickly. And this can be uncomfortable, or even potentially dangerous for individuals who suffer from inflammatory bowel disease as the bowel will stretch to accommodate the gas, which can trigger further inflammation.[107]

Of course, there is only one exit point for that gas. Although flatulence may be viewed as a socially unacceptable embarrassment, it is a sign that your digestive tract and its inhabitants are working well, and that your diet contains plenty of the right kind of fibre. Most fruit, vegetables, nuts, seeds, pulses and whole grains contain a combination of different types of fibres which feed and increase the diversity and numbers of probiotic bacteria.[108] Even breast milk contains prebiotic fibres, called human milk oligosaccharides, which support the development of the infant microbiome.[109]

SHORT CHAIN FATTY ACIDS

When the microbes in our gut ferment the fibre we eat, they produce short chain fatty acids (SCFAs), particularly acetate, propionate, and butyrate, with acetate being the most abundant.[110,111]

For substances that most people have never heard of, SCFAs pack a mighty big punch and they have multiple functions all over the body. All cells are covered in surface receptors which function as message "inboxes" for communications carried by a range of messenger molecules including hormones, neurotransmitters and SCFAs. SCFAs are known to bind to these receptors and work is ongoing to determine which SCFAs bind to which cells, and what this may trigger.[112]

SCFAs are the fuel of choice for the cells lining the gut, providing most of their energy needs and maintaining the tight junctions needed to ensure selective permeability.[113] They regulate the production, inhibition, and activation of inflammatory chemicals.[114] They promote the production of some immune factors, including T cells.[115] They increase the absorption of calcium, iron and magnesium and manage the homeostasis of bone mass.[116] They are involved in the regulation of appetite and metabolic processes, particularly glucose metabolism and insulin sensitivity.[117,118] They may mitigate some of the risk of cardiovascular disease.[119] They are central to the synthesis of cholesterol, they may stimulate apoptosis in colorectal cancer cells, and they facilitate communication between the gut and the brain.[120,121,122]

And they seem to be involved in the development and progression of neurological disorders. Dysbiosis and unbalanced levels of SCFAs occur in both Alzheimer's and Parkinson's diseases as well as in individuals on the autistic spectrum disorders and people suffering from depression.[112] Recent work indicates that increasing levels of the SCFA butyrate may even alleviate some of the symptoms of Alzheimer's and Parkinson's diseases.[123]

So, eating a diet rich in fibre supports probiotic bacteria and stimulates the production of health supporting processes and chemicals. But what about putting probiotics back into the system?

FERMENTED FOODS

There are dozens of fermented foods from all over the world. Some of the more well-known are kefir, live yoghurt, sauerkraut, kimchi, soya sauce, kombucha and miso. The fermentation processes of these foods are undertaken by probiotic bacteria and, in some cases, yeasts. These bacteria and yeasts ferment the fibres and sugars in the base food, for example cabbage, in sauerkraut. In that fermentation process probiotics proliferate and, when we eat fermented foods, they populate our gut.[124]

There are thousands of years of traditional use of such foods from all over the world and, whilst there is empirical evidence for their health-giving properties, the fermentation of food was probably originally developed as a food preservation method.[125] However, interest in the health benefits of fermented foods has been growing for the last few decades.[126] There is growing evidence for beneficial effects of fermented foods in weight maintenance; improved glucose metabolism, reduced risk of Type II Diabetes, and reduced risk of cardiovascular disease.[127] And eating fermented foods not only rapidly increases microbiome biodiversity, it also reduces inflammatory markers.[128]

A healthy microbiome is about maintaining diversity and balance. Every type of fermented food contains different types of microorganisms; you cannot make yoghurt with a kombucha scoby (a Symbiotic Colony Of Bacteria and Yeast) or sauerkraut with bread yeast. To keep the microbiome happy, it is advisable to eat a range of fermented foods as well as a wide variety of different fibres.

Of course, there are also a wide selection of probiotic food supplements available from good health-food stores and chemists and these can be particularly useful to suggest to patients following antibiotic use or after any GI upset.

THE SECOND BRAIN

As if digestion, absorption, immunity and providing living space for colonies of extraordinary health-promoting microorganisms wasn't enough, the gut is increasingly being recognised as a second brain. The complexities of the physical and chemical connections between the gut and the brain have generated so much interest that a whole new area of study has opened up, looking at the gut-brain axis. Recently, this has been expanded to include the influence of the microbiome. This complex multidirectional communication network is now referred to as the microbiota-gut-brain axis.

There are multiple connections between the GI tract and our nervous systems.

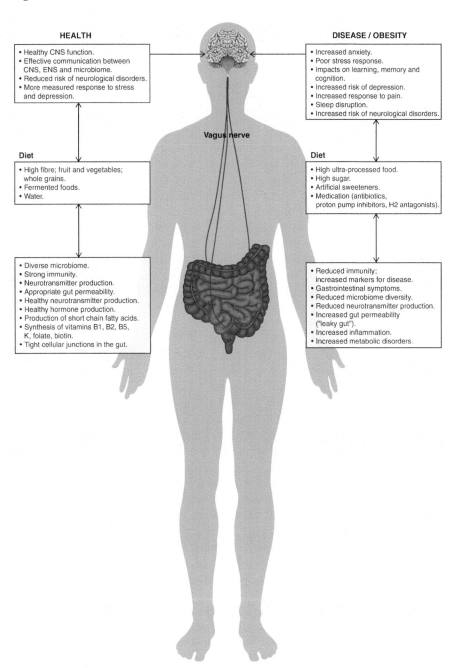

HEALTH

- Healthy CNS function.
- Effective communication between CNS, ENS and microbiome.
- Reduced risk of neurological disorders.
- More measured response to stress and depression.

DISEASE / OBESITY

- Increased anxiety.
- Poor stress response.
- Impacts on learning, memory and cognition.
- Increased risk of depression.
- Increased response to pain.
- Sleep disruption.
- Increased risk of neurological disorders.

Vagus nerve

Diet

- High fibre; fruit and vegetables; whole grains.
- Fermented foods.
- Water.

Diet

- High ultra-processed food.
- High sugar.
- Artificial sweeteners.
- Medication (antibiotics, proton pump inhibitors, H2 antagonists).

- Diverse microbiome.
- Strong immunity.
- Neurotransmitter production.
- Appropriate gut permeability.
- Healthy neurotransmitter production.
- Healthy hormone production.
- Production of short chain fatty acids.
- Synthesis of vitamins B1, B2, B5, K, folate, biotin.
- Tight cellular junctions in the gut.

- Reduced immunity; increased markers for disease.
- Gastrointestinal symptoms.
- Reduced microbiome diversity.
- Reduced neurotransmitter production.
- Increased gut permeability ("leaky gut").
- Increased inflammation.
- Increased metabolic disorders.

The Microbiota-Gut-Brain Axis.

THE NERVOUS SYSTEMS IN THE GUT

The sympathetic nervous system is usually connected with fight or flight but, in the GI tract, it slows things down, inhibits muscle contractions and stops the secretion of the various fluids the GI tract needs to function. This slowing down allows blood to move away from the GI tract and towards other organs that have more relevance to running away or fighting to survive.[129]

The parasympathetic nervous system, sometimes called the rest and digest system, controls unconscious body functions. This includes the movement of food through the GI tract, digestion and the secretion of necessary fluids, enzymes and other chemicals. It also regulates the function of the vagus nerve which sends and receives signals to and from the brain, the heart, the lungs, and the GI tract.

The vagus nerve sends information about hunger, fullness, metabolism, stress, and inflammation in the gut, to the brain.[130] We now know that the microbiome also uses the vagus nerve to send signals to the brain. Metabolites produced by the microbiome trigger vagal nerve transmissions to the central nervous system.[131] And the brain responds through the same pathway, sending signals through the vagus nerve to the gut, for example stimulating the cells lining the gut to shuffle up more closely, reinforcing the tight junctions.[132] There is increasing evidence that if this two-way communication goes wrong, it can have a significant impact on gut health, mental health and neurological health.[133]

The enteric nervous system (ENS) is a self-contained system that has both sensory and motor functions. It operates independently of the central nervous system and governs the GI tract.[134] The ENS has around half a billion neurons, as many as the spinal cord, and is similar to the brain in its size, complexity and production of neurotransmitters, hormones, and other messenger chemicals.[135] But do the processes of digestion really need that much neural input?

The ENS is the office manager for the whole of the GI tract. It looks after the real estate (the organs, their functions, repair and maintenance). It organises meetings and get-togethers (the action of digestion). It makes sure the supply of energy (metabolism) and lines of communication (the production of and response to neurotransmitters and hormones) continue to function. It pays the bills (co-ordinating the absorption of nutrients and energy generation) and keeps security tight (regulating the intestinal immune system).[136] And it acts as a two-way communication conduit (through the synthesis of neurotransmitters and hormones) between senior management (the body and central nervous system) and the staff (the microbiome).[136,137]

On top of all of that, the ENS is capable of learning in response to different stimuli, for example tailoring responses to any stretching of the stomach or gut, as well as stress, inflammation and infection.[138] And it appears the ENS has even more up its sleeve. It is being linked to neurodegenerative disorders like Alzheimer's and Parkinson's previously believed to be specific to the central nervous system.[139] A possible link between autistic spectrum disorders and the relationship between the ENS, the brain, and the microbiome is also being investigated.[140,141] And there is evidence that the depression and anxiety which was thought to trigger IBS, may actually be driven by irritation within the GI tract, rather than the other way around.[142]

Although the vagus nerve carries two-way communication between the ENS and the central nervous system, amazingly, the gut can continue to function without that exchange.[130]

NEUROTRANSMITTERS

The other key components of second brain function are chemicals, including neurotransmitters.

It is only relatively recently that the relevance of neurotransmitters to the function of the GI tract has become apparent. We now know that neurotransmitters help to regulate the movement of the gut and the absorption of nutrients, as well as systemic immunity, and inflammation.[143]

Over 90% of the serotonin in the body is synthesised in the gut by specialist cells which are coached by specific bacteria in the microbiome.[144] Serotonin was previously thought of as a chemical that stabilises mood and supports feelings of wellbeing and happiness. But we now know it has functions within the gut, including the stimulation of peristaltic motion to maintain gut motility, the secretion of mucus, nutrient absorption, and the regulation of metabolic homeostasis.[145,146]

It is also involved in immunity and inflammation. Almost all immune cells have serotonin receptors although the response to serotonin varies between the type of immune cells. In some it seems to be pro-inflammatory whilst in others it appears to be anti-inflammatory.[147] It plays a role in some autoimmune diseases including inflammatory bowel disease, Type I Diabetes, rheumatoid diseases, and multiple sclerosis.[148] It also seems to work directly on some pathogens, recent work has found that serotonin in the gut inhibits the pathogen enterohemorrhagic *E. coli*, decreasing its virulence and slowing its multiplication.[149]

GLUTAMATE AND GABA

Glutamate is one of the most abundant amino acids in the body. All protein containing foods, and any food with a strong umami flavour such as mushrooms, soy sauce, and monosodium glutamate are sources of glutamate.[150] It has a role in our sense of taste, particularly to the savoury sensation umami.[151] It is one of the favourite fuel sources for the cells lining the gut and is essential in maintaining the integrity of the gut and its mucosa.[152] And it is used in the production of many other molecules.[153]

In fact, glutamate is so important that we cannot rely on dietary sources alone and it is synthesised by the microbiome as well as the neurons and glial cells in the ENS.[154] Because glutamate is key to both the stimulation and the damping down of neural activity.

It is one of the main excitatory neurotransmitters which stimulate neural activity in the central nervous system and in the gut.[155] Within the gut, glutamate helps regulate both sensory and motor functions and stimulates two-way communication between the ENS and the CNS.[156] Glutamate's interaction in the microbiota-gut-brain axis may also impact on overall mental health.[150]

And glutamate is also a key substrate in the synthesis of the primary inhibitory neurotransmitter gamma-aminobutyric acid (GABA). GABA reduces the likelihood that neurons will act and decreases activity in the central nervous system.[157]

However, in the gut, GABA has multiple roles that go far beyond the calming of neuronal responses. It works as a modulator, regulating peristalsis and mucous secretion, and as a communication molecule, carrying messages between the microbiome, the ENS and the CNS.[158,159] It improves the integrity of the gut by stimulating the cells lining the gut to maintain tight junctions between each other.[160] It increases concentrations of SCFAs which in turn supports diversity in the microbiome.[161] And there is increasing evidence that GABA plays a role in immune cell activity in the gut, particularly those associated with inflammation.[162]

THE CENTRALITY OF THE GUT TO HEALTH

It is not possible to separate out the ENS, the chemical components such as neurotransmitters, and the microbiome and its metabolites, because all are so closely inter-related. Considering the action of the microbiome in modulating the function of the ENS, neurotransmitters and hormones, it is no surprise that research has found that supplementing with specific species of probiotic bacteria can change behaviour, reduce stress, depression, and anger, and improve memory.[163,164,165] And the evidence that a healthy microbiome helps to maintain overall metabolic health grows almost daily.[166] However, the relationships between all of these elements is complex and full of confounding and contradictory factors and the study of how the microbiome and its metabolites influences the gut and the brain is still very much in its infancy.

Whilst the gut may not be smart enough to help you pass a driving test, it is more than enough to trigger a "gut feeling" on which many of us base our actions. Historically, doctors knew that the digestive system was central to the health and wellbeing of their patients, and they viewed "the stomach" as being strongly linked to physical and emotional health.[167] Whilst modern healthcare practitioners may not wish to start examining the contents of a patient's chamber pot, it may be time to start giving more time, attention, and understanding to the digestive system and its outputs.

REFERENCES

1 Marsh, P.D., Do, T., Beighton, D., & Devine, D.A. (2016). Influence of saliva on the oral microbiota. *Periodontology, 2000, 70*(1), 80–92. https://doi.org/10.1111/prd.12098

2 Frenkel, E.S., & Ribbeck, K. (2015). Salivary mucins in host defense and disease prevention. *Journal of Oral Microbiology, 7,* 29759. https://doi.org/10.3402/jom.v7.29759

3 Humphrey, S.P., & Williamson, R.T. (2001). A review of saliva: Normal composition, flow and function. *The Journal of Prosthetic Dentistry, 85*(2), 162–169. https://doi.org/10.1067/mpr.2001.113778

4 Carreira, L., Castelo, P.M., Simões, C., Silva, F., Viegas, C., & Lamy, E. (2020). Changes in salivary proteome in response to bread odour. *Nutrients, 12*(4), 1002. https://doi.org/10.3390/nu12041002

5 Goodman, B.E. (2010). Insights into digestion and absorption of major nutrients in humans. *Advances in Physiology Education, 34*(2), 44–53. https://doi.org/10.1152/advan.00094.2009

6 Peyrot des Gachons, C., & Breslin, P.A. (2016). Salivary amylase: Digestion and metabolic syndrome. *Current Diabetes Reports, 16*(10), 102. https://doi.org/10.1007/s11892-016-0794-7

7 Kulkarni, B.V., & Mattes, R.D. (2014). Lingual lipase activity in the orosensory detection of fat by humans. *American Journal of Physiology. Regulatory, Integrative and Comparative Physiology, 306*(12), R879–R885. https://doi.org/10.1152/ajpregu.00352.2013

8 Keast, R.S.J., & Costanzon A. (2015). Is fat the sixth taste primary? Evidence and implications. *Flavour, 4*(5). https://doi.org/10.1186/2044-7248-4-5

9 Siebert, A.K., Obeid, R., Weder, S., Awwad, H.M., Sputtek, A., Geisel, J., & Keller, M. (2017). Vitamin B-12 fortified toothpaste improves vitamin status in vegans: A 12-wk randomized placebo-controlled study. *The American Journal of Clinical Nutrition, 105*(3), 618–625. https://doi.org/10.3945/ajcn.116.141978

10 Satia, M.C., Mukim, A.G., Tibrewala, K.D., & Bhavasr, M.S. (2015). A randomized two way cross over study for comparison of absorption of vitamin D3 buccal spray and soft gelatin capsule formulation in healthy subjects and in patients with intestinal malabsorption. *Nutrition Journal, 14*, 114. https://doi.org/10.1186/s12937-015-0105-1

11 Del Bo', C., Riso, P., Gardana, C., Brusamolino, A., Battezzati, A., & Ciappellano, S. (2019). Effect of two different sublingual dosages of vitamin B_{12} on cobalamin nutritional status in vegans and vegetarians with a marginal deficiency: A randomized controlled trial. *Clinical Nutrition, 38*(2), 575–583. https://doi.org/10.1016/j.clnu.2018.02.008

12 Žmitek, K., Hribar, M., Hristov, H., & Pravst, I. (2020). Efficiency of vitamin D supplementation in healthy adults is associated with body mass index and baseline serum 25-hydroxyvitamin D level. *Nutrients, 12*(5), 1268. https://doi.org/10.3390/nu12051268

13 Vanuytsel, T., Tack, J., & Farre, R. (2021). The role of intestinal permeability in gastrointestinal disorders and current methods of evaluation. *Frontiers in Nutrition, 8*, 717925. https://doi.org/10.3389/fnut.2021.717925

14 Iqbal, J., & Hussain, M.M. (2009). Intestinal lipid absorption. *American Journal of Physiology, Endocrinology and Metabolism, 296*(6), E1183–E1194. https://doi.org/10.1152/ajpendo.90899.2008

15 Giammanco, A., Cefalù, A.B., Noto, D., & Averna, M.R. (2015). The pathophysiology of intestinal lipoprotein production. *Frontiers in Physiology, 6*, 61. https://doi.org/10.3389/fphys.2015.00061

16 Dixon J.B. (2010). Mechanisms of chylomicron uptake into lacteals. *Annals of the New York Academy of Sciences, 1207, Suppl 1*(Suppl 1), E52–E57. https://doi.org/10.1111/j.1749-6632.2010.05716.x

17 Green, A.S., & Fascetti, A.J. (2016). Meeting the vitamin A requirement: The efficacy and importance of β-carotene in animal species. *The Scientific World Journal, 2016*, 7393620. https://doi.org/10.1155/2016/7393620

18 Borel, P., & Desmarchelier, C. (2017). Genetic variations associated with vitamin A status and vitamin A bioavailability. *Nutrients, 9*(3), 246. https://doi.org/10.3390/nu9030246

19 Pressman, P., Clemens, R.A., & Hayes, A.W. (2017). Bioavailability of micronutrients obtained from supplements and food: A survey and case study of the polyphenols. *Toxicology Research and Application, 1*. https://doi.org/10.1177/2397847317696366

20 Lattimer, J.M., & Haub, M.D. (2010). Effects of dietary fiber and its components on metabolic health. *Nutrients, 2*(12), 1266–1289. https://doi.org/10.3390/nu2121266

21 White, W.S., Zhou, Y., Crane, A., Dixon, P., Quadt, F., & Flendrig, L.M. (2017). Modeling the dose effects of soybean oil in salad dressing on carotenoid and fat-soluble vitamin bioavailability in salad vegetables. *The American Journal of Clinical Nutrition, 106*(4), 1041–1051. https://doi.org/10.3945/ajcn.117.153635

22 Woudstra, T., & Thomson, A.B.R. (2002). Nutrient absorption and intestinal adaptation with ageing. *Best Practice & Research Clinical Gastroenterology, 16*(1), 1–15. https://doi.org/10.1053/bega.2001.0262

23 Frommherz, L., Bub, A., Hummel, E., Rist, M.J., Roth, A., Watzl, B., & Kulling, S.E. (2016). Age-related changes of plasma bile acid concentrations in healthy adults – Results from the cross-sectional KarMeN study. *PloS One, 11*(4), e0153959. https://doi.org/10.1371/journal.pone.0153959

24 Granado-Lorencio, F., Blanco-Navarro, I., Pérez-Sacristán, B., Millán, I., Donoso-Navarro, E., & Silvestre-Mardomingo, R.A. (2013). Determinants of fat-soluble vitamin status in patients aged 65 years and over. *European Journal of Clinical Nutrition, 67*(12), 1325–1327. https://doi.org/10.1038/ejcn.2013.198

25 Goncalves, A., & Amiot, M.J. (2017). Fat-soluble micronutrients and metabolic syndrome. *Current Opinion in Clinical Nutrition and Metabolic Care, 20*(6), 492–497. https://doi.org/10.1097/MCO.0000000000000412

26 Paes-Silva, R.P., Gadelha, P., Lemos, M., Castro, C., Arruda, I., & Diniz, A. (2019). Adiposity, inflammation and fat-soluble vitamins in adolescents. *Jornal de Pediatria, 95*(5), 575–583. https://doi.org/10.1016/j.jped.2018.05.008

27 Heck, A.M., Yanovski, J.A., & Calis, K.A. (2000). Orlistat, a new lipase inhibitor for the management of obesity. *Pharmacotherapy, 20*(3), 270–279. https://doi.org/10.1592/phco.20.4.270.34882

28 Stancu, C., & Sima, A. (2001). Statins: Mechanism of action and effects. *Journal of Cellular and Molecular Medicine, 5*(4), 378–387. https://doi.org/10.1111/j.1582-4934.2001.tb00172.x

29 Said H.M. (2011). Intestinal absorption of water-soluble vitamins in health and disease. *The Biochemical Journal, 437*(3), 357–372. https://doi.org/10.1042/BJ20110326

30 Nielsen, M.J., Rasmussen, M.R., Andersen, C.B., Nexø, E., & Moestrup, S.K. (2012). Vitamin B12 transport from food to the body's cells – A sophisticated, multistep pathway. *Nature Reviews. Gastroenterology & Hepatology, 9*(6), 345–354. https://doi.org/10.1038/nrgastro.2012.76

31 Pawlak, R., Lester, S.E., & Babatunde, T. (2014). The prevalence of cobalamin deficiency among vegetarians assessed by serum vitamin B12: A review of literature. *European Journal of Clinical Nutrition, 68*(5), 541–548. https://doi.org/10.1038/ejcn.2014.46

32 Festen H.P. (1991). Intrinsic factor secretion and cobalamin absorption. Physiology and pathophysiology in the gastrointestinal tract. *Scandinavian Journal of Gastroenterology. Supplement, 188*, 1–7. https://doi.org/10.3109/00365529109111222

33 Kiela, P.R., & Ghishan, F.K. (2016). Physiology of intestinal absorption and secretion. *Best Practice & Research. Clinical Gastroenterology, 30*(2), 145–159. https://doi.org/10.1016/j.bpg.2016.02.007

34 Goff J.P. (2018). *Invited review:* Mineral absorption mechanisms, mineral interactions that affect acid-base and antioxidant status, and diet considerations to improve mineral status. *Journal of Dairy Science, 101*(4), 2763–2813. https://doi.org/10.3168/jds.2017-13112

35 Yang, L.P., Dong, Y.P., Luo, W.T., Zhu, T., Li, Q.W., et al. (2018). Tissue-specific regulatory effects of vitamin D and its receptor on Calbindin-D28K and Calbindin-D9K. *Biochemistry and Molecular Biology Journal, 4*(3), 23 https://doi.org/10.21767/2471-8084.100072

36 Knöpfel, T., Pastor-Arroyo, E.M., Schnitzbauer, U., Kratschmar K.V., Odermatt A., Pellegrini A., Hernando N., & Wagner C.A., (2017). The intestinal phosphate transporter NaPi-IIb (Slc34a2) is required to protect bone during dietary phosphate restriction. *Scientific Reports, 7,* 11018. https://doi.org/10.1038/s41598-017-10390-2

37 Gulec, S., Anderson, G. J., & Collins, J. F. (2014). Mechanistic and regulatory aspects of intestinal iron absorption. *American Journal of Physiology, Gastrointestinal and Liver Physiology, 307*(4), G397–G409. https://doi.org/10.1152/ajpgi.00348.2013

38 Nishito, Y., & Kambe, T. (2018). Absorption mechanisms of iron, copper, and zinc: An overview. *Journal of Nutritional Science and Vitaminology, 64*(1), 1–7. https://doi.org/10.3177/jnsv.64.1

39 Anderson, G. J., & Frazer, D. M. (2017). Current understanding of iron homeostasis. *The American Journal of Clinical Nutrition, 106*(Suppl 6), 1559S–1566S. https://doi.org/10.3945/ajcn.117.155804

40 Wolff, N.A., Garrick, M.D., Zhao, L., Garrick, L.M., Ghio, A.J., & Thévenod, F. (2018). A role for divalent metal transporter (DMT1) in mitochondrial uptake of iron and manganese. *Scientific Reports, 8*(1), 211. https://doi.org/10.1038/s41598-017-18584-4

41 Young, I., Parker, H.M., Rangan, A., Prvan, T., Cook, R.L., Donges, C.E., Steinbeck, K. S., O'Dwyer, N.J., Cheng, H.L., Franklin, J.L., & O'Connor, H.T. (2018). Association between haem and non-haem iron intake and serum ferritin in healthy young women. *Nutrients, 10*(1), 81. https://doi.org/10.3390/nu10010081

42 Arredondo, M., Martínez, R., Núñez, M.T., Ruz, M., & Olivares, M. (2006). Inhibition of iron and copper uptake by iron, copper and zinc. *Biological Research, 39*(1), 95–102. https://doi.org/10.4067/s0716-97602006000100011

43 Menon, A.V., Chang, J., & Kim, J. (2016). Mechanisms of divalent metal toxicity in affective disorders. *Toxicology, 339,* 58–72. https://doi.org/10.1016/j.tox.2015.11.001

44 Wu, R.Q., Zhang, D.F., Tu, E., Chen, Q.M., & Chen, W. (2014). The mucosal immune system in the oral cavity-an orchestra of T cell diversity. *International Journal of Oral Science, 6*(3), 125–132. https://doi.org/10.1038/ijos.2014.48

45 Abusleme, L., & Moutsopoulos, N.M. (2017). IL-17: Overview and role in oral immunity and microbiome. *Oral Diseases, 23*(7), 854–865. https://doi.org/10.1111/odi.12598

46 Hunt, R.H., Camilleri, M., Crowe, S.E., El-Omar, E.M., Fox, J.G., Kuipers, E.J., Malfertheiner, P., McColl, K.E., Pritchard, D.M., Rugge, M., Sonnenberg, A., Sugano, K., & Tack, J. (2015). The stomach in health and disease. *Gut, 64*(10), 1650–1668. https://doi.org/10.1136/gutjnl-2014-307595

47 Martinsen, T.C., Bergh, K., & Waldum, H.L. (2005). Gastric juice: A barrier against infectious diseases. *Basic & Clinical Pharmacology & Toxicology, 96*(2), 94–102. https://doi.org/10.1111/j.1742-7843.2005.pto960202.x

48 Beasley, D.E., Koltz, A.M., Lambert, J.E., Fierer, N., & Dunn, R.R. (2015). The evolution of stomach acidity and its relevance to the human microbiome. *PloS One, 10*(7), e0134116. https://doi.org/10.1371/journal.pone.0134116

49 Martinsen, T.C., Fossmark, R., & Waldum, H.L. (2019). The phylogeny and biological function of gastric juice-microbiological consequences of removing gastric acid. *International Journal of Molecular Sciences, 20*(23), 6031. https://doi.org/10.3390/ijms20236031

50 Warren, J.R., & Marshall, B. (1983). Unidentified curved bacilli on gastric epithelium in active chronic gastritis. *The Lancet, 1*(8336), 1273–1275. https://doi.org/10.1016/S0140-6736

51 Ohno, H., & Satoh-Takayama, N. (2020). Stomach microbiota, Helicobacter pylori, and group 2 innate lymphoid cells. *Experimental & Molecular Medicine, 52*(9), 1377–1382. https://doi.org/10.1038/s12276-020-00485-8

52 Yang, J., Zhou, X., Liu, X., Ling, Z., & Ji, F. (2021). Role of the gastric microbiome in gastric cancer: From carcinogenesis to treatment. *Frontiers in Microbiology, 12*, 641322. https://doi.org/10.3389/fmicb.2021.641322

53 Gorkiewicz, G., & Moschen, A. (2018). Gut microbiome: A new player in gastro-intestinal disease. *Virchows Archiv: European Journal of Pathology, 472*(1), 159–172. https://doi.org/10.1007/s00428-017-2277-x

54 Bik, E.M., Eckburg, P.B., Gill, S.R., Nelson, K.E., Purdom, E.A., Francois, F., Perez-Perez, G., Blaser, M.J., & Relman, D.A. (2006). Molecular analysis of the bacterial microbiota in the human stomach. *Proceedings of the National Academy of Sciences of the United States of America, 103*(3), 732–737. https://doi.org/10.1073/pnas.0506655103

55 Nie, S., & Yuan, Y. (2020). The role of gastric mucosal immunity in gastric diseases. *Journal of Immunology Research, 2020*, 7927054. https://doi.org/10.1155/2020/7927054

56 Da Silva C., Wagner C., Bonnardel J., Gorvel J.P., & Lelouard H., (2017). The Peyer's patch mononuclear phagocyte system at steady state and during infection. *Frontiers in Immunology, 8*, 1254 https://doi.org/10.3389/fimmu.2017.01254

57 Kobayashi, N., Takahashi, D., Takano, S., Kimura, S., & Hase, K. (2019). The roles of Peyer's patches and microfold cells in the gut immune system: Relevance to auto-immune diseases. *Frontiers in Immunology, 10*, 2345. https://doi.org/10.3389/fimmu.2019.02345

58 Jung, C., Hugot, J.P., & Barreau, F. (2010). Peyer's patches: The immune sensors of the intestine. *International Journal of Inflammation, 2010*, 823710. https://doi.org/10.4061/2010/823710

59 Vancamelbeke, M., & Vermeire, S. (2017). The intestinal barrier: A fundamental role in health and disease. *Expert Review of Gastroenterology & Hepatology, 11*(9), 821–834. https://doi.org/10.1080/17474124.2017.1343143

60 Johansson, M.E., Sjövall, H., & Hansson, G.C. (2013). The gastrointestinal mucus system in health and disease. *Nature Reviews. Gastroenterology & Hepatology, 10*(6), 352–361. https://doi.org/10.1038/nrgastro.2013.35

61 Johansson, M.E., & Hansson, G.C. (2016). Immunological aspects of intestinal mucus and mucins. *Nature Reviews. Immunology, 16*(10), 639–649. https://doi.org/10.1038/nri.2016.88

62 Lathrop, S.K., Bloom, S.M., Rao, S.M., Nutsch, K., Lio, C.W., Santacruz, N., Peterson, D.A., Stappenbeck, T.S., & Hsieh, C.S. (2011). Peripheral education of the immune system by colonic commensal microbiota. *Nature, 478*(7368), 250–254. https://doi.org/10.1038/nature10434

63 Dheilly, N.M., Bolnick, D., Bordenstein, S., Brindley, P.J., Figuères, C., Holmes, E.C., Martínez Martínez, J., Phillips, A.J., Poulin, R., & Rosario, K. (2017). Parasite microbiome project: Systematic investigation of microbiome dynamics within and across parasite-host interactions. *mSystems, 2*(4), e00050–17. https://doi.org/10.1128/mSystems.00050-17

64 Altveş, S., Yildiz, H.K., & Vural, H.C. (2020). Interaction of the microbiota with the human body in health and diseases. *Bioscience of Microbiota, Food and Health, 39*(2), 23–32. https://doi.org/10.12938/bmfh.19-023

65 Hill, C., Guarner, F., Reid, G., Gibson, G. R., Merenstein, D.J., Pot, B., Morelli, L., Canani, R.B., Flint, H.J., Salminen, S., Calder, P.C., & Sanders, M.E. (2014). Expert consensus document. The International Scientific Association for Probiotics and Prebiotics consensus statement on the scope and appropriate use of the term probiotic. *Nature reviews. Gastroenterology & Hepatology, 11*(8), 506–514. https://doi.org/10.1038/nrgastro.2014.66

66 Khan, R., Petersen, F.C., & Shekhar, S. (2019). Commensal bacteria: An emerging player in defense against respiratory pathogens. *Frontiers in Immunology, 10*, 1203. https://doi.org/10.3389/fimmu.2019.01203

67 Kilian, M., Chapple, I.L., Hannig, M., Marsh, P.D., Meuric, V., Pedersen, A.M., Tonetti, M.S., Wade, W.G., & Zaura, E. (2016). The oral microbiome – an update for oral healthcare professionals. *British Dental Journal, 221*(10), 657–666. https://doi.org/10.1038/sj.bdj.2016.865

68 Cross, B., Faustoferri, R.C., & Quivey, R.G., Jr. (2016). What are we learning and what can we learn from the Human Oral Microbiome Project?. *Current Oral Health Reports, 3*(1), 56–63. https://doi.org/10.1007/s40496-016-0080-4

69 Schairer, D.O., Chouake, J.S., Nosanchuk, J.D., & Friedman, A.J. (2012). The potential of nitric oxide releasing therapies as antimicrobial agents. *Virulence, 3*(3), 271–279. https://doi.org/10.4161/viru.20328

70 Bryan, N.S., Tribble, G., & Angelov, N. (2017). Oral microbiome and nitric oxide: The missing link in the management of blood pressure. *Current Hypertension Reports, 19*(4), 33. https://doi.org/10.1007/s11906-017-0725-2

71 Cornejo Ulloa, P., van der Veen, M.H., & Krom, B.P. (2019). Review: Modulation of the oral microbiome by the host to promote ecological balance. *Odontology, 107*(4), 437–448. https://doi.org/10.1007/s10266-019-00413-x

72 Tribble, G.D., Angelov, N., Weltman, R., Wang, B.Y., Eswaran, S.V., Gay, I.C., Parthasarathy, K., Dao, D.V., Richardson, K.N., Ismail, N.M., Sharina, I.G., Hyde, E.R., Ajami, N.J., Petrosino, J.F., & Bryan, N.S. (2019). Frequency of tongue cleaning impacts the human tongue microbiome composition and enterosalivary circulation of nitrate. *Frontiers in Cellular and Infection Microbiology, 9*, 39. https://doi.org/10.3389/fcimb.2019.00039

73 Sansores-España, D., Carrillo-Avila, A., Melgar-Rodriguez, S., Díaz-Zuñiga, J., & Martínez-Aguilar, V. (2021). Periodontitis and Alzheimer´s disease. *Medicina Oral, Patologia Oral y Cirugia Bucal, 26*(1), e43–e48. https://doi.org/10.4317/medoral. 23940

74 Li, B.Z., Zhou, H.Y., Guo, B., Chen, W.J., Tao, J.H., Cao, N.W., Chu, X.J., & Meng, X. (2020). Dysbiosis of oral microbiota is associated with systemic lupus erythematosus. *Archives of Oral Biology, 113*, 104708. https://doi.org/10.1016/j.archoralbio.2020. 104708

75 Akazawa H. (2018). Periodontitis and diabetes mellitus: Be true to your teeth. *International Heart Journal, 59*(4), 680–682. https://doi.org/10.1536/ihj.18-410

76 Chhibber-Goel, J., Singhal, V., Bhowmik, D., Vivek, R., Parakh, N., Bhargava, B., & Sharma, A. (2016). Linkages between oral commensal bacteria and atherosclerotic plaques in coronary artery disease patients. *NPJ Biofilms and Microbiomes, 2*, 7. https://doi.org/10.1038/s41522-016-0009-7

77 Mascitti, M., Togni, L., Troiano, G., Caponio, V., Gissi, D.B., Montebugnoli, L., Procaccini, M., Lo Muzio, L., & Santarelli, A. (2019). Beyond head and neck cancer: The relationship between oral microbiota and tumour development in distant organs. *Frontiers in Cellular and Infection Microbiology, 9*, 232. https://doi.org/10.3389/fcimb.2019.00232

78 Walker, R.W., Clemente, J.C., Peter, I., & Loos, R. (2017). The prenatal gut microbiome: Are we colonized with bacteria in utero? *Pediatric Obesity, 12 Suppl 1*(Suppl 1), 3–17. https://doi.org/10.1111/ijpo.12217

79 Cresci, G.A., & Bawden, E. (2015). Gut microbiome: What we do and don't know. *Nutrition in Clinical Practice, 30*(6), 734–746. https://doi.org/10.1177/0884533615 609899

80 Rampelli, S., Turroni, S., Mallol, C., Hernandez, C., Galván, B., Sistiaga, A., Biagi, E., Astolfi, A., Brigidi, P., Benazzi, S., Lewis, C. M., Jr, Warinner, C., Hofman, C.A., Schnorr, S.L., & Candela, M. (2021). Components of a Neanderthal gut microbiome recovered from fecal sediments from El Salt. *Communications Biology, 4*(1), 169. https://doi.org/10.1038/s42003-021-01689-y

81 Berg, G., Rybakova, D., Fischer, D., Cernava, T., Vergès, M.C., Charles, T., Chen, X., Cocolin, L., Eversole, K., Corral, G.H., Kazou, M., Kinkel, L., Lange, L., Lima, N., Loy, A., Macklin, J.A., Maguin, E., Mauchline, T., McClure, R., Mitter, B., & Schloter, M. (2020). Microbiome definition re-visited: Old concepts and new challenges. *Microbiome, 8*(1), 103. https://doi.org/10.1186/s40168-020-00875-0

82 Moeller, A.H. (2017). The shrinking human gut microbiome. *Current Opinion in Microbiology, 38*, 30–35. https://doi.org/10.1016/j.mib.2017.04.002

83 Watanabe, F., & Bito, T. (2018). Vitamin B$_{12}$ sources and microbial interaction. *Experimental Biology and Medicine, 243*(2), 148–158. https://doi.org/10.1177/15353 70217746612

84 Said H.M., (2013). Recent advances in transport of water-soluble vitamins in organs of the digestive system: A focus on the colon and the pancreas. *American Journal of Physiology. Gastrointestinal and Liver Physiology, 305*(9), G601–10. https://doi.org/10.1152/ajpgi.00231.2013

85 Zinöcker, M.K., & Lindseth, I.A. (2018). The western diet-microbiome-host interaction and its role in metabolic disease. *Nutrients, 10*(3), 365. https://doi.org/10.3390/nu10030365

86 Gibney M.J. (2018). Ultra-processed foods: Definitions and policy issues. *Current Developments in Nutrition, 3*(2), nzy077. https://doi.org/10.1093/cdn/nzy077

87 Rauber, F., Louzada, M., Martinez Steele, E., Rezende, L., Millett, C., Monteiro, C.A., & Levy, R.B. (2019). Ultra-processed foods and excessive free sugar intake in the UK: A nationally representative cross-sectional study. *BMJ Open, 9*(10), e027546. https://doi.org/10.1136/bmjopen-2018-027546

88 Shaw L.P., Bassam H., Barnes C.P., Walker A.S., Klien N., & Balloux F., (2019). Modelling microbiome recovery after antibiotics using a stability landscape framework. *The ISME Journal, 13*(7), 1845–1856. https://doi.org/10.1038/s41396-019-0392-1

89 Kim, S., Covington, A., & Pamer, E. G. (2017). The intestinal microbiota: Antibiotics, colonization resistance, and enteric pathogens. *Immunological Reviews, 279*(1), 90–105. https://doi.org/10.1111/imr.12563

90 Karl, J.P., Margolis, L.M., Madslien, E.H., Murphy, N.E., Castellani, J.W., Gundersen, Y., Hoke, A.V., Levangie, M.W., Kumar, R., Chakraborty, N., Gautam, A., Hammamieh, R., Martini, S., Montain, S.J., & Pasiakos, S.M. (2017). Changes in intestinal microbiota composition and metabolism coincide with increased intestinal permeability in young adults under prolonged physiological stress. *American Journal of Physiology, Gastrointestinal and Liver Physiology, 312*(6), G559–G571. https://doi.org/10.1152/ajpgi.00066.2017

91 Sun, Y., Li, L., Xie, R., Wang, B., Jiang, K., & Cao, H. (2019). Stress triggers flare of inflammatory bowel disease in children and adults. *Frontiers in Pediatrics, 7*, 432. https://doi.org/10.3389/fped.2019.00432

92 Tetel, M.J., de Vries, G.J., Melcangi, R.C., Panzica, G., & O'Mahony, S.M. (2018). Steroids, stress and the gut microbiome-brain axis. *Journal of Neuroendocrinology, 30*(2), e12548. https://doi.org/10.1111/jne.12548

93 Weiss, G.A., & Hennet, T. (2017). Mechanisms and consequences of intestinal dysbiosis. *Cellular and Molecular Life Sciences, 74*(16), 2959–2977. https://doi.org/10.1007/s00018-017-2509-x

94 Yang, T., Santisteban, M.M., Rodriguez, V., Li, E., Ahmari, N., Carvajal, J. M., Zadeh, M., Gong, M., Qi, Y., Zubcevic, J., Sahay, B., Pepine, C.J., Raizada, M.K., & Mohamadzadeh, M. (2015). Gut dysbiosis is linked to hypertension. *Hypertension, 65*(6), 1331–1340. https://doi.org/10.1161/HYPERTENSIONAHA.115.05315

95 Horta-Baas, G., Romero-Figueroa, M., Montiel-Jarquín, A.J., Pizano-Zárate, M.L., García-Mena, J., & Ramírez-Durán, N. (2017). Intestinal dysbiosis and rheumatoid arthritis: A link between gut microbiota and the pathogenesis of rheumatoid arthritis. *Journal of Immunology Research, 2017*, 4835189. https://doi.org/10.1155/2017/4835189

96 Visser, M., Kell, D.B., & Pretorius, E. (2019). Bacterial dysbiosis and translocation in psoriasis vulgaris. *Frontiers in Cellular and Infection Microbiology*, 9, 7. https://doi.org/10.3389/fcimb.2019.00007

97 Saus, E., Iraola-Guzmán, S., Willis, J.R., Brunet-Vega, A., & Gabaldón, T. (2019). Microbiome and colorectal cancer: Roles in carcinogenesis and clinical potential. *Molecular Aspects of Medicine*, 69, 93–106. https://doi.org/10.1016/j.mam.2019.05.001

98 Wilkins, L.J., Monga, M., Miller, A.W., (2019). Defining dysbiosis for a cluster of chronic diseases. *Nature Scientific Reports*, 9, 12918. https://doi.org/10.1038/s41598-019-49452-y

99 Pickard, J.M., Zeng, M.Y., Caruso, R., & Núñez, G. (2017). Gut microbiota: Role in pathogen colonization, immune responses, and inflammatory disease. *Immunological Reviews*, 279(1), 70–89. https://doi.org/10.1111/imr.12567

100 Manor, O., Dai, C.L., Kornilov, S.A., Smith, B., Price, N.D., Lovejoy, J.C., Gibbons, S.M., & Magis, A.T. (2020). Health and disease markers correlate with gut microbiome composition across thousands of people. *Nature Communications*, 11(1), 5206. https://doi.org/10.1038/s41467-020-18871-1

101 Public Health England and the Food Standards Agency (2020). National Diet and Nutrition Survey Rolling programme Years 9 to 11 (2016/2017 to 2018/2019) https://assets.publishing.service.gov.uk/government/uploads/system/uploads/attachment_data/file/943114/NDNS_UK_Y9-11_report.pdf

102 Barber, T.M., Kabisch, S., Pfeiffer, A., & Weickert, M.O. (2020). The health benefits of dietary fibre. *Nutrients*, 12(10), 3209. https://doi.org/10.3390/nu12103209

103 Reynolds, A., Mann, J., Cummings, J., Winter, N., Mete, E., & Te Morenga, L. (2019). Carbohydrate quality and human health: A series of systematic reviews and meta-analyses. *The Lancet*, 393(10170), 434–445. https://doi.org/10.1016/S0140-6736(18)31809-9

104 Holscher, H.D. (2017). Dietary fiber and prebiotics and the gastrointestinal microbiota. *Gut Microbes*, 8(2), 172–184. https://doi.org/10.1080/19490976.2017.1290756

105 Harvey, R., Ferrieres, D. (2011). In: Biochemistry, Lippincott's Illustrated Reviews, Lippincott Williams and Wilkins (Publisher) 5th ed. Harvey R.A., editor. Lippincott Williams, & Wilkins; Baltimore, MD, USA.

106 DeMartino, P., & Cockburn, D.W. (2020). Resistant starch: Impact on the gut microbiome and health. *Current Opinion in Biotechnology*, 61, 66–71. https://doi.org/10.1016/j.copbio.2019.10.008

107 Gibson, P.R. (2017). Use of the low-FODMAP diet in inflammatory bowel disease. *Journal of Gastroenterology and Hepatology*, 32 Suppl 1, 40–42. https://doi.org/10.1111/jgh.13695

108 Myhrstad, M., Tunsjø, H., Charnock, C., & Telle-Hansen, V.H. (2020). Dietary fiber, gut microbiota, and metabolic regulation – Current status in human randomized trials. *Nutrients*, 12(3), 859. https://doi.org/10.3390/nu12030859

109 Wiciński, M., Sawicka, E., Gębalski, J., Kubiak, K., & Malinowski, B. (2020). Human milk oligosaccharides: Health benefits, potential applications in infant formulas, and pharmacology. *Nutrients*, 12(1), 266. https://doi.org/10.3390/nu12010266

110 Blaak, E.E., Canfora, E.E., Theis, S., Frost, G., Groen, A.K., Mithieux, G., Nauta, A., Scott, K., Stahl, B., van Harsselaar, J., van Tol, R., Vaughan, E.E., & Verbeke, K. (2020). Short chain fatty acids in human gut and metabolic health. *Beneficial Microbes*, 11(5), 411–455. https://doi.org/10.3920/BM2020.0057

111 Morrison, D.J., & Preston, T. (2016). Formation of short chain fatty acids by the gut microbiota and their impact on human metabolism. *Gut Microbes*, 7(3), 189–200. https://doi.org/10.1080/19490976.2015.1134082

112 Silva, Y.P., Bernardi, A., & Frozza, R.L. (2020). The role of short-chain fatty acids from gut microbiota in gut-brain communication. *Frontiers in Endocrinology*, *11*, 25. https://doi.org/10.3389/fendo.2020.00025

113 Parada Venegas, D., De la Fuente, M.K., Landskron, G., González, M.J., Quera, R., Dijkstra, G., Harmsen, H., Faber, K.N., & Hermoso, M.A. (2019). Short Chain Fatty Acids (SCFAs)-mediated gut epithelial and immune regulation and its relevance for inflammatory bowel diseases. *Frontiers in Immunology*, *10*, 277. https://doi.org/10.3389/fimmu.2019.00277

114 He, J., Zhang, P., Shen, L., Niu, L., Tan, Y., Chen, L., Zhao, Y., Bai, L., Hao, X., Li, X., Zhang, S., & Zhu, L. (2020). Short-Chain Fatty Acids and their association with signalling pathways in inflammation, glucose and lipid metabolism. *International Journal of Molecular Sciences*, *21*(17), 6356. https://doi.org/10.3390/ijms21176356

115 Yang, W., Yu, T., Huang, X., Bilotta, A.J., Xu, L., Lu, Y., Sun, J., Pan, F., Zhou, J., Zhang, W., Yao, S., Maynard, C.L., Singh, N., Dann, S. M., Liu, Z., & Cong, Y. (2020). Intestinal microbiota-derived short-chain fatty acids regulation of immune cell IL-22 production and gut immunity. *Nature Communications*, *11*(1), 4457. https://doi.org/10.1038/s41467-020-18262-6

116 Lucas, S., Omata, Y., Hofmann, J., Böttcher, M., Iljazovic, A., Sarter, K., Albrecht, O., Schulz, O., Krishnacoumar, B., Krönke, G., Herrmann, M., Mougiakakos, D., Strowig, T., Schett, G., & Zaiss, M. M. (2018). Short-chain fatty acids regulate systemic bone mass and protect from pathological bone loss. *Nature Communications*, *9*(1), 55. https://doi.org/10.1038/s41467-017-02490-4

117 Frost, G., Sleeth, M.L., Sahuri-Arisoylu, M., Lizarbe, B., Cerdan, S., Brody, L., Anastasovska, J., Ghourab, S., Hankir, M., Zhang, S., Carling, D., Swann, J.R., Gibson, G., Viardot, A., Morrison, D., Louise Thomas, E., & Bell, J.D. (2014). The short-chain fatty acid acetate reduces appetite via a central homeostatic mechanism. *Nature Communications*, *5*, 3611. https://doi.org/10.1038/ncomms4611

118 Hernández, M., Canfora, E.E., Jocken, J., & Blaak, E.E. (2019). The Short-Chain Fatty Acid Acetate in body weight control and insulin sensitivity. *Nutrients*, *11*(8), 1943. https://doi.org/10.3390/nu11081943

119 Chambers, E.S., Preston, T., Frost, G., & Morrison, D.J. (2018). Role of Gut Microbiota-Generated Short-Chain Fatty Acids in metabolic and cardiovascular health. *Current Nutrition Reports*, *7*(4), 198–206. https://doi.org/10.1007/s13668-018-0248-8

120 Markowiak-Kopeć, P., & Śliżewska, K. (2020). The effect of probiotics on the production of Short-Chain Fatty Acids by human intestinal microbiome. *Nutrients*, *12*(4), 1107. https://doi.org/10.3390/nu12041107

121 Donohoe, D.R., Collins, L.B., Wali, A., Bigler, R., Sun, W., & Bultman, S.J. (2012). The Warburg effect dictates the mechanism of butyrate-mediated histone acetylation and cell proliferation. *Molecular Cell*, *48*(4), 612–626. https://doi.org/10.1016/j.molcel.2012.08.033

122 Dalile, B., Van Oudenhove, L., Vervliet, B., & Verbeke, K. (2019). The role of short-chain fatty acids in microbiota-gut-brain communication. *Nature Reviews. Gastroenterology & Hepatology*, *16*(8), 461–478. https://doi.org/10.1038/s41575-019-0157-3

123 Walker, A.C., Bhargava, R., Vaziriyan-Sani, A.S., Pourciau, C., Donahue, E.T., Dove, A.S., Gebhardt, M.J., Ellward, G.L., Romeo, T., & Czyż, D.M. (2021). Colonization of the Caenorhabditis elegans gut with human enteric bacterial pathogens leads to proteostasis disruption that is rescued by butyrate. *PLoS Pathogens*, *17*(5), e1009510. https://doi.org/10.1371/journal.ppat.1009510

124 Stiemsma L.T., Nakamura R.E., Nguyen J.G., & Michels K.B., (2020). Does consumption of fermented foods modify the human gut microbiota? *The Journal of Nutrition*, *150*(7), 1680–1693 https://doi.org/10.1093/jn/nxaa077

125 Şanlier, N., Gökcen, B.B., & Sezgin, A.C. (2019). Health benefits of fermented foods. *Critical Reviews in Food Science and Nutrition, 59*(3), 506–527. https://doi.org/10.1080/10408398.2017.1383355

126 Dimidi, E., Cox, S.R., Rossi, M., & Whelan, K. (2019). Fermented foods: Definitions and characteristics, impact on the gut microbiota and effects on gastrointestinal health and disease. *Nutrients, 11*(8), 1806. https://doi.org/10.3390/nu11081806

127 Marco, M.L., Heeney, D., Binda, S., Cifelli, C.J., Cotter, P.D., Foligné, B., Gänzle, M., Kort, R., Pasin, G., Pihlanto, A., Smid, E.J., & Hutkins, R. (2017). Health benefits of fermented foods: Microbiota and beyond. *Current Opinion in Biotechnology, 44*, 94–102. https://doi.org/10.1016/j.copbio.2016.11.010

128 Wastyk, H.C., Fragiadakis, G.K., Perelman, D., Dahan, D., Merrill, B.D., Yu, F. B., Topf, M., Gonzalez, C.G., Van Treuren, W., Han, S., Robinson, J.L., Elias, J.E., Sonnenburg, E.D., Gardner, C.D., & Sonnenburg, J.L. (2021). Gut-microbiota-targeted diets modulate human immune status. *Cell, 184*(16), 4137–4153.e14. https://doi.org/10.1016/j.cell.2021.06.019

129 Browning, K.N., & Travagli, R.A. (2014). Central nervous system control of gastro-intestinal motility and secretion and modulation of gastrointestinal functions. *Comprehensive Physiology, 4*(4), 1339–1368. https://doi.org/10.1002/cphy.c130055

130 Breit, S., Kupferberg, A., Rogler, G., & Hasler, G. (2018). Vagus nerve as modulator of the brain-gut axis in psychiatric and inflammatory disorders. *Frontiers in Psychiatry, 9*, 44. https://doi.org/10.3389/fpsyt.2018.00044

131 Bonaz, B., Bazin, T., & Pellissier, S. (2018). The vagus nerve at the interface of the microbiota-gut-brain axis. *Frontiers in Neuroscience, 12*, 49. https://doi.org/10.3389/fnins.2018.00049

132 Zhou, H., Liang, H., Li, Z. F., Xiang, H., Liu, W., & Li, J.G. (2013). Vagus nerve stimulation attenuates intestinal epithelial tight junctions disruption in endotoxemic mice through α7 nicotinic acetylcholine receptors. *Shock, 40*(2), 144–151. https://doi.org/10.1097/SHK.0b013e318299e9c0

133 Mohajeri, M.H., La Fata, G., Steinert, R.E., & Weber, P. (2018). Relationship between the gut microbiome and brain function. *Nutrition Reviews, 76*(7), 481–496. https://doi.org/10.1093/nutrit/nuy009

134 Rao M., Gershon M.D. (2016). The bowel and beyond: the enteric nervous system in neurological disorders. *Nature Reviews Gastroenterology & Hepatology,* 13(9), 517–528. https://doi.org/10.1038/nrgastro.2016.107

135 Mayer, E.A. (2011). Gut feelings: The emerging biology of gut-brain communication. *Nature Reviews. Neuroscience, 12*(8), 453–466. https://doi.org/10.1038/nrn3071

136 Schneider, S., Wright, C.M., & Heuckeroth, R.O. (2019). Unexpected roles for the second brain: Enteric nervous system as master regulator of bowel function. *Annual Review of Physiology, 81*, 235–259. https://doi.org/10.1146/annurev-physiol-021317-121515

137 Fung, C., Vanden Berghe, P. (2020) Functional circuits and signal processing in the enteric nervous system. *Cellular and Molecular Life Sciences, 77*(22), 4505–4522. https://doi.org/10.1007/s00018-020-03543-6

138 Schemann, M., Frieling, T., & Enck, P. (2020). To learn, to remember, to forget-How smart is the gut?. *Acta Physiologica, 228*(1), e13296. https://doi.org/10.1111/apha.13296

139 Chalazonitis, A., & Rao, M. (2018). Enteric nervous system manifestations of neuro-degenerative disease. *Brain Research, 1693*(Pt B), 207–213. https://doi.org/10.1016/j.brainres.2018.01.011

140 Cryan, J.F., O'Riordan, K.J., Cowan, C., Sandhu, K.V., Bastiaanssen, T., Boehme, M., Codagnone, M.G., Cussotto, S., Fulling, C., Golubeva, A.V., Guzzetta, K.E., Jaggar, M., Long-Smith, C.M., Lyte, J.M., Martin, J.A., Molinero-Perez, A., Moloney, G.,

Morelli, E., Morillas, E., O'Connor, R., & Dinan, T.G. (2019). The microbiota-gut-brain axis. *Physiological Reviews*, *99*(4), 1877–2013. https://doi.org/10.1152/physrev. 00018.2018

141 Saurman, V., Margolis, K.G., & Luna, R.A. (2020). Autism spectrum disorder as a brain-gut-microbiome axis disorder. *Digestive Diseases and Sciences*, *65*(3), 818–828. https://doi.org/10.1007/s10620-020-06133-5

142 Jahng, J., & Kim, Y.S. (2016). Irritable bowel syndrome: Is it really a functional disorder? A new perspective on alteration of enteric nervous system. *Journal of Neurogastroenterology and Motility*, *22*(2), 163–165. https://doi.org/10.5056/jnm16043

143 Mittal, R., Debs, L.H., Patel, A.P., Nguyen, D., Patel, K., O'Connor, G., Grati, M., Mittal, J., Yan, D., Eshraghi, A.A., Deo, S.K., Daunert, S., & Liu, X.Z. (2017). Neurotransmitters: The critical modulators regulating gut-brain axis. *Journal of Cellular Physiology*, *232*(9), 2359–2372. https://doi.org/10.1002/jcp.25518

144 Yano, J.M., Yu, K., Donaldson, G.P., Shastri, G.G., Ann, P., Ma, L., Nagler, C.R., Ismagilov, R.F., Mazmanian, S.K., & Hsiao, E.Y. (2015). Indigenous bacteria from the gut microbiota regulate host serotonin biosynthesis. *Cell*, *161*(2), 264–276. https://doi.org/10.1016/j.cell.2015.02.047

145 Mawe, G.M., & Hoffman, J.M. (2013). Serotonin signalling in the gut – functions, dysfunctions and therapeutic targets. *Nature Reviews. Gastroenterology & Hepatology*, *10*(8), 473–486. https://doi.org/10.1038/nrgastro.2013.105

146 Jones, L.A., Sun, E.W., Martin, A.M., & Keating, D.J. (2020). The ever-changing roles of serotonin. *The International Journal of Biochemistry & Cell Biology*, *125*, 105776. https://doi.org/10.1016/j.biocel.2020.105776

147 Sochocka, M., Donskow-Łysoniewska, K., Diniz, B.S., Kurpas, D., Brzozowska, E., & Leszek, J. (2019). The gut microbiome alterations and inflammation-driven pathogenesis of Alzheimer's Disease – A critical review. *Molecular Neurobiology*, *56*(3), 1841–1851. https://doi.org/10.1007/s12035-018-1188-4

148 Wan, M., Ding, L., Wang, D., Han, J., & Gao, P. (2020). Serotonin: A potent immune cell modulator in autoimmune diseases. *Frontiers in Immunology*, *11*, 186. https://doi.org/10.3389/fimmu.2020.00186

149 Kumar, A., Russell, R.M., Pifer, R., Menezes-Garcia, Z., Cuesta, S., Narayanan, S., MacMillan, J.B., & Sperandio, V. (2020). The serotonin neurotransmitter modulates virulence of enteric pathogens. *Cell Host & Microbe*, *28*(1), 41–53.e8. https://doi.org/10.1016/j.chom.2020.05.004

150 Kraal, A.Z., Arvanitis, N.R., Jaeger, A.P., & Ellingrod, V.L. (2020). Could dietary glutamate play a role in psychiatric distress?. *Neuropsychobiology*, *79*(1), 13–19. https://doi.org/10.1159/000496294

151 Vandenbeuch, A., & Kinnamon, S.C. (2016). Glutamate: Tastant and neuromodulator in taste buds. *Advances in Nutrition*, *7*(4), 823S–7 S. https://doi.org/10.3945/an.115. 011304

152 Rao, R., & Samak, G. (2012). Role of glutamine in protection of intestinal epithelial tight junctions. *Journal of Epithelial Biology & Pharmacology*, *5*(Suppl 1-M7), 47–54. https://doi.org/10.2174/1875044301205010047

153 Tomé, D. (2018). The roles of dietary glutamate in the intestine. *Annals of Nutrition & Metabolism*, *73 Suppl 5*, 15–20. https://doi.org/10.1159/000494777

154 Baj, A., Moro, E., Bistoletti, M., Orlandi, V., Crema, F., & Giaroni, C. (2019). Glutamatergic signaling along the microbiota-gut-brain axis. *International Journal of Molecular Sciences*, *20*(6), 1482. https://doi.org/10.3390/ijms20061482

155 Julio-Pieper, M., O'Connor, R.M., Dinan, T.G., & Cryan, J.F. (2013). Regulation of the brain-gut axis by group III metabotropic glutamate receptors. *European Journal of Pharmacology*, *698*(1–3), 19–30. https://doi.org/10.1016/j.ejphar.2012. 10.027

156 Filpa, V., Moro, E., Protasoni, M., Crema, F., Frigo, G., & Giaroni, C. (2016). Role of glutamatergic neurotransmission in the enteric nervous system and brain-gut axis in health and disease. *Neuropharmacology*, *111*, 14–33. https://doi.org/10.1016/j. neuropharm.2016.08.024

157 Bhat, R., Axtell, R., Mitra, A., Miranda, M., Lock, C., Tsien, R.W., & Steinman, L. (2010). Inhibitory role for GABA in autoimmune inflammation. *Proceedings of the National Academy of Sciences of the United States of America*, *107*(6), 2580–2585. https://doi.org/10.1073/pnas.0915139107

158 Krantis, A. (2000). GABA in the mammalian enteric nervous system. *Physiology*, *15*, 284–290. https://doi.org/10.1152/physiologyonline.2000.15.6.284

159 Mazzoli R., & Pessione E. (2016). The neuro-endocrinological role of microbial glutamate and GABA signalling. *Frontiers in Microbiology 7*, 1934. https://doi.org/10. 3389/fmicb.2016.01934

160 Sokovic Bajic, S., Djokic, J., Dinic, M., Veljovic, K., Golic, N., Mihajlovic, S., & Tolinacki, M. (2019). GABA-producing natural dairy isolate from artisanal zlatar cheese attenuates gut inflammation and strengthens gut epithelial barrier *in vitro*. *Frontiers in Microbiology*, *10*, 527. https://doi.org/10.3389

161 Ngo, D.H., & Vo, T.S. (2019). An updated review on pharmaceutical properties of gamma-aminobutyric acid. *Molecules*, *24*(15), 2678. https://doi.org/10.3390/molecules 24152678

162 Auteri, M., Zizzo, M.G., & Serio, R. (2015). GABA and GABA receptors in the gastrointestinal tract: From motility to inflammation. *Pharmacological Research*, *93*, 11–21. https://doi.org/10.1016/j.phrs.2014.12.001

163 Allen, A.P., Hutch, W., Borre, Y.E., Kennedy, P.J., Temko, A., Boylan, G., Murphy, E., Cryan, J.F., Dinan, T.G., & Clarke, G. (2016). Bifidobacterium longum 1714 as a translational psychobiotic: Modulation of stress, electrophysiology and neurocognition in healthy volunteers. *Translational Psychiatry*, *6*(11), e939. https://doi.org/10.1038/tp. 2016.191

164 Pinto-Sanchez, M.I., Hall, G.B., Ghajar, K., Nardelli, A., Bolino, C., Lau, J.T., Martin, F.P., Cominetti, O., Welsh, C., Rieder, A., Traynor, J., Gregory, C., De Palma, G., Pigrau, M., Ford, A.C., Macri, J., Berger, B., Bergonzelli, G., Surette, M.G., Collins, S.M., … Bercik, P. (2017). Probiotic Bifidobacterium longum NCC3001 reduces depression scores and alters brain activity: A pilot study in patients with irritable bowel syndrome. *Gastroenterology*, *153*(2), 448–459.e8. https://doi.org/10.1053/j.gastro. 2017.05.003

165 Messaoudi, M., Violle, N., Bisson, J.F., Desor, D., Javelot, H., & Rougeot, C. (2011). Beneficial psychological effects of a probiotic formulation (Lactobacillus helveticus R0052 and Bifidobacterium longum R0175) in healthy human volunteers. *Gut Microbes*, *2*(4), 256–261. https://doi.org/10.4161/gmic.2.4.16108

166 Fan, Y., & Pedersen, O. (2021). Gut microbiota in human metabolic health and disease. *Nature Reviews. Microbiology*, *19*(1), 55–71. https://doi.org/10.1038/s41579-020-0433-9

167 Miller, I. (2018). The gut-brain axis: Historical reflections. *Microbial Ecology in Health and Disease*, *29*(1), 1542921. https://doi.org/10.1080/16512235.2018.1542921

4 Obesity

Obesity carries risks to our health, and those risks add costs to our already overburdened health services. The risks and diseases associated with obesity will not be discussed in detail here; primary care practitioners are already all too well aware of what they are. Instead, this chapter will highlight things that go beyond "eat less, move more" which will, hopefully, be useful in devising other ways of managing or even reducing obesity.

There is ongoing debate about whether obesity should be recognised as a disease.[1] If obesity is a disease, it could persuade people to seek help. But equally, it could discourage individuals to take action by suggesting that external treatment is the only answer to reducing obesity.[2] Probably the most important thing to remember is that there is nothing simple about obesity.

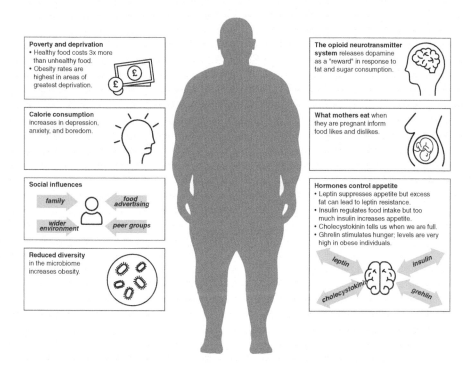

Obesity is far more complex than calories in/calories out.

The NHS states that obesity is generally caused by eating too much and moving too little, but this is too simplistic. Obesity is not a straightforward calories in/calories out calculation. It is a complex tangle of issues which include our mental

DOI: 10.1201/b22900-5

health and wellbeing; how our bodies (and their inhabitants) function; how we view activity; our genetic makeup and predispositions; and our relationships with food and eating, both directly, and within wider society. Modern life and the built environment that we live in heavily encourage a lack of activity. And there is an almost endless variety of cheap, highly processed foods available, at far lower cost than healthier options. A pack of five apples is more expensive than a pack of five doughnuts in most supermarkets.

The most recent statistics on overweight and obesity in the UK are frankly, terrifying. The NHS publishes yearly updates on obesity-related data, including hospital admissions linked to obesity.[3] In England in 2019, 64.2% of adults were either overweight or obese. The pictures in Scotland (66%), Wales (60%), and Northern Ireland (65%) are just as grim.[4] On average, 63.8% of the adult population of the UK is either obese or overweight.

OBESITY AND POVERTY

Although obesity rates are highest in areas of deprivation and lowest in areas of affluence, not everyone living in an area of deprivation will be obese, nor will everyone living in an affluent area be a healthy weight.

Obesity and poverty are both public health issues and poverty's impact on obesity is profound. The road to obesity is not necessarily one of greed or indulgence; at a fundamental level, poverty reduces choice and forces hard decisions. A recent report found that healthy foods cost three times more than unhealthy foods.[5] Too often people need to decide if they pay for food or pay for heating. Should they pay for apples, or pay for doughnuts? Being unable to access or afford sufficient nutritious food is called "food insecurity".

Two decades ago, there were very few food banks in the UK; now there are more than 2,200.[6] Often, for those living in poverty, eating healthy food is secondary to eating at all. And food banks have advised that people are now refusing to accept potatoes, because recipients simply cannot afford the fuel costs to cook them.[7] The Trussell Trust reports that 16% of adults in the UK (over 10 million people) are food insecure, and families with children are twice as likely to be food insecure.[8] Food insecurity means that residents in affluent UK households eat more fruit and vegetables whilst those living in less well-off circumstances consume cheaper, poorer quality foods.[9]

Whilst the government states that it is concerned about the increase in obesity, particularly in childhood, it is taking little effective action to tackle it. Increasing social spending on children reduces childhood obesity.[10] Yet spending on public health and social care in the UK has fallen by 13% in real terms over the last decade and welfare payments for the poorest in our society have been slashed by £37 billion.[11,12] These cuts have had the biggest impact on families with children, particularly those who are eligible for free school meals.[13]

Primary care practitioners cannot do much about the socioeconomic circumstances of patients. However, understanding the impact that a lack of financial resources can have, and a judicious use of social prescribing, may be useful in helping patients modify some aspects of their lives.

ULTRA-PROCESSED FOOD

In the early 2000s, Carlos Monteiro, a Brazilian scientist, noticed that consumption of highly processed foods and obesity in Brazil seemed to be rising at the same rate.[14] In 2010 he published a paper describing a new class of food – ultra-processed foods (UPFs).[15]

The evidence against UPF in relation to the obesity epidemic that is swamping the globe is stacking up. A lot of UPF is what used to be termed "junk food", but these days quite a lot of it claims to be healthy. Because, along with sugar, salt, ultra-processed fat, and additives, some may have added nutrients. Like fibre being added to sugary breakfast cereals, or vitamins to sugar-laden drinks.

UPFs are made in factories from ingredients which have been created out of other foods, things like high-fructose corn syrup, hydrolysed protein, and modified starch. These types of ingredients would not be used in home cooking or eaten as stand-alone foods.

Examples of Ultra-Processed Food Ingredients

Ingredient	Example Wording in an Ingredients List on Packaging
Salt	Salt
	Any additive with "sodium" in its name
Sugar	Dextrose; corn dextrose
	Glucose syrup; glucose-fructose syrup
	Fructose; high-fructose corn syrup
	Partially inverted refiners syrup
Fats and oils	Hydrogenated fat
	Partially hydrogenated fat
	Vegetable fat (saturated and unsaturated plant fats (usually palm and rapeseed) chemically combined at a molecular level)
Hydrolysed protein (protein split into its component amino acids and peptides)	Disodium inosinate
	Flavour enhancer
	Hydrolysed vegetable protein
	Monosodium glutamate
Modified starch	Modified corn starch
	Modified maize starch
	Modified potato starch
Food colourants	E110 Sunset yellow
	E129 Allura Red AC
	E131 Patent Blue V
	E150c Ammonia caramel
	E172 Iron oxides and hydroxides
Flavours	Flavouring
	Nature identical flavouring
	Natural flavouring

(Continued)

Ingredient	Example Wording in an Ingredients List on Packaging
Non-sugar sweeteners	Acesulfame K
	Aspartame
	Isomalt; maltitol; mannitol; sorbitol; xylitol
	Sucralose
Emulsifiers	Alginate (sodium, potassium, ammonium, calcium)
	Guar gum
	Locust bean gum
	Xanthan gum
Humectants	Glucose syrup
	Glycerine
	Lactic acid esters of mono- and diglycerides of fatty acids
Sequestrants	Calcium chloride
	Calcium disodium ethylene diamine tetra-acetate
	Sodium gluconate
	Sodium hexametaphosphate
Firming agents	Calcium chloride
	Calcium citrate
	Magnesium chloride
	Magnesium sulphate
Bulking agents	Inulin
	Konjak
	Maltodextrin
	Xanthan gum
Antifoaming agents	Polyethylene glycol
	Polyglycerol esters of fatty acids
	Polysorbates
	Silicon dioxide
Anticaking agents	Cellulose
	Potassium aluminium silicate
	Polydimethylsioxane
	Silicon dioxide
Glazing agents	Carnauba wax
	Microcrystalline wax
	Shellac
	Stearic acid

UPFs are calorie dense, nutrient poor, and often high in sugars, cheap oils, and salt. They also contain a range of additives used to make non-food ingredients highly palatable. UPF is generally low cost, tasty, convenient, sold in bright shiny packaging that makes it look attractive, and aggressively advertised.

Between 2008 and 2014, UPFs made up 56.8% of the calories consumed in the UK.[16] That figure is likely to have increased in the intervening years, particularly as the UK has the highest consumption of UPF in 19 European countries.[17] The more UPF consumed within a nation, the greater the increase in obesity.[18]

For every percentage point increase in consumption of UPFs, there is an increase of a 0.25% in the prevalence of obesity.[17]

In ways that are not yet fully understood, when we eat UPF, the mechanisms that tell us we are hungry or full are bypassed. People eating diets high in UPFs consume more calories than people eating diets made up of less processed foods, even where diets have been specifically designed to match each other in calories, sugar, fat, salt, fibre, carbohydrates, and protein.[19] And it seems that when we eat UPF, we eat faster.[20]

One of the ways in which UPFs may make us eat more is that they require little chewing (apple vs doughnut again). Hunger and satiety (feeling full) are both influenced by chewing. Increased chewing reduces feelings of hunger and our food intake, whilst at the same time increasing satiation.[21,22] So if we don't need to chew something, it is unlikely to make us feel full.

Added to which, fat, salt, and sugar, all significant components of UPFs, are increasingly being acknowledged as being addictive.[23,24,25] It is well recognised that some people show addictive behaviours for foods, and food cravings, like those seen in drug addiction, have been noted in obese individuals.[26,27,28] And it seems that easily digested and assimilated carbohydrate could also be addictive, although the biochemistry behind this is not yet fully understood.[29]

UPFs, which present little resistance to chewing and which are loaded with fat, salt, and sugar, appear intentionally designed to drive over consumption.

There may be a link between the addictive nature of some foods and human evolution. Humanity spent hundreds of thousands of years actively seeking out high-calorie foods, because being underweight was far more of a threat to survival than being overweight.[30] In an experimental maze setting, people remembered the locations of high-calorie foods more often, and more accurately, than they did for low-calorie foods.[31]

As with all things obesity related, there are no easy answers. But a really good take-away would be to suggest patients steer clear of the ultra-processed food.

THE GLYCAEMIC INDEX

This is probably a good point to talk about the glycaemic index (GI). The GI classifies carbohydrate-containing foods by how fast our digestion will convert them into glucose, and therefore blood sugar, in our bodies. The lower the food is on the GI, the slower it is to convert to glucose. Glucose and white bread have a GI score of 100, yet there are foods which are higher on the GI scale.

Chana dal has a GI of 5.[32] In a 50 g serving it contains 21 g of carbohydrates, 13 g of protein, and 2.40 g of fat. Much of the carbohydrate is actually made up of dietary fibre which cannot be broken down by our digestion. And protein and fat both slow the breakdown of carbohydrate content in digestion. Dates, which are incredibly sweet, have a GI of 55, which puts them into the low GI category, because they also contain a large amount of fibre which slows down the release of sugar[32]

Kellogg's corn flakes on the other hand have a GI of 132.[32] In a 30 g serving they contain 25 g of carbohydrates, only 2.1 g of protein, and virtually no fibre or fat. This means there is very little to slow the breakdown of carbohydrate into glucose.

Unsurprisingly, UPFs tend to be high GI.[33]

Sample of Foods and their GI. Data from Glycemic Index Research[32]

Food	GI	Carbohydrate
Hummus	6	5 g per 30 g
Full fat milk	11	12 per 250 ml
Carrots, raw	16	8 per 80 g
Mixed nuts, salt roasted	24	17 per 50 g
Spaghetti, boiled	34	48 per 180 g
Baked beans (UK)	40	20 per 150 g
Apple, raw	44	13 per 120 g
Carrots, peeled, diced, boiled	49	5 per 80 g
Wholemeal pitta bread	56	14 per 30 g
Basmati rice, boiled	65	39 per 150 g
Sainsbury's Cornflakes (UK)	65	25 per 30 g
Mashed potato	73	18 per 150 g
Watermelon	80	6 per 150 g
Sultana Bran (UK)	90	38 per 50 g
Kellogg's cornflakes (UK)	93	25 per 30 g
Jasmine rice	109	42 per 150 g
Kellogg's cornflakes (USA)	132	25 per 30 g

The "GI Diet" is big business, there are dozens of books out there telling us how to lose weight by controlling the types of carbohydrates we eat. But whilst "diets" may lead to weight loss, they do not necessarily address the underlying issues that led to weight increase or obesity in the first place. A lot of diets are difficult to adhere to long term and as soon as "dieting" stops, habitual eating patterns re-assert themselves and weight begins to creep up again.

HOW OUR RELATIONSHIP WITH FOOD IMPACTS OBESITY

What we eat, when we eat, why we eat, and how much we eat are known as "eating behaviours". These are a complex bundle of internal and external factors including, among other things, neural reward systems, what our mothers ate when they were pregnant, a range of social influences, how much money we can afford to spend, our constantly changing state of mind, and our personal likes and dislikes.[34,35]

Foods containing high levels of fat and sugar stimulate the release of dopamine, triggering feelings of "reward" in rats and mice, and the same seems to be true for humans.[36,37] High-fat food triggers a reward response through the opioid neurotransmitter system whilst sugar fulfils many of the criteria which determine whether a substance is addictive.[38,39] As with drug addiction, the neural reward response from fat and sugar diminishes over time so that more and more of the food providing the response needs to be eaten.[40] It is no wonder that we love eating foods that are high fat and high sugar!

The flavours of the foods that women eat when pregnant have been shown to inform the likes and dislikes of infants and, as they grow, children begin to copy their parents eating behaviours.[41,42] Eating habits developed during childhood tend to continue throughout life and if those eating patterns are less than healthy, the risk of obesity and other health issues will increase.[43] Not only does obesity in parents increase the risk of children being overweight, but the children of overweight parents also have a particularly strong reward response to food.[44]

Our relationship with food is also linked with social factors. As children we generally eat with our families and that can influence how we eat for the rest of our lives.[45] As adolescents the influence of peers, both close friends and those in the wider social environment, becomes more important and can have a significant effect on dietary choices, not all of them positive.[46] As adults we eat differently depending on whether we eat in company, with family or friends, or if we eat alone.[47] And at all stages and ages of life, the impact of food advertising needs to be considered. The days of advertising that suggests that drinking Martini will make the consumer one of the beautiful people are thankfully long gone. But the influence of advertising on food choices remains significant.[48,49,50]

Mental health also has an impact on what, when, why, and how we eat. Depression, anxiety, and boredom have all been linked with both higher calorie consumption and obesity.[51] Obesity can also lead to depression, and that depression may trigger higher calorie consumption, thereby creating a feedback loop leading to further weight gain.[52]

Given the complex multifaceted nature of our relationship with food, it is no wonder that changing the way we eat is far from straightforward. It is one of the most difficult things to do because there are so many layers to it, and it is made even more difficult by the easy availability, and societal acceptability, of potentially addictive, calorie-dense, nutrient-poor foods.

Although the role of social support is not fully understood, it does appear that external support providing positive reinforcement and encouragement helps effective weight loss. And that support can come from a health care practitioner, family, friends, social media, or even an app![53]

INSULIN AND CARBOHYDRATE

The carbohydrate-insulin model has been the predominant theory for the cause of obesity for many years. This states that a high-carbohydrate diet stimulates an excessive release of insulin after eating. High levels of insulin stimulate the deposit of fat (calories) into fat cells, instead of using them to create energy. This slows the metabolic rate, decreasing energy expenditure, but increasing hunger, which results in a gradual accumulation of body fat.[54] The carbohydrate-insulin model is one of the theories behind the rise in popularity of the "keto" diet, which advocates low-carbohydrate, high-fat diets.

However, a somewhat contentious new theory suggests that the carbohydrate-insulin model is too simplistic. Whilst recognising that insulin plays a key role in regulating body fat, some recent studies have found no significant differences in weight loss between higher carbohydrate diet models and higher fat diet models.[55]

The new theory suggests that insulin's functions in blood sugar management and weight gain or loss should be considered as part of a body-wide network that controls energy balance.[56] Because insulin does not work alone.

HUNGER AND APPETITE

Complex interrelated physical and chemical mechanisms have evolved to regulate our food intake.[57] When we eat our stomach expands, triggering sensors which give us a sense of fullness.[58] At the same time, a range of hormones are secreted by enteroendocrine cells which line the GI tract from mouth to anus.[59] More than 30 different hormones have been identified and many of them send signals to the hypothalamus in our brain about satiation.[60] Satiation is the opposite of hunger; it tells us when we have eaten enough and that we do not want to eat any more.[61]

The hormone leptin, which is manufactured by fat cells, tells the brain how much fat (and therefore available energy) is stored in the body. If there is enough fat in the body, leptin tells the hypothalamus to inhibit hunger and so we stop eating. But the more fat cells there are in the body, the more leptin is produced.[62] And high levels of leptin make the brain less receptive to the hormone, so leptin's function of suppressing appetite becomes less effective. Appetite and food intake increase, leading to more body fat being laid down, which in turn produces more leptin.[63]

Insulin, produced in the pancreas, is also an appetite regulator. Levels increase sharply as we eat and when circulating insulin reaches the hypothalamus it causes a loss of appetite, inhibiting food intake.[64] Consistently high levels of circulating insulin create insulin resistance, where body cells do not respond to the hormone and therefore cannot access glucose for energy production.[65] And just like with leptin, insulin resistance can create increased hunger which can result in a vicious cycle of weight gain and increased appetite driving each other.[66]

Other hormones which are key in the regulation of hunger and satiety, are cholecystokinin (CCK), ghrelin, and glucagon-like peptide 1 (GLP-1).

CCK is released by cells lining the duodenum when they sense the presence of sugars and amino acids in the GI tract.[67] It is involved with gut motility, gastric and gallbladder emptying, and the secretion of pancreatic enzymes.[68] It is also a neurotransmitter that sends satiety signals to the brain via the vagus nerve, inhibiting further food intake.[69] Providing additional pharmaceutical CCK can reduce individual meal sizes, but it does not necessarily reduce overall daily intake of food because people tend to simply eat more frequently to compensate for lower food intake.[70]

Ghrelin is sometimes called "the hunger hormone" because one of its main functions is to stimulate hunger. It is also involved in the secretion of growth hormone, the regulation of gut motility, circadian sleep/wake rhythms, taste sensations, reward-seeking behaviour, and glucose metabolism regulation.[71] It is secreted by the stomach and production seems to be linked to normal meal routines as it increases before regular meal times, and then slows after eating.[72] In obese people, ghrelin levels are consistently high, even after eating.[73] A lack of sleep stimulates increased ghrelin production but reduces production of leptin which may be one of the reasons behind the link between obesity and sleep.[74]

GLP-1 is secreted by enteroendocrine cells in the gut in response to calorie consumption and the release of bile acids.[75,76] It actively reduces blood sugar by stimulating insulin synthesis and release.[77] It also reduces appetite, slowing gastric acid secretion and delaying gastric emptying, so the stomach feels full for longer.[78]

SATIETY VALUE

Another factor to consider in weight gain or loss is the "satiety value" of foods; how satisfied and full a person feels after eating a particular food. Unlike the GI, where a high score is considered negative because the food causes blood sugar to increase rapidly, the more satisfying a food is, the higher its number on the satiety index.[79] So, potatoes, with a score of 323, are more satisfying than white bread, which has a score of 100; and fish, with a score of 225 makes us feel full more rapidly than red lentils, which have a score of 133.[80] Unsurprisingly UPF is low scoring on the satiety index.

We are generally oblivious to the intricate choreography that controls the interactions of hormones, neural signalling, and physical cues, we just know when we are hungry, or when we feel full. Unfortunately UPF seems to be able to bypass many of the mechanisms we have in place to stop us overeating. Individuals eating a diet dominated by UPF consume significantly more food, by both weight and calorie content, a lot faster, than people eating a largely unprocessed diet.[81]

The pleasure and reward of food clearly goes far beyond metabolic need.

FAT IS NOT THE ENEMY

Having discussed the issues of UPF at length and noting that UPF often contains high levels of fat, it is perhaps surprising that much of the nutrition world does not view fat as a "bad" thing. It is the nature and quality of the fat that is the issue, rather than "fat" as a whole. Interestingly, overall fat intakes in the UK have fallen over the last decade, as have total energy intakes, yet the epidemic of obesity continues to increase.[82]

Some fats, like the omega-3 fats, are really good for us. Some, like trans fats are really bad for us. And some (including saturated fats) are somewhere in the middle; we need some but too much is not a great idea.

In the early days of the 20th century, scientists were starting to understand that cholesterol was somehow involved in heart disease, particularly in the formation of atherosclerotic plaques. To find the connection, studies were done, feeding saturated fats and cholesterol to rabbits. This didn't turn out so well for the rabbits. Because, as herbivores, rabbits have virtually no cholesterol or saturated fat in their natural diet so, not surprisingly, feeding them high cholesterol foods created atherosclerotic plaques in abundance.[83] This work formed the basis of the "lipid hypothesis".

A key study (the Seven Countries Study) based on the lipid hypothesis was published in 1984.[84] It found that replacing saturated fat with unsaturated vegetable oils resolved the issues of cholesterol, atherosclerosis, and heart disease. The results from this study have directed nutrition and diet policy in the UK, and in many other countries, for decades. Yet despite that, the issues of cholesterol, atherosclerosis, and heart disease have continued to get bigger and bigger.

Recently, evidence was found that the Seven Countries Study cherry-picked its data.[85] So, for decades, multiple countries have based their national dietary guidelines on fat consumption on data that were essentially falsified. A revised analysis shows that the skewed data significantly overestimated the impact of replacing saturated fat intake with unsaturated vegetable oils.[86] There really does not seem to be much benefit from swapping saturated fats for unsaturated fats and oils.[87]

SATURATED FAT – REALLY NOT SO BAD

Which begs the questions: Does saturated fat consumption lead to an increase in cholesterol, atherosclerotic plaques, and heart disease in humans? And will replacing saturated fat with unsaturated vegetable oils reduce the incidence of morbidity and mortality from heart attacks and strokes?

The answer to both questions is "no".

The general view of saturated fats is, at last, changing. They are no longer considered to be the root of all health evil and there are even calls being made to change national dietary guidelines.[88] Although high saturated fat consumption does increase total cholesterol, the types of cholesterol formed are not those which are linked with heart disease.[89] Evidence now shows that saturated fat does not clog arteries.[90] Nor does it cause cardiovascular disease, increase the risk of developing type II diabetes, or increase the risk of stroke.[91,92,93]

This is not to say that eating huge quantities of saturated fat is good; consuming huge amounts of anything is not a great idea. But many of the foods which were demonised as being "high cholesterol" or "bad for you" are being rehabilitated. High on that list are eggs and full-fat dairy products.

Two decades ago, advice on eggs was "don't eat more than three a week because they cause heart disease". This has now changed, and there is broad recognition that eggs are nutritional powerhouses. An average UK egg provides a good amount of vitamins A, D, B2, and B12; folate, biotin, pantothenic acid, and choline; the minerals phosphorus, iodine and selenium; a healthy chunk of complete protein and some fat.[94,95] The fat content of an egg is found in the yolk and is made up of a mixture of different saturated, monounsaturated, and polyunsaturated fatty acids, including some omega-6 and omega-3 fatty acids.[96] Eggs do contain cholesterol, but egg consumption does not affect cholesterol concentrations in the blood.[97]

Eggs are affordable, widely available, easy to cook, and fantastically versatile. What's not to love?

The nutrition world has also been re-evaluating full-fat dairy products. Unfortunately, UK government dietary advice does not appear to have kept up with this revised view and continues to push the outdated low-fat milk, cheese and yoghurt message. Full-fat dairy contains the fat-soluble vitamins A, D, and E. Semi-skimmed milk contains a very little vitamin A and no vitamins D or E, whilst skimmed milk contains no fat-soluble vitamins.[98]

Taking the fat out of milk does not impact its mineral content. All milk contains potassium, calcium, magnesium, and phosphorus, but without vitamin D (absent from both semi-skimmed and skimmed milk), the calcium and phosphorus cannot be absorbed. And whilst full-fat milk does contain saturated fat, there is no evidence of harm from that fat content. Instead, there is evidence that consumption of full-fat dairy products reduces the risk of developing cardiovascular disease and type II diabetes.[99,100]

Do full fat dairy. It's good for you. And it tastes way better than the low-fat stuff.

What about those serried ranks of seed oils on the supermarket shelves, promoted as being better for your health? Well, they may not necessarily be all that good for you. A recently published study of nearly 200,000 participants found that substituting polyunsaturated vegetable oils for saturated fats actually increased the risk of developing cardiovascular disease.[101]

Unless a seed oil states "extra virgin" or "cold pressed" on the label, it will have undergone a series of processes which alter the structure and nature of the oil, removing substances that makes them healthy (vitamins, minerals, fibre, and substances like lecithin and chlorophyl) and gaining a load of toxic substances, including rancidity products and trans fats. Seed oils are easily damaged by heat, light, and oxygen and it is expensive to exclude these from the processes that extract oil from seeds (which is why extra virgin or cold-pressed oils cost a lot more than standard oils). Most seed oils are exposed to heat, light and oxygen during refining. In addition, some seriously toxic chemicals, like heptane and hexane (by-products of the petroleum industry), sodium hydroxide (also known as caustic soda or drain cleaner), and acid-treated activated clays, are used when seed oils are made. Although most of these substances will be removed during processing, there is no guarantee that the oils sold in supermarkets have had all traces eliminated.[102] These highly processed seed oils are used in food manufacture, including margarines and UPFs.

TRANS FATS AND OMEGA-3

Two other fats that need to be considered are trans fats and omega-3 fats.

A tiny proportion of trans fats occur naturally in products derived from cows and sheep but the majority are present due to industrial food processing.[103] Trans fats shift the balance in cholesterol, decreasing the more beneficial high-density lipoprotein (HDL) and increasing the less desirable low-density lipoprotein (LDL).[104] This shift has been linked to the formation of arterial plaques and an increased risk of all forms of cardiovascular disease.[105,106] Trans fats also interfere with the alpha-6 desaturase enzyme which converts omega-3 fats into usable forms.[107] Alterations to alpha-6 desaturase increases the risk of metabolic and inflammatory disorder.[108] This may be why trans fats have been linked to increased risk of ischemic stroke, type II diabetes, poor word recall, and all-cause mortality.[109] Trans-fat consumption has been linked to increased weight gain, particularly abdominal fat deposits.[110]

Trans fats have different chemical bonds from naturally occurring fats which makes them rigid and inflexible. This means the body cannot break them down in the same way that naturally occurring fats are metabolised for energy, through β-oxidation. So they get stashed in cell membranes, supposedly out of the way.[111] But this makes the cell membranes they sit in more rigid than they should be and this has significant detrimental effects on all manner of cellular functions, from transport of substances in and out of cells, to cell signalling, energy production, and apoptosis.[112]

The negative health impacts of trans fats were first noted in the 1980s but it wasn't until the early-2000s that research really started ramping up around them. In 2015, an article in the *BMJ* called for trans fats to be banned in the UK.[113] The UK government has not yet taken any action to prohibit, or even reduce their use. Although industry agreed to a voluntary reduction in 2011, intakes in the UK remain high.[114]

The other key fats to consider in relation to obesity are the essential fatty acids, omega-3 and omega-6. The key omega-3 fats are eicosapentaenoic acid (EPA), docosahexaenoic acid (DHA), and alpha-linolenic acid (ALA), whilst the key omega-6 fats are linoleic acid (LA), gamma linolenic acid (GLA), and arachidonic acid (AA). The human body cannot synthesise the omega fats in the quantities needed to support health and so they must come from the diet. Although we can synthesise some of the omega-3 fats from omega-6 fats, the process is slow and inefficient.[102]

Omega-3 fatty acids are found in oily fish, particularly salmon, mackerel, tuna, herring, and sardines. They are also found in seaweed, marine algae, and nuts and seeds like walnuts, chia, flax, and hemp.

Omega-6 fatty acids are found in seeds, particularly those which are used to make the seed oils which have become so ubiquitous in our diets. They are also found in meat, poultry, and eggs where animals are fed on grains. Grass-fed animals have far higher levels of omega-3, and lower levels of omega-6.[115]

The current view in nutrition science is that we need at least 250 mg/d of a combination of EPA and DHA; however the UK government has not actually made that recommendation.[116] Instead, they recommend that everyone should eat at least one portion of oily fish a week, despite being fully aware that oily fish consumption in this country falls far below that.[117] There are no intake recommendations for omega-6 fats, but most of us get far more than we need because they occur in the vegetable oils which now dominate our fat intake.

The omega-3 fatty acids are used as structural components in cell membranes where they enable flexibility and permeability. They facilitate cell signalling pathways and have potent anti-inflammatory effects because they are used to create anti-inflammatory eicosanoids.[118,119,120] In recent years, omega-3 fatty acids have been found to be protective against developing metabolic disease and there is growing evidence that high intakes may be useful in reducing obesity although the mechanisms behind these functions are not yet fully understood.[121,122]

Some of the omega-6 fatty acids are used as energy substrate but most work alongside the omega-3s as structural components of cell membranes, allowing fluidity and flexibility, and in cell signalling.[123] They are also metabolised into a range of pro-inflammatory prostaglandins, thromboxanes, and leukotrienes – eicosanoids that our bodies use in the management of injury and infection.[124]

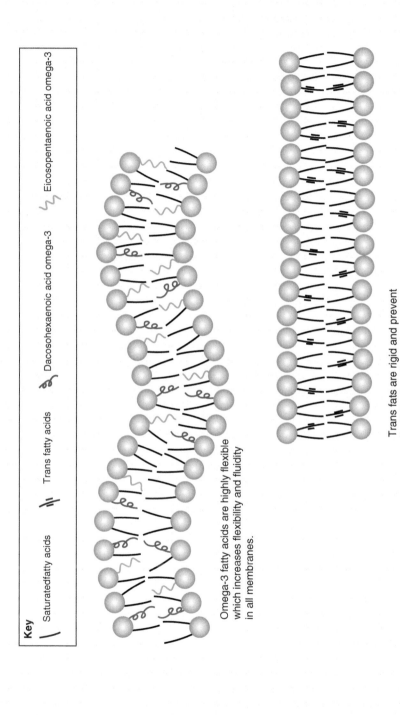

Key

| Saturated fatty acids | Trans fatty acids | Dacosohexaenoic acid omega-3 | Eicosopentaenoic acid omega-3 |

Omega-3 fatty acids are highly flexible which increases flexibility and fluidity in all membranes.

Trans fats are rigid and prevent flexibility and permeability in cell membranes.

Omega-3 fatty acids enable cell membrane flexibility and permeability.

Our modern diets have tipped the balance between these two essential elements; we now consume far too much omega-6 and nowhere near enough omega-3. Evidence suggests that we evolved consuming a 1:1 ratio of these fats, however today the ratio in Western diets is more like 20:1 omega-6/omega-3 and this creates health issues, not least of which is an increased risk of obesity.[125]

Omega-6 fatty acids encourage fat accumulation and increase the risk of insulin and leptin resistance.[126,127] They impact on what type of fat is laid down, promoting the accumulation of white fat cells which store energy in the form of triglycerides, whilst inhibiting brown fat cells which actively burn triglycerides to produce heat.[125,128] High intakes of omega-6 fatty acids are also associated with the development of non-alcoholic fatty liver disease, an independent risk factor for cardiovascular disease often found in obese individuals.[129]

On the other hand, omega-3 fats promote brown fat cell formation, the fats our bodies prefer to use in energy metabolism.[130] Higher concentrations of omega-3 also reduce the overall size of fat cells.[131] They actively block the pro-inflammatory effects of omega-6 fatty acids and significantly reduce insulin resistance.[132,133] And a higher omega-3 to omega-6 ratio has been associated with reduced obesity and smaller waist circumference.[134,135]

Fat certainly needs to be considered in relation to obesity, but perhaps not in the way that policy makers have been advocating for the last 60 years. It is time to flip the message around, particularly as there is so much evidence that consumption of vegetable seed oils can actually increase your risk of obesity, chronic disease, and death.[136]

OBESITY AND THE MICROBIOME

In the early 2000s, interest and research in the microbiome and its impact on our health and wellbeing started to increase.[137] We now know that every centimetre of our body, both inside and out, hosts complex ecosystems of bacteria, viruses, protozoa, fungi, symbionts, and parasites. We also know that our microbiome is as unique and individual as we are.[138]

Work in germ-free mice over the last two decades has shown that obesity and systemic inflammation are closely linked to a reduced diversity of the gut microbiome.[139] This work has stimulated a huge amount of research looking at how the microbiome may impact on obesity in humans.

Ideally the microbiome is made up a broad mix of beneficial microorganisms, neutral commensals, and pathogens. The good guys and the commensals generally keep the bad guys in check. However, a range of internal and external factors, including diet, stress, the use of antibiotics, exercise, age, hormones, and inflammatory status can tip the balance of the gut ecosystem, reducing diversity and allowing pathogens to flourish.[140]

As our understanding of the microbiome has developed, it has become increasingly apparent that it is one of the most significant factors influencing our health and wellbeing.[141] This influence may extend to a causative role in the development of obesity.[142] Although the mechanisms are still not fully understood, research is beginning to find links between specific bacterial species and metabolic risk factors for obesity.[143]

Many of the species of microorganism in our gut have not yet been identified, partially because there are so many different species, but also because it has been difficult to culture many of the species outside of the gut.[144] One recently identified bacterium (*Dysosmobacter welbionis*) has been found at lower levels in the gut of obese individuals and at higher levels in leaner individuals.[145] It has not yet been tested on humans, but mice treated with the bacteria appear to be protected against weight gain, have better glucose tolerance, and lower insulin resistance.[145] This is not the only instance where the microbiome of obese individuals has been found to be significantly different from that of leaner individuals. When obese mice were supplemented with the bacteria *Bacteroides thetaiotaomicron*, their levels of obesity reduced; this bacterium has been found to be significantly lower in obese humans than in leaner people.[146]

What we eat does not just impact our own metabolism. Our Western diet is high in refined sugar, a substance known to have a negative impact on the environment of the gut. Diets high in refined sugar reduce the diversity of the microbiome, particular impacting beneficial bacterial species, and increase the production of pro-inflammatory chemicals in the gut.[147]

Eating a wide range of plant foods, and healthy animal-based foods like oily fish and dairy, promotes the growth of bacteria associated with better metabolic health and lower inflammation.[148] And a diet rich in omega-3 fats derived from fish supports microbial diversity and reduces obesity-associated inflammation.[149] On the flip side, eating a diet high in omega-6 fatty acids (found in the seed oils that proponents of the low-fat myth advocate) reduces the diversity of the microbiome and increases adipose tissue inflammation more than eating a diet high in saturated fats.[150]

Changing what we eat can have a rapid impact on the microbiome, often within 48 hours of dietary changes. The diversity of the microbiome decreases where a diet has a majority of animal-derived foods and increases if a higher amount of plant-derived foods are added.[151] But changes to the microbiome following dietary shifts are not consistent. Some people see significant changes to levels of some bacteria, others may have changes to different species of bacteria, and some individuals may see no change at all.[152]

Plant-based foods provide a range of essential nutrients, but one of the most important, and potentially most overlooked, is fibre. Sometimes known as prebiotics, fibre is fermented by the microbiome to produce short-chain fatty acids, the preferred fuel for the cells lining the gut. Fibre also increases satiety, increases faecal bulk, reduces lipid absorption, improves glucose tolerance, and promotes insulin sensitivity.[153,154]

The microbiome is a constantly changing thing; not only do the inhabitants reproduce rapidly, but they are also expelled on a regular basis via bowel emptying. The importance of a healthy and diverse microbiome to overall health, and its positive effect on obesity needs to be recognised. Obese individuals with a diverse microbiome who eat a diet high in fibre and whole grains have better health outcomes than obese individuals who have less diversity within their microbiome.[155]

THERE IS NO SINGLE "BEST WAY" TO LOSE WEIGHT

Different things work for different people.

There are two medications available for weight loss in the UK; Orlistat which is available on prescription but also over the counter (OTC) as Alli, and XLS Medical which is a medical device and is only available OTC.

Orlistat inhibits the enzymes that allow for the digestion and absorption of fats.[156] There are concerns that this may have a negative impact on the absorption of the fat-soluble vitamins, particularly vitamin D.[157]

The active ingredient in XLS Medical is Clavitanol which claims to reduce the production of enzymes used in the breakdown and absorption of fats, carbohydrates, and proteins and actively binds to dietary fat molecules, preventing their absorption. As a medical device XLS Medical is not listed on the Electronic Medicines Compendium or within the British National Formulary, nor is there any peer-reviewed literature available on the product.

There are also surgery-based options, however these can have unintended consequences with negative impacts on both the microbiome and micronutrient status.[158,159]

Of course, before contemplating either surgery or medicine, what people are eating needs to be considered. There are plenty of diet-based programmes available for people who want to lose weight. But some are more difficult to stick to than others. Whilst some programmes seek to amend an individual's relationship with food, many are highly restrictive, being based on self-control and will power.[160] And once the weight is lost, maintaining changes to eating behaviours can be difficult; eating patterns often revert to what they were before dieting occurred, along with rapid weight gain.[161]

Only about 20% of overweight or obese people who lose weight manage to maintain that loss in the long term. It takes a lot of hard work to keep the weight off, requiring daily physical activity, a continuation of calorie restriction, ongoing monitoring of weight, and maintaining a consistent pattern of eating.[162]

For any weight loss programme to work, it must be easy to stick to. Any diet that is too restrictive around what can or cannot be eaten, or the amount of calories that can be consumed is unlikely to be successful. This can then set up a constantly repeated cycle of attempt, failure, and weight gain.[163]

A key issue in successful weight loss is support, from both professionals and peers. Where a programme includes supportive behavioural change elements, weight loss is more long term.[164] Where that support takes the form of personalised nutrition advice, success is even greater.[165]

Motivation and support are as important as how easy a diet is to stick to. Extrinsic motivation comes from external things, like how friends and family view being overweight and how supportive they are about weight loss. Intrinsic motivation comes from within the individual and is often about autonomy and deriving satisfaction from the activity itself.[166] Either one is essential in achieving effective weight loss, but every person is different; some may need extrinsic motivation, some intrinsic. And some may need a combination of the two.

Finally, setting clearly defined, achievable goals, which can evolve over time is essential. Those goals are best if they are self-defined and personalised, but additional externally defined goals can provide guidance and support. Goals need to be able to change in response to all manner of factors, and if they are set by a healthcare professional, they may be too inflexible to work effectively. This does not mean that any goals cannot be discussed with a healthcare professional, but if goals are set with the aid of someone else, then both parties need to agree to the meaning of those goals and the goals are "owned" by the individual seeking to lose weight.[167]

Make it easy – suggest a gradual change, slowly reducing intakes of highly processed and high sugar food and replacing them with an increased intake of whole grain, high-fibre carbohydrates, good-quality protein, and healthy (including saturated!) fats.

Support your patients – through social prescribing, through counselling, or setting aside time for patients to come and see you every few weeks to talk about their journey.

Talk to them about their motivation – why do they want to lose weight? Is it just because you, as a healthcare practitioner have told them they need to? Or is it because they want to do it for themselves, for whatever reason.

Help them to set the kind of goals they want – in diet, in exercise, in feeling in control of their weight loss.

Above all, listen and be supportive.

REFERENCES

1 Christensen S. (2020). Recognizing obesity as a disease. *Journal of the American Association of Nurse Practitioners, 32*(7), 497–503. https://doi.org/10.1097/JXX. 0000000000000482

2 Wilding J.P.H., & Pile R. (2019). Should obesity be recognised as a disease? *BMJ, 366,* l4858. doi: https://doi.org/10.1136/bmj.l4258

3 Health and Social Care Information Center. (2021). Statistics on Obesity, Physical Activity and Diet, England 2021. *Government Statistical Service, Lifestyles Team, NHS Digital* https://digital.nhs.uk/data-and-information/publications/statistical/statistics-on-obesity-physical-activity-and-diet/england-2021

4 House of Commons Library. (2021). Obesity Statistics. https://researchbriefings.files. parliament.uk/documents/SN03336/SN03336.pdf

5 The Food Foundation. (2021). The Broken Plate 2021. https://foodfoundation.org.uk/ wp-content/uploads/2021/07/FF-Broken-Plate-2021.pdf

6 House of Commons Library. (2021). Food Banks in the UK. https://commonslibrary. parliament.uk/research-briefings/cbp-8585/

7 Sweney, M. (March 2022). Food bank users declining potatoes as cooking costs too high, says Iceland boss. *The Guardian.* https://www.theguardian.com/business/2022/mar/23/ food-bank-users-declining-potatoes-as-cooking-costs-too-high-says-iceland-boss

8 The Trussell Trust. (2021). Scale of food insecurity demands long-term plan to end the need for food banks. https://www.trusselltrust.org/2021/03/19/scale-of-food-insecurity-demands-long-term-plan-to-end-the-need-for-food-banks/

9 Adams J. (2020). Addressing socioeconomic inequalities in obesity: Democratising access to resources for achieving and maintaining a healthy weight. *PLoS Medicine, 17*(7), e1003243. https://doi.org/10.1371/journal.pmed.1003243

10 Miyawaki, A., Evans, C., Lucas, P. J., & Kobayashi, Y. (2021). Relationships between social spending and childhood obesity in OECD countries: An ecological study. *BMJ Open, 11*(2), e044205. https://doi.org/10.1136/bmjopen-2020-044205

11 The Kings Fund. (2021). Spending on public health. https://www.kingsfund.org.uk/projects/nhs-in-a-nutshell/spending-public-health

12 Butler, P. (2018). Welfare spending for UK's poorest shrinks by £37bn. *The Guardian* https://www.theguardian.com/politics/2018/sep/23/welfare-spending-uk-poorest-austerity-frank-field

13 Human Rights Watch. (2019). Nothing Left in the Cupboards; Austerity, Welfare Cuts, and the Right to Food in the UK. https://www.hrw.org/report/2019/05/20/nothing-left-cupboards/austerity-welfare-cuts-and-right-food-uk

14 Wilson, B. (2020). How ultra-processed food took over your shopping basket. *The Guardian.* https://www.theguardian.com/food/2020/feb/13/how-ultra-processed-food-took-over-your-shopping-basket-brazil-carlos-monteiro

15 Monteiro, C.A., Levy, R.B., Claro, R.M., Castro, I.R., & Cannon, G. (2010). A new classification of foods based on the extent and purpose of their processing. *Cadernos de Saude Publica, 26*(11), 2039–2049. https://doi.org/10.1590/s0102-311x2010001100005

16 Rauber, F., Louzada, M., Martinez Steele, E., Rezende, L., Millett, C., Monteiro, C.A., & Levy, R.B. (2019). Ultra-processed foods and excessive free sugar intake in the UK: A nationally representative cross-sectional study. *BMJ Open, 9*(10), e027546. https://doi.org/10.1136/bmjopen-2018-027546

17 Monteiro, C., Moubarac, J., Levy, R., Canella, D., Louzada, M., & Cannon, G. (2018). Household availability of ultra-processed foods and obesity in nineteen European countries. *Public Health Nutrition, 21*(1), 18–26. https://doi.org/10.1017/S1368980017001379

18 Rauber, F., Steele, E.M., Louzada, M., Millett, C., Monteiro, C.A., & Levy, R.B. (2020). Ultra-processed food consumption and indicators of obesity in the United Kingdom population (2008–2016). *PloS One, 15*(5), e0232676. https://doi.org/10.1371/journal.pone.0232676

19 Hall, K.D., Ayuketah, A., Brychta, R., Cai, H., Cassimatis, T., Chen, K.Y., Chung, S.T., Costa, E., Courville, A., Darcey, V., Fletcher, L.A., Forde, C.G., Gharib, A.M., Guo, J., Howard, R., Joseph, P.V., McGehee, S., Ouwerkerk, R., Raisinger, K., Rozga, I., & Zhou, M. (2019). Ultra-processed diets cause excess calorie intake and weight gain: An inpatient randomized controlled trial of ad libitum food intake. *Cell Metabolism, 30*(1), 67–77.e3. https://doi.org/10.1016/j.cmet.2019.05.008

20 Robinson, E., Almiron-Roig, E., Rutters, F., de Graaf, C., Forde, C.G., Tudur Smith, C., Nolan, S.J., & Jebb, S.A. (2014). A systematic review and meta-analysis examining the effect of eating rate on energy intake and hunger. *The American Journal of Clinical Nutrition, 100*(1), 123–151. https://doi.org/10.3945

21 Miquel-Kergoat, S., Azais-Braesco, V., Burton-Freeman, B., & Hetherington, M.M. (2015). Effects of chewing on appetite, food intake and gut hormones: A systematic review and meta-analysis. *Physiology & Behavior, 151*, 88–96. https://doi.org/10.1016/j.physbeh.2015.07.017

22 Krop, E.M., Hetherington, M.M., Nekitsing, C., Miquel, S., Postelnicu, L., & Sarkar, A. (2018). Influence of oral processing on appetite and food intake - A systematic review and meta-analysis. *Appetite, 125*, 253–269. https://doi.org/10.1016/j.appet.2018.01.018

23 Sarkar, S., Kochhar, K.P., & Khan, N.A. (2019). Fat addiction: Psychological and physiological trajectory. *Nutrients, 11*(11), 2785. https://doi.org/10.3390/nu11112785

24 Morris, M.J., Na, E.S., & Johnson, A.K. (2008). Salt craving: The psychobiology of pathogenic sodium intake. *Physiology & Behavior, 94*(5), 709–721. https://doi.org/10.1016/j.physbeh.2008.04.008

25 DiNicolantonio, J.J., O'Keefe, J.H., & Wilson, W.L. (2018). Sugar addiction: Is it real? A narrative review. *British Journal of Sports Medicine, 52*(14), 910–913. https://doi.org/10.1136/bjsports-2017–097971

26 Gearhardt, A.N., & Hebebrand, J. (2021). The concept of "food addiction" helps inform the understanding of overeating and obesity: Debate Consensus. *The American Journal of Clinical Nutrition, 113*(2), 274–276. https://doi.org/10.1093/ajcn/nqaa345

27 Oginsky, M.F., Goforth, P.B., Nobile, C.W., Lopez-Antiago L.F., & Ferrario C.R. (2016). Eating 'junk-food' produces rapid and long-lasting increases in NAC CP-AMPA receptors: Implications for enhanced cue-induced motivation and food addiction. *Neuropsychopharmacology, 41*, 2977–2986. https://doi.org/10.1038/npp.2016.111

28 Schulte, E.M., Smeal, J.K., & Gearhardt, A.N. (2017). Foods are differentially associated with subjective effect report questions of abuse liability. *PloS One, 12*(8), e0184220. https://doi.org/10.1371/journal.pone.0184220

29 Lennerz, B., & Lennerz, J.K. (2018). Food addiction, high-glycemic-index carbohydrates, and obesity. *Clinical Chemistry, 64*(1), 64–71. https://doi.org/10.1373/clinchem.2017.273532

30 Higginson, A.D., McNamara, L.M., & Houston, A.I. (2016). Fatness and fitness: Exposing the logic of evolutionary explanations for obesity. *Proceedings of the Royal Society B, 283,* 20152443. http://doi.org/10.1098/rspb.2015.2443

31 de Vries, R., Morquecho-Campos, P., de Vet, E. de Rijk M., Postma E., de Graaf K., Engel B., & Boesveldt, S. (2020). Human spatial memory implicitly prioritizes high-calorie foods. *Nature Scientific Reports, 10*, 1517. https://doi.org/10.1038/s41598-020-72570-x

32 Glycemic Index Research and GI News. The University of Sydney. https://glycemicindex.com/gi-search/

33 Fardet, A. (2016). Minimally processed foods are more satiating and less hyperglycemic than ultra-processed foods: A preliminary study with 98 ready-to-eat foods. *Food & Function, 7*(5), 2338–2346. https://doi.org/10.1039/c6fo00107f

34 Gahagan, S. (2012). Development of eating behavior: biology and context. *Journal of Developmental and Behavioral Pediatrics: JDBP, 33*(3), 261–271. https://doi.org/10.1097/DBP.0b013e31824a7baa

35 Meule, A., & Vögele, C. (2013). The psychology of eating. *Frontiers in Psychology, 4*, 215. https://doi.org/10.3389/fpsyg.2013.00215

36 Fritz, B.M., Muñoz, B., Yin, F., Bauchle, C., & Atwood, B.K. (2018). A high-fat, high-sugar 'Western' diet alters dorsal striatal glutamate, opioid, and dopamine transmission in mice. *Neuroscience, 372*, 1–15. https://doi.org/10.1016/j.neuroscience.2017.12.036

37 Hartmann, H., Pauli, L.K., Janssen, L.K., Huhn, S., Ceglarek, U., & Horstmann, A. (2020). Preliminary evidence for an association between intake of high-fat high-sugar diet, variations in peripheral dopamine precursor availability and dopamine-dependent cognition in humans. *Journal of Neuroendocrinology, 32*(12), e12917. https://doi.org/10.1111/jne.12917

38 Reyes, T.M. (2012). High-fat diet alters the dopamine and opioid systems: Effects across development. *International Journal of Obesity Supplements, 2*(Suppl 2), S25–S28. https://doi.org/10.1038/ijosup.2012.18

39 Wiss, D.A, Avena, N., Rada, P. (2018). Sugar addiction: From evolution to revolution. *Frontiers in Psychiatry, 9*, 545. https://doi.org/10.3389/fpsyt.2018.00545

40 Stice, E., Yokum, S., Blum, K., & Bohon, C. (2010). Weight gain is associated with reduced striatal response to palatable food. *The Journal of Neuroscience, 30*(39), 13105–13109. https://doi.org/10.1523/JNEUROSCI.2105–10.2010

41 Mennella, J.A., Jagnow, C.P., & Beauchamp, G.K. (2001). Prenatal and postnatal flavor learning by human infants. *Pediatrics, 107*(6), E88. https://doi.org/10.1542/peds.107.6.e88

42 Yelverton, C.A., Geraghty, A.A., O'Brien, E.C., Killeen S.L. Horan M.K., Donnelly, J.M., Larkin, E., Mehegan, J., & McAuliffe, F.M. (2020). Breastfeeding and maternal eating behaviours are associated with child eating behaviours: Findings from the ROLO Kids Study. *European Journal of Clinical Nutrition, 75*, 670–679. https://doi.org/10.1038/s41430-020-00764-7

43 Scaglioni, S., De Cosmi, V., Ciappolino, V., Parazzini, F., Brambilla, P., & Agostoni, C. (2018). Factors influencing children's eating behaviours. *Nutrients, 10*(6), 706. https://doi.org/10.3390/nu10060706

44 Stice, E., Yokum, S., Burger, K.S., Epstein, L.H., & Small, D.M. (2011). Youth at risk for obesity show greater activation of striatal and somatosensory regions to food. *The Journal of Neuroscience, 31*(12), 4360–4366. https://doi.org/10.1523

45 Raine, K.D. (2005). Determinants of healthy eating in Canada: An overview and synthesis. *Canadian Journal of Public Health, 96 Suppl 3*(Suppl 3), S8–S15. https://doi.org/10.1007/BF03405195

46 Ragelienė, T., & Grønhøj, A. (2020). The influence of peers' and siblings' on children's and adolescents' healthy eating behavior. A systematic literature review. *Appetite, 148*, 104592. https://doi.org/10.1016/j.appet.2020.104592

47 Higgs S., & Thomas J. (2016). Social influences on eating. *Current Opinion in Behavioral Sciences, 9*, 1–6. https://doi.org/10.1016/j.cobeha.2015.10.005

48 Ponce-Blandón, J.A., Pabón-Carrasco, M., Romero-Castillo, R., Romero-Martín, M., Jiménez-Picón, N., & Lomas-Campos, M. (2020). Effects of advertising on food consumption preferences in children. *Nutrients, 12*(11), 3337. https://doi.org/10.3390/nu12113337

49 Delfino, L.D., Tebar, W.R., Silva, D., Gil, F., Mota, J., & Christofaro, D. (2020). Food advertisements on television and eating habits in adolescents: A school-based study. *Revista de Saude Publica, 54*, 55. https://doi.org/10.11606/s1518–8787.2020054001558

50 Harris, J.L., Bargh, J.A., & Brownell, K.D. (2009). Priming effects of television food advertising on eating behavior. *Health Psychology, 28*(4), 404–413. https://doi.org/10.1037/a0014399

51 Braden, A., Musher-Eizenman, D., Watford, T., & Emley, E. (2018). Eating when depressed, anxious, bored, or happy: Are emotional eating types associated with unique psychological and physical health correlates? *Appetite, 125*, 410–417. https://doi.org/10.1016/j.appet.2018.02.022

52 Rajan, T.M., & Menon, V. (2017). Psychiatric disorders and obesity: A review of association studies. *Journal of Postgraduate Medicine, 63*(3), 182–190. https://doi.org/10.4103/jpgm.JPGM_712_16

53 Chang, L., Chattopadhyay, K., Li, J., Xu, M., & Li, L. (2021). Interplay of support, comparison, and surveillance in social media weight management interventions: Qualitative study. *JMIR mHealth and uHealth, 9*(3), e19239. https://doi.org/10.2196/19239

54 Ludwig, D.S., & Ebbeling, C.B. (2018). The Carbohydrate-Insulin Model of Obesity: Beyond "Calories In, Calories Out". *JAMA Internal Medicine, 178*(8), 1098–1103. https://doi.org/10.1001/jamainternmed.2018.2933

55 Hall, K.D., Guo, J., Courville, A.B., Boring, J., Brychta, R., Chen, K.Y., Darcey, V., Forde, C.G., Gharib, A.M., Gallagher, I., Howard, R., Joseph, P.V., Milley, L., Ouwerkerk, R., Raisinger, K., Rozga, I., Schick, A., Stagliano, M., Torres, S., Walter, M., Chung, S.T. (2021). Effect of a plant-based, low-fat diet versus an animal-based, ketogenic diet on ad libitum energy intake. *Nature Medicine, 27*(2), 344–353. https://doi.org/10.1038/s41591-020-01209-1

56 Speakman, J.R., & Hall, K.D. (2021). Carbohydrates, insulin, and obesity. *Science, 372*(6542), 577–578. https://doi.org/10.1126/science.aav0448

57 Abdalla, M.M. (2017). Central and peripheral control of food intake. *Endocrine Regulations*, *51*(1), 52–70. https://doi.org/10.1515/enr-2017-0006

58 Bluemel, S., Menne, D., Milos, G., Goetze, O., Fried, M., Schwizer, W., Fox, M., & Steingoetter, A. (2017). Relationship of body weight with gastrointestinal motor and sensory function: Studies in anorexia nervosa and obesity. *BMC Gastroenterology*, *17*(1), 4. https://doi.org/10.1186/s12876-016-0560-y

59 Gunawardene, A.R., Corfe, B.M., & Staton, C.A. (2011). Classification and functions of enteroendocrine cells of the lower gastrointestinal tract. *International Journal of Experimental Pathology*, *92*(4), 219–231. https://doi.org/10.1111/j.1365-2613.2011.00767.x

60 Woods, S.C., & D'Alessio, D.A. (2008). Central control of body weight and appetite. *The Journal of Clinical Endocrinology and Metabolism*, *93*(11 Suppl 1), S37–S50. https://doi.org/10.1210/jc.2008-1630

61 Bellisle, F., Drewnowski, A., Anderson, G.H., Westerterp-Plantenga, M., & Martin, C.K. (2012). Sweetness, satiation, and satiety. *The Journal of Nutrition*, *142*(6), 1149S–54 S. https://doi.org/10.3945/jn.111.149583

62 Ahima, R.S., & Antwi, D.A. (2008). Brain regulation of appetite and satiety. *Endocrinology and Metabolism Clinics of North America*, *37*(4), 811–823. https://doi.org/10.1016/j.ecl.2008.08.005

63 Liu, J., Yang, X., Yu, S., & Zheng, R. (2018). The leptin resistance. *Advances in Experimental Medicine and Biology*, *1090*, 145–163. https://doi.org/10.1007/978-981-13-1286-1_8

64 Al-Zubaidi, A., Heldmann, M., Mertins, A., Brabant, G., Nolde, J.M., Jauch-Chara, K., & Münte, T.F. (2019). Impact of hunger, satiety, and oral glucose on the association between insulin and resting-state human brain activity. *Frontiers in Human Neuroscience*, *13*, 162. https://doi.org/10.3389/fnhum.2019.00162

65 Brown, A.E., & Walker, M. (2016). Genetics of insulin resistance and the metabolic syndrome. *Current Cardiology Reports*, *18*(8), 75. https://doi.org/10.1007/s11886-016-0755-4

66 Ono, H. (2019). Molecular mechanisms of hypothalamic insulin resistance. *International Journal of Molecular Sciences*, *20*(6), 1317. https://doi.org/10.3390/ijms20061317

67 Wauson, E.M., Lorente-Rodríguez, A., & Cobb, M.H. (2013). Minireview: Nutrient sensing by G protein-coupled receptors. *Molecular Endocrinology*, *27*(8), 1188–1197. https://doi.org/10.1210/me.2013-1100

68 Rehfeld, J.F. (2017). Cholecystokinin – From local gut hormone to ubiquitous Messenger. *Frontiers in Endocrinology*, *8*, 47. https://doi.org/10.3389/fendo.2017.00047

69 Desai, A.J., Dong, M., Harikumar, K.G., & Miller, L.J. (2016). Cholecystokinin-induced satiety, a key gut servomechanism that is affected by the membrane micro-environment of this receptor. *International Journal of Obesity Supplements*, *6*(Suppl 1), S22–S27. https://doi.org/10.1038/ijosup.2016.5

70 Andermann, M.L., & Lowell, B.B. (2017). Toward a wiring diagram understanding of appetite control. *Neuron*, *95*(4), 757–778. https://doi.org/10.1016/j.neuron.2017.06.014

71 Poher, A.L., Tschöp, M.H., & Müller, T.D. (2018). Ghrelin regulation of glucose metabolism. *Peptides*, *100*, 236–242. https://doi.org/10.1016/j.peptides.2017.12.015

72 Cummings, D.E., Purnell, J.Q., Frayo, R.S., Schmidova, K., Wisse, B.E., & Weigle, D.S. (2001). A prandial rise in plasma ghrelin levels suggests a role in meal initiation in humans. *Diabetes*, *50*(8), 1714–1719. https://doi.org/10.2337/diabetes.50.8.1714

73 Perry, B., & Wang, Y. (2012). Appetite regulation and weight control: The role of gut hormones. *Nutrition and Diabetes*, *2*(1), e26. https://doi.org/10.1038/nutd.2011.21

74 Beccuti, G., & Pannain, S. (2011). Sleep and obesity. *Current Opinion in Clinical Nutrition and Metabolic Care, 14*(4), 402–412. https://doi.org/10.1097/MCO.0b013e32 83479109

75 Paternoster, S., & Falasca, M. (2018). Dissecting the physiology and pathophysiology of glucagon-like peptide-1. *Frontiers in Endocrinology, 9*, 584. https://doi.org/10.3389/fendo.2018.00584

76 MacLean, P.S., Blundell, J.E., Mennella, J.A., & Batterham, R.L. (2017). Biological control of appetite: A daunting complexity. *Obesity, 25* Suppl 1, S8–S16. https://doi.org/10.1002/oby.21771

77 Pizarroso, N.A., Fuciños, P., Gonçalves, C., Pastrana, L., & Amado, I.R. (2021). A review on the role of food-derived bioactive molecules and the microbiota-gut-brain axis in satiety regulation. *Nutrients, 13*(2), 632. https://doi.org/10.3390/nu13020632

78 Weltens, N., Iven, J., Van Oudenhove, L., & Kano, M. (2018). The gut-brain axis in health neuroscience: Implications for functional gastrointestinal disorders and appetite regulation. *Annals of the New York Academy of Sciences, 1428*(1), 129–150. https://doi.org/10.1111/nyas.13969

79 Holt, S.H., Miller, J.C., Petocz, P., & Farmakalidis, E. (1995). A satiety index of common foods. *European Journal of Clinical Nutrition, 49*(9), 675–690. https://5y1.org/download/b7cbe05a2a520b4b4cfba62a959dc7c4.pdf

80 Buckland, N.J., James Stubbs, R., & Finlayson, G. (2015). Towards a satiety map of common foods: Associations between perceived satiety value of 100 foods and their objective and subjective attributes. *Physiology & Behavior, 152*(Pt B), 340–346. https://doi.org/10.1016/j.physbeh.2015.07.001

81 Forde, C.G., Mars, M., & de Graaf, K. (2020). Ultra-processing or oral processing? A role for energy density and eating rate in moderating energy intake from processed foods. *Current Developments in Nutrition, 4*(3), nzaa019. https://doi.org/10.1093/cdn/nzaa019

82 Derbyshire, E. (2019). UK dietary changes over the last two decades: A focus on vitamin & mineral intakes. *Journal of Vitamins and Minerals, 2,* 104. https://www.gavinpublishers.com/articles/research-article/Journal-of-Vitamins-Minerals/uk-dietary-changes-over-the-last-two-decades-a-focus-on-vitamin-mineral-intakes

83 Fan, J., Kitajima, S., Watanabe, T., Xu, J., Zhang, J., Liu, E., & Chen, Y.E. (2015). Rabbit models for the study of human atherosclerosis: From pathophysiological mechanisms to translational medicine. *Pharmacology & Therapeutics, 146*, 104–119. https://doi.org/10.1016/j.pharmthera.2014.09.009

84 Keys, A., Menotti, A., Aravanis, C., Blackburn, H., Djordevic, B.S., Buzina, R., Dontas, A.S., Fidanza, F., Karvonen, M.J., & Kimura, N. (1984). The seven countries study: 2,289 deaths in 15 years. *Preventive Medicine, 13*(2), 141–154. https://doi.org/10.1016/0091-7435

85 Begley, S. (2017). Records Found in Dusty Basement Undermine Decades of Dietary Advice. *Scientific American* https://www.scientificamerican.com/article/records-found-in-dusty-basement-undermine-decades-of-dietary-advice/

86 Ramsden, C.E., Zamora, D., Majchrzak-Hong, S., Faurot, K.R., Broste, S.K., Frantz, R.P., Davis, J.M., Ringel, A., Suchindran, C.M., & Hibbeln, J.R. (2016). Re-evaluation of the traditional diet-heart hypothesis: Analysis of recovered data from Minnesota Coronary Experiment (1968–73). *BMJ, 353*, i1246. https://doi.org/10.1136/bmj.i1246

87 Veerman, J.L. (2016). Dietary fats: A new look at old data challenges established wisdom. *BMJ, 353*, i1512. https://doi.org/10.1136/bmj.i1512

88 Astrup, A., Magkos, F., Bier, D.M., Brenna, J.T., de Oliveira Otto, M.C., Hill, J. O., King, J.C., Mente, A., Ordovas, J.M., Volek, J.S., Yusuf, S., & Krauss, R.M. (2020). Saturated fats and health: A reassessment and proposal for food-based recommendations: JACC

state-of-the-art review. *Journal of the American College of Cardiology*, *76*(7), 844–857. https://doi.org/10.1016/j.jacc.2020.05.077

89 DiNicolantonio, J.J., & O'Keefe, J.H. (2018). Effects of dietary fats on blood lipids: A review of direct comparison trials. *Open Heart*, *5*(2), e000871. https://doi.org/10.1136/openhrt-2018-000871

90 Malhotra A., Redberg R.F., & Meier P. (2017). Saturated fat does not clog the arteries: coronary heart disease is a chronic inflammatory condition, the risk of which can be effectively reduced from healthy lifestyle interventions. *British Journal of Sports Medicine*, *51*(15), 1111–1112. https://doi.org/10.1136/bjsports-2016-097285

91 Zhu, Y., Bo, Y., & Liu, Y. (2019). Dietary total fat, fatty acids intake, and risk of cardiovascular disease: A dose-response meta-analysis of cohort studies. *Lipids in Health and Disease*, *18*(1), 91. https://doi.org/10.1186/s12944-019-1035-2

92 Schwab, U., Lauritzen, L., Tholstrup, T., Haldorssoni, T., Riserus, U., Uusitupa, M., & Becker, W. (2014). Effect of the amount and type of dietary fat on cardiometabolic risk factors and risk of developing type 2 diabetes, cardiovascular diseases, and cancer: A systematic review. *Food & Nutrition Research*, *58*, 10.3402/fnr.v58.25145. https://doi.org/10.3402/fnr.v58.25145

93 Kang, Z.Q., Yang, Y., & Xiao, B. (2020). Dietary saturated fat intake and risk of stroke: Systematic review and dose-response meta-analysis of prospective cohort studies. *Nutrition, Metabolism, and Cardiovascular Diseases*, *30*(2), 179–189. https://doi.org/10.1016

94 Egg nutrition information. (2020). *British Lion Eggs*. https://www.egginfo.co.uk/egg-nutrition-and-health/egg-nutrition-information

95 Réhault-Godbert, S., Guyot, N., & Nys, Y. (2019). The Golden Egg: Nutritional value, bioactivities, and emerging benefits for human health. *Nutrients*, *11*(3), 684. https://doi.org/10.3390/nu11030684

96 Zita, L., Okrouhlá, M., Krunt, O., Kraus, A., Stádník, L., Čítek, J., & Stupka, R. (2022). Changes in fatty acids profile, health indices, and physical characteristics of organic eggs from laying hens at the beginning of the first and second laying cycles. *Animals*, *12*(1), 125. https://doi.org/10.3390/ani12010125

97 Kim, J.E., & Campbell, W.W. (2018). Dietary cholesterol contained in whole eggs is not well absorbed and does not acutely affect plasma total cholesterol concentration in men and women: Results from 2 randomized controlled crossover studies. *Nutrients*, *10*(9), 1272. https://doi.org/10.3390/nu10091272

98 Public Health England. (2021). McCance and Widdowson's Composition of Foods Integrated Dataset (CoFID). https://www.gov.uk/government/publications/composition-of-foods-integrated-dataset-cofid

99 Astrup, A., Geiker, N., & Magkos, F. (2019). Effects of full-fat and fermented dairy products on cardiometabolic disease: Food is more than the sum of its parts. *Advances in Nutrition*, *10*(5), 924S–930 S. https://doi.org/10.1093/advances/nmz069

100 Hirahatake, K.M., Astrup, A., Hill, J.O., Slavin, J.L., Allison, D.B., & Maki, K.C. (2020). Potential cardiometabolic health benefits of full-fat dairy: The evidence base. *Advances in Nutrition*, *11*(3), 533–547. https://doi.org/10.1093/advances/nmz132

101 Ho, F.K., Gray, S.R., Welsh, P., Petermann-Rocha, F., Foster, H., Waddell, H., Anderson, J., Lyall, D., Sattar, N., Gill, J., Mathers, J.C., Pell, J.P., & Celis-Morales, C. (2020). Associations of fat and carbohydrate intake with cardiovascular disease and mortality: Prospective cohort study of UK Biobank participants. *BMJ*, *368*, m688. https://doi.org/10.1136/bmj.m688

102 Erasmus, U. (1993). Fats that Heal Fats that Kill; Section 3:16. *Alive Books* Burnaby BC Canada.

103 Dhaka, V., Gulia, N., Ahlawat, K.S., & Khatkar, B.S. (2011). Trans fats-sources, health risks and alternative approach – A review. *Journal of Food Science and Technology*, *48*(5), 534–541. https://doi.org/10.1007/s13197-010-0225-8

104 Oteng, A.B., & Kersten A. (2020). Mechanisms of action of *trans* fatty acids. *Advances in Nutrition, 11*(3), 697–708. https://doi.org/10.1093/advances/nmz125

105 Zapolska, D.D., Bryk, D., & Olejarz, W. (2015). Trans fatty acids and atherosclerosis-effects on inflammation and endothelial function. *Journal of Nutrition & Food Sciences, 5,* 426. https://doi.org/10.4172/2155-9600.1000426

106 Hadj Ahmed, S., Kharroubi, W., Kaoubaa, N., Zarrouk, A., Batbout, F., Gamra, H., Najjar, M.F., Lizard, G., Hininger-Favier, I., & Hammami, M. (2018). Correlation of trans fatty acids with the severity of coronary artery disease lesions. *Lipids in Health and Disease, 17*(1), 52. https://doi.org/10.1186/s12944-018-0699-3

107 Burns-Whitmore, B., Froyen, E., Heskey, C., Parker, T., & San Pablo, G. (2019). Alpha-linolenic and linoleic fatty acids in the vegan diet: Do they require Dietary Reference Intake/adequate intake special consideration? *Nutrients, 11*(10), 2365. https://doi.org/10.3390/nu11102365

108 Brown, K.M., Sharma, S., Baker, E., Hawkins, W., van der Merwe, M., & Puppa, M.J. (2019). Delta-6-desaturase (FADS2) inhibition and omega-3 fatty acids in skeletal muscle protein turnover. *Biochemistry and Biophysics Reports, 18,* 100622. https://doi.org/10.1016/j.bbrep.2019.100622

109 de Souza, R.J., Mente, A., Maroleanu, A., Cozma, A.I., Ha, V., Kishibe, T., Uleryk, E., Budylowski, P., Schünemann, H., Beyene, J., & Anand, S.S. (2015). Intake of saturated and trans unsaturated fatty acids and risk of all cause mortality, cardiovascular disease, and type 2 diabetes: Systematic review and meta-analysis of observational studies. *BMJ, 351,* h3978. https://doi.org/10.1136/bmj.h3978

110 Thompson, A.K., Minihane, A-M., & Williams, C.M. (2010). *Trans* fatty acids and weight gain. *International Journal of Obesity (2005), 35*(3), 315–324. https://doi.org/10.1038/ijo.2010.141

111 Tyler, A., Greenfield, J.L., Seddon, J.M., Brooks, N.J., & Purushothaman, S. (2019). Coupling phase behavior of fatty acid containing membranes to membrane bio-mechanics. *Frontiers in Cell and Developmental Biology, 7,* 187. https://doi.org/10.3389/fcell.2019.00187

112 Ibarguren, M., López, D.J., & Escribá, P.V. (2014). The effect of natural and synthetic fatty acids on membrane structure, microdomain organization, cellular functions and human health. *Biochimica et Biophysica Acta, 1838*(6), 1518–1528. https://doi.org/10.1016/j.bbamem.2013.12.021

113 Allen, K., Pearson-Stuttard, J., Hooton, W., Diggle, P., Capewell, S., & O'Flaherty, M. (2015). Potential of trans fats policies to reduce socioeconomic inequalities in mortality from coronary heart disease in England: Cost effectiveness modelling study. *BMJ, 351,* h4583. https://doi.org/10.1136/bmj.h4583

114 Wanders, A.J., Zock, P.L., & Brouwer, I.A. (2017). Trans fat intake and its dietary sources in general populations worldwide: A systematic review. *Nutrients, 9*(8), 840. https://doi.org/10.3390/nu9080840

115 Simopoulos, A.P., & DiNicolantonio, J.J. (2016). The importance of a balanced ω-6 to ω-3 ratio in the prevention and management of obesity. *Open Heart, 3*(2), e000385. https://doi.org/10.1136/openhrt-2015-000385

116 Derbyshire, E. (2019). Oily fish and omega-3s across the life stages: A focus on intakes and future directions. *Frontiers in Nutrition, 6,* 165. https://doi.org/10.3389/fnut.2019.00165

117 Public Health England. (2019). NDNS: Time trend and income analyses for Years 1 to 9. https://www.gov.uk/government/statistics/ndns-time-trend-and-income-analyses-for-years-1-to-9

118 Swanson, D., Block, R., & Mousa, S.A. (2012). Omega-3 fatty acids EPA and DHA: Health benefits throughout life. *Advances in Nutrition, 3*(1), 1–7. https://doi.org/10.3945/an.111.000893

119 Cholewski, M., Tomczykowa, M., & Tomczyk, M. (2018). A comprehensive review of chemistry, sources and bioavailability of omega-3 fatty acids. *Nutrients*, *10*(11), 1662. https://doi.org/10.3390/nu10111662

120 Haß, U., Herpich, C., & Norman, K. (2019). Anti-inflammatory diets and fatigue. *Nutrients*, *11*(10), 2315. https://doi.org/10.3390/nu11102315

121 Young, I.E., Parker, H.M., Cook, R.L., O'Dwyer, N.J., Garg, M.L., Steinbeck, K.S., Cheng, H.L., Donges, C., Franklin, J.L., & O'Connor, H.T. (2020). Association between obesity and omega-3 status in healthy young women. *Nutrients*, *12*(5), 1480. https://doi.org/10.3390/nu12051480

122 Albracht-Schulte, K., Kalupahana, N.S., Ramalingam, L., Wang, S., Rahman, S.M., Robert-McComb, J., & Moustaid-Moussa, N. (2018). Omega-3 fatty acids in obesity and metabolic syndrome: A mechanistic update. *The Journal of Nutritional Biochemistry*, *58*, 1–16. https://doi.org/10.1016/j.jnutbio.2018.02.012

123 Whelan, J., & Fritsche, K. (2013). Linoleic acid. *Advances in Nutrition*, *4*(3), 311–312. https://doi.org/10.3945/an.113.003772

124 Funk, C.D. (2001). Prostaglandins and leukotrienes: Advances in eicosanoid biology. *Science*, *294*(5548), 1871–1875. https://doi.org/10.1126/science.294.5548.1871

125 Simopoulos, A.P. (2016). An increase in the omega-6/Omega-3 fatty acid ratio increases the risk for obesity. *Nutrients*, *8*(3), 128. https://doi.org/10.3390/nu8030128

126 Tsurutani, Y., Inoue, K., Sugisawa, C., Saito, J., Omura, M., & Nishikawa, T. (2018). Increased serum dihomo-γ-linolenic acid levels are associated with obesity, body fat accumulation, and insulin resistance in Japanese patients with type 2 diabetes. *Internal Medicine*, *57*(20), 2929–2935. https://doi.org/10.2169/internalmedicine.0816-18

127 Phillips, C.M., Goumidi, L., Bertrais, S., Field, M. R., Ordovas, J.M., Cupples, L. A., Defoort, C., Lovegrove, J.A., Drevon, C.A., Blaak, E.E., Gibney, M.J., Kiec-Wilk, B., Karlstrom, B., Lopez-Miranda, J., McManus, R., Hercberg, S., Lairon, D., Planells, R., & Roche, H.M. (2010). Leptin receptor polymorphisms interact with polyunsaturated fatty acids to augment risk of insulin resistance and metabolic syndrome in adults. *The Journal of Nutrition*, *140*(2), 238–244. https://doi.org/10.3945/jn.109.115329

128 Smorlesi, A., Frontini, A., Giordano, A., & Cinti, S. (2012). The adipose organ: white-brown adipocyte plasticity and metabolic inflammation. *Obesity Reviews*, *13 Suppl 2*, 83–96. https://doi.org/10.1111/j.1467-789X.2012.01039.x

129 Patterson, E., Wall, R., Fitzgerald, G.F., Ross, R.P., & Stanton, C. (2012). Health implications of high dietary omega-6 polyunsaturated fatty acids. *Journal of Nutrition and Metabolism*, *2012*, 539426. https://doi.org/10.1155/2012/539426

130 Lund, J., Larsen, L.H., & Lauritzen, L. (2018). Fish oil as a potential activator of brown and beige fat thermogenesis. *Adipocyte*, *7*(2), 88–95. https://doi.org/10.1080/21623945.2018.1442980

131 Martínez-Fernández, L., Laiglesia, L.M., Huerta, A.E., Martínez, J.A., & Moreno-Aliaga, M.J. (2015). Omega-3 fatty acids and adipose tissue function in obesity and metabolic syndrome. *Prostaglandins & Other Lipid Mediators*, *121*(Pt A), 24–41. https://doi.org/10.1016/j.prostaglandins.2015.07.003

132 D'Angelo, S., Motti, M.L., & Meccariello, R. (2020). ω-3 and ω-6 Polyunsaturated fatty acids, obesity and cancer. *Nutrients*, *12*(9), 2751. https://doi.org/10.3390/nu12092751

133 Hernandez, J.D., Li, T., Rau, C. M., LeSuer, W.E., Wang, P., Coletta, D. K., Madura, J.A., 2nd, Jacobsen, E.A., De Filippis, E. (2021). ω-3PUFA supplementation ameliorates adipose tissue inflammation and insulin-stimulated glucose disposal in subjects with obesity: A potential role for apolipoprotein E. *International Journal of Obesity (2005)*, *45*(6), 1331–1341. https://doi.org/10.1038/s41366-021-00801-w

134 Micallef, M., Munro, I., Phang, M., & Garg, M. (2009). Plasma n-3 Polyunsaturated Fatty Acids are negatively associated with obesity. *The British Journal of Nutrition*, *102*(9), 1370–1374. https://doi.org/10.1017/S0007114509382173

135 Torres-Castillo, N., Silva-Gómez, J.A., Campos-Perez, W., Barron-Cabrera, E., Hernandez-Cañaveral, I., Garcia-Cazarin, M., Marquez-Sandoval, Y., Gonzalez-Becerra, K., Barron-Gallardo, C., & Martinez-Lopez, E. (2018). High dietary ω-6:ω-3 PUFA ratio is positively associated with excessive adiposity and waist circumference. *Obesity Facts*, *11*(4), 344–353. https://doi.org/10.1159/000492116

136 Ramsden, C.E., Zamora, D., Leelarthaepin, B., Majchrzak-Hong, S.F., Faurot, K.R., Suchindran, C.M., Ringel, A., Davis, J.M., & Hibbeln, J.R. (2013). Use of dietary linoleic acid for secondary prevention of coronary heart disease and death: Evaluation of recovered data from the Sydney Diet Heart Study and updated meta-analysis. *BMJ*, *346*, e8707. https://doi.org/10.1136/bmj.e8707

137 NIH Human Microbiome Portfolio Analysis Team. (2019). A review of 10 years of human microbiome research activities at the US National Institutes of Health, Fiscal Years 2007–2016. *Microbiome*, *7*(1), 31. https://doi.org/10.1186/s40168-019-0620-y

138 Gilbert, J.A. (2015). Our unique microbial identity. *Genome Biology*, *16*(1), 97. https://doi.org/10.1186/s13059-015-0664-7

139 Sonnenburg, J.L., & Bäckhed, F. (2016). Diet-microbiota interactions as moderators of human metabolism. *Nature*, *535*(7610), 56–64. https://doi.org/10.1038/nature18846

140 Weiss, G.A., & Hennet, T. (2017). Mechanisms and consequences of intestinal dysbiosis. *Cellular and Molecular Life Sciences: CMLS*, *74*(16), 2959–2977. https://doi.org/10.1007/s00018-017-2509-x

141 Kho, Z.Y., & Lal, S.K. (2018). The human gut microbiome – a potential controller of wellness and disease. *Frontiers in Microbiology*, *9*, 1835. https://doi.org/10.3389/fmicb.2018.01835

142 Tseng, C.H., & Wu, C.Y. (2019). The gut microbiome in obesity. *Journal of the Formosan Medical Association*, *118 Suppl 1*, S3–S9. https://doi.org/10.1016/j.jfma.2018.07.009

143 Maruvada, P., Leone, V., Kaplan, L.M., & Chang, E.B. (2017). The human microbiome and obesity: Moving beyond associations. *Cell Host & Microbe*, *22*(5), 589–599. https://doi.org/10.1016/j.chom.2017.10.005

144 Almeida, A., Mitchell, A.L., Boland, M., Forster, S.C., Gloor, G.B., Tarkowska, A., Lawley, T.D., & Finn, R.D. (2019). A new genomic blueprint of the human gut microbiota. *Nature*, *568*(7753), 499–504. https://doi.org/10.1038/s41586-019-0965-1

145 Le Roy, T., Moens de Hase, E., Van Hul, M., Paquot, A., Pelicaen, R., Régnier, M., Depommier, C., Druart, C., Everard, A., Maiter, D., Delzenne, N.M., Bindels, L. B., de Barsy, M., Loumaye, A., Hermans, M. P., Thissen, J. P., Vieira-Silva, S., Falony, G., Raes, J., Muccioli, G.G., & Cani, P.D. (2021). *Dysosmobacter welbionis* is a newly isolated human commensal bacterium preventing diet-induced obesity and metabolic disorders in mice. *Gut*, gutjnl-2020-323778. https://doi.org/10.1136/gutjnl-2020-323778

146 Ding, R.X., Goh, W.R., Wu, R. N., Yue, X. Q., Luo, X., Khine, W., Wu, J.R., & Lee, Y.K. (2019). Revisit gut microbiota and its impact on human health and disease. *Journal of Food and Drug Analysis*, *27*(3), 623–631. https://doi.org/10.1016/j.jfda.2018.12.012

147 Rinninella, E., Cintoni, M., Raoul, P., Lopetuso, L.R., Scaldaferri, F., Pulcini, G., Miggiano, G., Gasbarrini, A., & Mele, M.C. (2019). Food components and dietary habits: Keys for a healthy gut microbiota composition. *Nutrients*, *11*(10), 2393. https://doi.org/10.3390/nu11102393

148 Asnicar, F., Berry, S.E., Valdes, A.M., Nguyen, L.H., Piccinno, G., Drew, D.A., Leeming, E., Gibson, R., Le Roy, C., Khatib, H.A., Francis, L., Mazidi, M., Mompeo, O., Valles-Colomer, M., Tett, A., Beghini, F., Dubois, L., Bazzani, D., Thomas, A.M., Mirzayi, C., & Segata, N. (2021). Microbiome connections with host metabolism and habitual diet from 1,098 deeply phenotyped individuals. *Nature Medicine*, *27*(2), 321–332. https://doi.org/10.1038/s41591-020-01183-8

149 Caesar, R., Tremaroli, V., Kovatcheva-Datchary, P., Cani, P.D., & Bäckhed, F. (2015). Crosstalk between gut microbiota and dietary lipids aggravates Wat inflammation through TLR signaling. *Cell Metabolism, 22*(4), 658–668. https://doi.org/10.1016/j.cmet.2015.07.026

150 Huang, E.Y., Leone, V.A., Devkota, S., Wang, Y., Brady, M.J., & Chang, E.B. (2013). Composition of dietary fat source shapes gut microbiota architecture and alters host inflammatory mediators in mouse adipose tissue. *JPEN. Journal of Parenteral and Enteral Nutrition, 37*(6), 746–754. https://doi.org/10.1177/0148607113486931

151 David, L.A., Maurice, C.F., Carmody, R.N., Gootenberg, D.B., Button, J.E., Wolfe, B.E., Ling, A.V., Devlin, A.S., Varma, Y., Fischbach, M.A., Biddinger, S.B., Dutton, R.J., & Turnbaugh, P.J. (2014). Diet rapidly and reproducibly alters the human gut microbiome. *Nature, 505*(7484), 559–563. https://doi.org/10.1038/nature12820

152 Cotillard, A., Kennedy, S.P., Kong, L.C., Prifti, E., Pons, N., Le Chatelier, E., Almeida, M., Quinquis, B., Levenez, F., Galleron, N., Gougis, S., Rizkalla, S., Batto, J.M., Renault, P., ANR MicroObes consortium, Doré, J., Zucker, J.D., Clément, K., & Ehrlich, S.D. (2013). Dietary intervention impact on gut microbial gene richness. *Nature, 500*(7464), 585–588. https://doi.org/10.1038/nature12480

153 Barber, T.M., Kabisch, S., Pfeiffer, A., & Weickert, M.O. (2020). The health benefits of dietary fibre. *Nutrients, 12*(10), 3209. https://doi.org/10.3390/nu12103209

154 Martinez, K.B., Leone, V., & Chang, E.B. (2017). Western diets, gut dysbiosis, and metabolic diseases: Are they linked? *Gut Microbes, 8*(2), 130–142. https://doi.org/10.1080/19490976.2016.1270811

155 Hjorth, M.F., Roager, H.M., Larsen, T.M., Poulsen, S.K., Licht, T.R., Bahl, M. I., Zohar, Y., & Astrup, A. (2018). Pre-treatment microbial Prevotella-to-Bacteroides ratio, determines body fat loss success during a 6-month randomized controlled diet intervention. *International Journal of Obesity (2005), 42*(3), 580–583. https://doi.org/10.1038/ijo.2017.220

156 Electronic Medicines Compendium, Summary of Product Characteristics for Xenical 120 mg. https://www.medicines.org.uk/emc/product/2592/smpc

157 McDuffie, J.R., Calis, K.A., Booth, S.L., Uwaifo, G.I., & Yanovski, J.A. (2002). Effects of orlistat on fat-soluble vitamins in obese adolescents. *Pharmacotherapy, 22*(7), 814–822. https://doi.org/10.1592/phco.22.11.814.33627

158 Ciobârcă, D., Cătoi, A.F., Copăescu, C., Miere, D., & Crişan, G. (2020). Bariatric surgery in obesity: Effects on gut microbiota and micronutrient status. *Nutrients, 12*(1), 235. https://doi.org/10.3390/nu12010235

159 Kim, J., Ahn, C.W., Fang, S., Lee, H.S., & Park, J.S. (2019). Association between metformin dose and vitamin B12 deficiency in patients with type 2 diabetes. *Medicine, 98*(46), e17918. https://doi.org/10.1097/MD.0000000000017918

160 Gudzune, K.A., Doshi, R.S., Mehta, A.K., Chaudhry, Z.W., Jacobs, D.K., Vakil, R.M., Lee, C.J., Bleich, S.N., & Clark, J.M. (2015). Efficacy of commercial weight-loss programs: An updated systematic review. *Annals of Internal Medicine, 162*(7), 501–512. https://doi.org/10.7326/M14-2238

161 Bickel, W.K., Moody, L.N., Koffarnus, M., Thomas, J.G., & Wing, R. (2018). Self-control as measured by delay discounting is greater among successful weight losers than controls. *Journal of Behavioral Medicine, 41*(6), 891–896. https://doi.org/10.1007/s10865-018-9936-5

162 Wing, R.R., & Phelan, S. (2005). Long-term weight loss maintenance. *The American Journal of Clinical Nutrition, 82*(1 Suppl), 222S–225 S. https://doi.org/10.1093/ajcn/82.1.222S

163 Thom, G., & Lean, M. (2017). Is there an optimal diet for weight management and metabolic health? *Gastroenterology, 152*(7), 1739–1751. https://doi.org/10.1053/j.gastro.2017.01.056

164 Foster, G.D., Wyatt, H.R., Hill, J.O., Makris, A.P., Rosenbaum, D.L., Brill, C., Stein, R.I., Mohammed, B.S., Miller, B., Rader, D.J., Zemel, B., Wadden, T.A., Tenhave, T., Newcomb, C.W., & Klein, S. (2010). Weight and metabolic outcomes after 2 years on a low-carbohydrate versus low-fat diet: A randomized trial. *Annals of Internal Medicine*, *153*(3), 147–157. https://doi.org/10.7326/0003-4819-153-3-201008030-00005

165 Livingstone, K.M., Celis-Morales, C., Navas-Carretero, S., San-Cristobal, R., Forster, H., Woolhead, C., O'Donovan, C.B., Moschonis, G., Manios, Y., Traczyk, I., Gundersen, T.E., Drevon, C.A., Marsaux, C., Fallaize, R., Macready, A.L., Daniel, H., Saris, W., Lovegrove, J.A., Gibney, M., & Gibney, E.R. (2021). Personalised nutrition advice reduces intake of discretionary foods and beverages: Findings from the Food4Me randomised controlled trial. *The international Journal of Behavioral Nutrition and Physical Activity*, *18*(1), 70. https://doi.org/10.1186/s12966-021-01136-5

166 Poraj-Weder, M., Wąsowicz, G., & Pasternak, A. (2021). Why it is so hard to lose weight? An exploration of patients' and dietitians' perspectives by means of thematic analysis. *Health Psychology Open*, *8*(1), 20551029211024406. https://doi.org/10.1177/20551029211024406

167 Spreckley, M., Seidell, J., & Halberstadt, J. (2021). Perspectives into the experience of successful, substantial long-term weight-loss maintenance: A systematic review. *International Journal of Qualitative Studies on Health and Well-being*, *16*(1), 1862481. https://doi.org/10.1080/17482631.2020.1862481

5 Immunity

There are multiple aspects of the immune system, but at a top-line level, it is split into two sections, the innate immune system, and the acquired (or adaptive) immune system. And, like every other system of the body, each element of the immune system is underpinned by micronutrient sufficiency, or undercut by inadequate nutrition.[1]

Innate immunity is the immune system that we are born with. It is the first general response to any pathogen, it works swiftly, within minutes or hours, but it is non-specific and has limited power. It is made up of:[2]

- Physical barriers including the skin, cell membranes, and the linings of body cavities (lungs, gut, cardiovascular system).
- Biochemical barriers such as mucus, gastric acid, and tears.
- Defensins, proteins which have antimicrobial properties.
- The complement system which supports and enhances the function of other areas of the immune system.
- Cytokines, protein messengers produced by innate immune cells.
- Inflammation triggered by chemicals released by damaged cells; these chemicals signal other cells to come to the assistance of the site of inflammation.
- A range of leukocytes (white blood cells).
  - Phagocytes, including macrophages, neutrophils, and dendritic cells, which consume dead, dying, or damaged cells and pathogens.
  - Natural killer (NK) cells which target damaged host cells, for example, if they have been infected by a virus.
  - Mast cells which release histamine, triggering inflammation, and signalling neutrophils and macrophages.
  - Eosinophils and basophils which trigger inflammation during allergic reactions and parasitic infections.

Acquired or adaptive immunity develops immunological memory in response to any pathogens that are encountered. Because the response needs to be specifically tailored to a threat, the initial activation can be slow, and it may take several days to develop a first response.[3] But if these pathogens are ever encountered again, an effective defence can be swiftly mounted because memory cells are stored in anticipation of just such an encounter. The acquired immune system is primarily dependent on lymphocytes which initially develop in bone

DOI: 10.1201/b22900-6

marrow, but which may mature elsewhere. There are two different types of lymphocytes:

- T cells mature in the thymus gland and differentiate into two different types of cells: cytotoxic T cells which directly kill infected or damaged cells, and helper T cells which coordinate the response of other immune cells.
- B cells are produced in bone marrow. When they are exposed to a pathogen they develop antibodies which circulate in blood and plasma.

Both B and T cells have "memory" cells which are stored in epithelial linings, lymph nodes, and bone marrow.[4] This allows for rapid manufacture and deployment of pathogen-specific B and T cells if necessary.

There are also a number of factors which work across both innate and acquired immunity. Although the complement system is part of the innate immune system, it modulates the activity of T and B cells. Complement proteins are activated by infection. They recruit inflammatory cells and tag pathogens for other immune cells to eliminate.[5] Cytokines also work across the boundaries of the different sectors of the immune system. They facilitate communication with all of the different cells of the immune system and with the surrounding tissues. There are different types of cytokines including interferons, interleukins, and tumour necrosis factor and they are produced by cells within both the innate and acquired immune systems.[6]

IMMUNITY REQUIRES BOTH MICRONUTRIENTS AND MACRONUTRIENTS

As with all body systems, the immune system is dependent on the nutrients that we take in through our diet. Deficiency, or even insufficiency of any nutrient can reduce the operating efficiency of our immune system.[1] And evidence of the role of specific nutrients in the optimal functioning of the immune system is growing.[7,8]

When the immune system is activated by a pathogen it immediately starts to synthesise immune cells. It also triggers the generation of fever and begins work repairing tissues damaged by invading pathogens, or its own inflammatory responses.[9] All of this uses a huge amount of energy, which needs to be generated by our energy-producing metabolism.[10] So, as well as micronutrients, a well-functioning immune system needs enough calories to fund energy production (and the micronutrients that are needed in that production). It also needs a good supply of protein to provide the building blocks for enzymes, immune cells, and immune chemicals. A detailed discussion of the nutrients needed to fund our energy requirements can be found in Chapter 8.

No nutrient acts alone, all are interrelated and interlinked with many having synergistic roles with a range of substances. And, important thought they are, nutrition is more than a collection of micronutrients. It is also about food as a whole; when, why, who with, and how we eat, as well as how much and how often we eat. Our relationship with food and how it makes us feel has a powerful impact on immunity. Food and mood are interlinked through a complex network of factors and, whilst chocolate cake may make people transiently happy, poor diet is associated with low mood in a feedback loop where diet and mental health drive each other either up or down.[11] The immune system functions better when we are in a state of happiness or contentment, but unhappiness or depression has the opposite effect.[12,13]

Some of the specific micronutrients that have roles in maintaining and running an effective immune system are discussed below.

Nutrients Fund Immunity

Micronutrients Needed for the Effective Function of the Immune System

Vitamins	Minerals	Other Substances
Vitamin A	Iron	Omega-3 fatty acids
β carotene	Zinc	Omega-6 fatty acids
Vitamin D	Selenium	
Vitamin E		
B vitamins, particularly:		
B6, B12, folic acid, and vitamin C		

OMEGA-3 AND OMEGA-6

Our first line of defence is barriers; our skin, the epithelium, our mucous membranes, and our cell membranes. Nutrients which are key to the health of these are the long-chain polyunsaturated fatty acids (PUFAs) omega-3 and omega-6.

The PUFA fatty acids arachidonic acid (AA) (omega-6) and the omega-3 fatty acids EPA and DHA are essential in the formation of all cell membranes, where they influence both structure and function. Being highly unsaturated, these fatty acid chains have "bends" in their chains which means they cannot be tightly packed together. This allows greater fluidity and flexibility than would be possible if they were not present.[14] And this fluidity and flexibility enables permeability, allowing the passage of substances in and out of cells.[15] A diagram of how omega-3 fatty acids enable cell membrane flexibility can be found in Chapter 4.

We need an intake of both omega-3 and omega-6, but that intake needs to be balanced, preferably with a 1:1 ratio. Unfortunately, most Western diets have a ratio of omega-6 to omega-3 between 10:1 and 20:1.[16] This unbalanced ratio may well be having a negative impact on our health. Current evidence suggests that a ratio of high omega-6 to low omega-3 actively promotes the development of some diseases, including cardiovascular disease, some inflammatory diseases, and various cancers.[17]

Omega-3 fatty acids have a broadly anti-inflammatory impact which has raised concerns that overly high intakes could damp down immune responses that rely on inflammatory factors.[18] Omega-6 fatty acids have a broadly pro-inflammatory impact, with a role in the regulation of inflammatory responses.[19]

There are vegetable sources of omega-3, primarily in the form of alpha-linolenic acid (ALA). Unfortunately, human conversion of ALA to EPA and DHA is extremely inefficient and our bodies really need omega-3 in the forms of EPA and DHA.[20] The best sources of EPA and DHA are fresh oily fish. Tinned and smoked fish do not provide good sources of omega-3 fatty acids because the processing exposes them to prolonged heat which damages the fragile long-chain fatty acids. Although the UK government recommends everyone should consume 140 g of oily fish a week, most people do not consume fish of any kind, let alone oily fish.[21]

Some eggs are "fortified" with omega-3 through the feeding of hens with high omega-3 seeds such as flax, chia, and hemp. Unlike humans, hens are pretty good at converting the ALA found in these seeds to the EPA and DHA that humans need.[22] However, although egg consumption in the UK is growing, it still equates to only 1.9 eggs per person per week.[23] And omega-3 enriched eggs are not particularly common in the UK.

Sources of omega-6 are plentiful, both in animal and vegetable form, most often in the forms of linoleic acid (LA), gamma-linolenic acid (GLA), and AA which can be found in meat, poultry, eggs, nuts, and most vegetable oils.

Omega-3 fatty acids increase macrophage and neutrophil production, upregulate the function of immune cells, and modulate both T- and B-cell activity.[18] And both omega-3 and omega-6 are used to produce eicosanoids, highly bioactive molecules that have roles in the regulation of multiple physiological processes.[24]

Prostaglandins are eicosanoids, which are derived from both omega-6 AA and omega-3 EPA. Both are involved in regulating the inflammatory response and can be either pro- or anti-inflammatory, at different points in the inflammatory cycle.[18,25]

Leukotrienes are eicosanoids derived from omega-6 AA and omega-3 EPA. Those synthesised from AA are pro-inflammatory and stimulate factors in innate immunity which are reliant on inflammatory responses.[26] Those derived from EPA are anti-inflammatory, but they have far lower potency than those which are made from omega-6.[27]

Thromboxanes are eicosanoids which derive from omega-6 AA. They are pro-inflammatory mediators that stimulate platelet aggregation and vasoconstriction in response to tissue injury.[28]

Maresins are recently identified eicosanoids which derive from the omega-3 DHA. They are potent anti-inflammatory mediators that counter-regulate pro-inflammatory cytokines and stimulate phagocytosis to remove pathogens.[29]

Protectins are part of a sub-family of eicosanoids derived from the omega-3 DHA. They are specialist mediators which regulate the action of neutrophils and macrophages and promote tissue homeostasis.[30]

Resolvins are eicosanoids which derive from the omega-3 fatty acids EPA and DHA. They are generated in response to inflammation, helping to regulate macrophage functions by controlling the production of cytokines.[31]

Although both omega-3 and omega-6 are essential for our health and wellbeing, the unbalanced intake of excessive omega-6 to insufficient omega-3 may well be a significant factor in the prevalence of chronic inflammatory disease in the western world. To help redress that balance, everyone would be well advised to take a daily supplement either of fish oil or one of the algal sources of omega-3. However, the omega fatty acids do not work alone. Many other micronutrients also work to support our immune system.

VITAMINS

VITAMIN A

Vitamin A is really several related compounds, some of animal origin (retinoids), and some of vegetable origin (β-Carotene and other carotenoids) which are converted into retinoids in the body. Dietary sources of vitamin A and β-Carotene can be found in the nutrient cheat sheet in the last section of the book.

Vitamin A is key in the formation and function of epithelial cells, including the skin, and the mucosal cells that line the airways, the digestive tract, and the urinary tract. It supports our first line of defence (barriers) by enhancing the tight junctions between cells.[32] Deficiency in vitamin A leads to changes in epithelial tissues, making them dry, fragile, and prone to cracking, reducing the integrity of barriers, and increasing the likelihood of successful invasion by pathogens.[33] Vitamin A is extremely important to the immune system; serum levels of vitamin A fall during infection and the greater the severity of infection, the greater the decrease in vitamin A.[34]

Vitamin A regulates dendritic cells, leukocytes that are part of the innate immune system. Dendritic cells identify antigens, capture them, and present them to T and B cells, which then produce antibodies.[35] It also enhances T- and B-cell proliferation and activation and inhibits B-cell apoptosis (programmed cell death).[36]

There is very little research looking at the impact of vitamin A supplementation on populations other than infants and young children. Vitamin A sufficiency through supplementation has been shown to be protective against measles.[37] It reduces the severity of the disease in children; if a child diagnosed with measles is given two doses of 30,000 µg (100,000 IU) of vitamin A, 24 hours apart, mortality is significantly reduced.[38,39] Vitamin A sufficiency also inhibits the development of mumps, a virus closely related to measles.[40] Indeed, supplementing children with vitamin A is linked to a clinically meaningful reduction in all-cause morbidity and mortality in children.[41] Given the relevance of vitamin A to the immune system, it is not unreasonable to extrapolate a similar clinically meaningful reduction in adults.

Nearly 20 years ago, a study found that 15% of people in the UK aged 19–24 had vitamin A intakes below the Lower Reference Nutrient Intake, the level which puts most people at risk of deficiency.[42] And vitamin A intakes in the UK have fallen over the last two decades, which suggests that a significant proportion of the UK population are deficient in vitamin A.[43]

Vitamin A (in the retinol form) is one of the few vitamins with significant safety issues if consumed in excess. The UK has taken a precautionary approach to safe intakes and advises that retinol intakes from supplementation should not exceed 800 µg a day (the equivalent of 2,666 IU).[44] However intake levels associated with toxicity are far higher than this. Current evidence suggests that toxicity occurs only at intakes more than three times this amount: 3,000 µg a day (equivalent to 9,999 IU).[45]

β-carotene does not have the same safety concerns. The body converts β-carotene to retinol only as needed, but there is huge variability in this conversion. It is impacted by the food matrix in which it is found, how that food may have been prepared and the amount of β-carotene, dietary fibre, and dietary fat that happens to be in the food. The health and function of the gut are also important, parasites, inflammation, infection, and fever all reduce the conversion of β-carotene to retinol. And the minerals iron and zinc, as well as dietary protein, are needed for conversion, but both iron and zinc are nutrients of concern in the UK.[46] Depending on all of the above, conversion can be as low as 5%, or as high as 65%.[47]

Because of toxicity risks vitamin A is not widely found in stand-alone supplements, although it is often included in multi-vitamin and mineral products, particularly products which are intended to support immunity.

Vitamin D

Vitamin D is so important to so many aspects of health that Chapter 6 is entirely dedicated to this nutrient. Rather than simply repeat that information, here the focus is solely on vitamin D's role within the immune system. Dietary sources of vitamin D can be found in the nutrient cheat sheet in the last section of the book.

Although vitamin D is most commonly associated with bone health, it is being increasingly recognised as a central molecule in the immune system. Deficiency of vitamin D has been linked to an increased risk of developing autoimmune diseases, as well as an increased risk of contracting viral, respiratory, and urinary tract infections.[48,49]

The active form of vitamin D, 1α,25-dihydroxyvitamin D, strengthens the physical barrier function of epithelial tissues, working with vitamin A to maintain the tight junctions between cells.[32] Vitamin D increases the antimicrobial activity of macrophages, reduces the release of pro-inflammatory cytokines and stimulates dendritic cells to activate T cells.[50] Low levels of vitamin D are strongly associated with increased susceptibility to sepsis.[51] It also stimulates the production of cathelicidins, antimicrobial peptides secreted by neutrophils.[52] High levels of cathelicidins have been linked with a reduced risk of death from infection during dialysis.[53]

The gut is central to the health of the body and vitamin D appears to be one of the key substances in the complex environment within the digestive system. The simple and necessary act of eating can expose us to risk through the ingestion of pathogens or allergens. Along with vitamin A, vitamin D's role in maintaining the integrity of the epithelial barrier helps to prevent the passage of pathogens from the gut into the body.[54] Vitamin D status even impacts the gut microbiome; high levels of circulating vitamin D shifts the profile of intestinal bacteria away from dysbiosis, associated with some autoimmune diseases, and towards a healthier balance of microorganisms.[55]

The UK population is largely deficient in vitamin D for much of the year.[56] UK government advice on vitamin D supplementation is ineffectual. It suggests that "everyone should consider taking a daily vitamin D supplement of 10 μg during the autumn and winter."[57] But 10 μg will only ensure that patients who are not already deficient will maintain a plasma level of 25 nmol/L, a level which the rest of the world views as deficient.[58] Any patient with immune issues should be advised to take at least 25 μg (equivalent to 1,000 IU) a day, all year round. Vitamin D has been shown to be safe up to 100 μg (4,000 IU) per day for long-term consumption and therefore, depending on the judgement of the practitioner, a higher dose would be both safe, and potentially, life changing.

Vitamin E

Vitamin E, or α-tocopherol, is a fat-soluble substance that scavenges free radicals and prevents the oxidation of lipids, particularly PUFAs within cell membranes.[59] Dietary sources of vitamin E can be found in the nutrient cheat sheet in the last section of the book.

Immune cell signalling is dependent on the composition and integrity of their membranes. They contain high concentrations of PUFAs in the lipid bilayer of their membranes and are highly metabolically active, and this makes them extremely vulnerable to oxidative damage (peroxidation).

Fortunately, many immune cells contain high levels of vitamin E, which helps to protect them from peroxidation.[60] Vitamin E also supports cell signalling and facilitates the production of some key immune mediators.[61]

Supplementation with vitamin E has been found to increase T- and B-cell differentiation, proliferation, and function.[62] It reduces levels of C-reactive protein and pro-inflammatory cytokines, including cyclooxygenase-2 (COX-2), and inhibits the release of histamine from mast cells.[63,64] And supplementing with vitamin E also protects and increases the selenium-dependent glutathione family of enzymes.[65] These antioxidant enzymes help to regulate the inflammatory aspect of innate immunity and the proliferation and function of lymphocytes.[66]

The effects of vitamin E on immune cells may explain why vitamin E insufficiency can impair immunity, particularly in relation to antibody production and T- and B-cell functions and increased inflammatory responses.

As with all fat-soluble vitamins, vitamin E absorption is increased in the presence of dietary fats; the higher fat the food, the more vitamin E is absorbed, and any fat malabsorption disorder can lead to deficiency. Vitamin E in supplement form is best consumed with a meal to facilitate absorption.

The B Vitamins

The B complex of vitamins consists of eight substances, thiamine (B1), riboflavin (B2), niacin (B3), pantothenic acid (B5), pyridoxin (B6), biotin, folate (sometimes known as folic acid), and cobalamin (B12). Choline is also considered to be part of the complex; although it has not been classified as a vitamin, it is an essential nutrient that must be obtained from the diet to maintain health. The B complex works synergistically and many of the substances within it have interdependent relationship functions, often as cofactors in enzymes within energy metabolism and the synthesis of organic molecules such as DNA, neurotransmitters, and cytokines.

Dietary sources of the B vitamins can be found in the nutrient cheat sheet in the last section of the book.

The immune system uses a lot of energy, in fact, energy use can increase by up to 25% during infection.[67] Therefore, the role of B vitamins within energy metabolism can be said to support overall immunity. The nutrition behind energy metabolism is discussed in detail in Chapter 8. However, three B vitamins do have specific roles within the immune system: B6, B12, and folic acid.[68]

One of vitamin B6's key functions is as a coenzyme in protein synthesis. This makes it central to the proliferation, maturation, and function of multiple immune cells including lymphocytes and NK cells as well as the production of cytokines.[69] B6 is also involved in the regulation of inflammation, and in antibody production.[70]

Although folic acid is best known for reducing the risk of neural tube defects in foetal development, it has many other functions. It is essential for the proliferation and survival of regulatory T cells which modify inappropriate immune responses.[71] It is used in the production of cytokines, particularly interleukins.[69] And it works with B12 in maintaining and enhancing NK cells, as well as in antibody production and function.[72]

Vitamin B12 facilitates the production and function of T cells.[68] It modulates the production of pro- and anti-inflammatory cytokines.[73] It stimulates NK cell activity.[74] And it is essential in folate metabolism, resetting folate, from its "used" methylated form (methyltetrahydrofolate) back to its active tetrahydrofolate form.[75]

Vitamins B6, B12, and folic acid also collaborate in another key function, the management of homocysteine. Whilst not strictly related to the immune system, the amino acid homocysteine is generated as an intermediate substance in the breakdown of protein. It is linked to an increased risk of stroke and cardiovascular and arterial diseases.[76] Homocysteine is strongly pro-inflammatory, and it seems to negatively influence immune responses in both innate and acquired immunity.[77,78]

There currently do not appear to be any concerns around intakes for vitamin B6. However, a significant percentage of the population fail to achieve the Lower Reference Nutrient Intake for folic acid.[46] And many vegetarians and vegans have levels of vitamin B12 at the low/deficient end of the reference range.[79,80]

VITAMIN C

Also known as L-ascorbic acid, vitamin C is one of the water-soluble vitamins and it has been linked with immune function for almost a century. Most animals synthesise their own vitamin C through an enzymatic process, but humans, along with the other great apes (and guinea pigs) have lost the capacity to make their own.[81] It is a powerful antioxidant and a co-factor in a wide range of enzymatic processes.[82] Dietary sources of vitamin C can be found in the nutrient cheat sheets in the last section of the book.

Vitamin C is essential in the synthesis of collagen, the protein which maintains the integrity of all epithelial tissues, and therefore a key defence against pathogens.[83] The symptoms of scurvy (vitamin C deficiency) are the result of an inability to synthesise and stabilise the collagen which provides strength and integrity to blood vessels, connective tissues, and bone.[84] Supplementing with vitamin C can speed wound healing time, a function that is enhanced by vitamin C's action in the function and differentiation of keratinocytes and fibroblasts, cells which support the structural framework of our tissues and help create scar tissue.[85,86]

But the action of vitamin C goes much further. It increases phagocytosis and stimulates the generation of reactive oxygen species (ROS) in some leukocytes, particularly monocytes, macrophages, and neutrophils.[87] ROS, sometimes known as free radicals, are used by leukocytes to kill pathogens.[88] This creates oxidative damage, but fortunately, vitamin C's antioxidant function protects these cells. This may be one of the reasons that plasma vitamin C levels decline so sharply during infections.[89] Vitamin C also stimulates the development, proliferation and function of T cells and NK cells.[90]

Vitamin C is found in fresh fruit and vegetables, but intake of these in the UK is disturbingly low. 77% of adults and 91% of children under the age of 16 eat less than 3.5 portions per day.[91] Only 31% of adults and 8% of teenagers eat the government recommended five portions of fruit and vegetables a day.[43] And a significant number of women have plasma levels of vitamin C so low that it puts them at risk of deficiency.[92] Whilst scurvy may not yet be widespread, it is increasing. In 2008, the NHS registered 61 cases of scurvy as a primary or secondary diagnosis; in 2021, there were 171.[93] But insufficiency does not need to get as far as an outright deficiency to have a negative impact on immune function.

UK reference nutrient intakes are set solely on the basis of preventing deficiency, not on the basis of supporting health. The RNI for vitamin C is set at 40 mg/day which is only just enough, in most people, for the prevention of scurvy.[94] It is certainly not optimum in terms of the multiple functions that vitamin C has. The level of vitamin C which appears to have a beneficial effect on the immune system ranges from 500 mg to 4,000 mg/day.[88] As vitamin C is water soluble it is safe to consume at high levels, the only adverse effect being that at very high levels an individual may develop what is known as "bowel tolerance" as vitamin C is osmotic and pulls water into the bowel, resulting in temporarily loose stools.

MINERALS

IRON

Most commonly thought of as a component of haemoglobin, which transports oxygen, and myoglobin, which binds and stores oxygen within muscle tissues, iron also forms a key part of the immune system. Dietary sources of iron can be found in the nutrient cheat sheets in the last section of the book.

Iron is integral to hundreds of proteins and enzymes involved in energy production, DNA replication and repair, as well as both antioxidant and pro-oxidant functions.[95] A significant proportion of iron is found in macrophages. Macrophages scavenge dead and damaged cells of all kinds, and the iron contained in them is recycled for re-use.[96] This scavenging accounts for around 90% of the daily need for iron.[97]

All immune cells are high-energy users and iron is needed for the basic biochemistry of energy metabolism.[98] Iron is also essential in the synthesis of many of the weapons within the arsenal of immune cells. It is used in the manufacture of the metalloprotein enzyme myeloperoxidase which is used by neutrophils and monocytes to generate ROS.[99] Iron also regulates NK cell activity, the proliferation, differentiation and activation of T cells, and the antibody response in B cells.[100] Low levels of iron are therefore not only a concern because of poor oxygenation, it also means that immune cells are less able to fight infections.[101]

Unfortunately, iron is also used by invading microbes, to support DNA replication, for energy metabolism, and as a defence against ROS. Therefore, as part of innate immunity, the body uses pro-inflammatory cytokines as well as hepcidin (the hormone that regulates iron levels), ferroportin (a key iron transporter), and ferritin (the iron storage protein), to sequester iron.[102] This means that there is limited free iron available for pathogens to access.[103] This strategy is known as nutritional immunity.[104]

While most of the population in the UK do not have issue with iron levels, 32% of teenagers and 27% of women fail to achieve the LRNI for iron, putting them at risk of deficiency.[43] Because of toxicity issues, supplementation should be approached with care, particularly among males and post-menopausal women who do not lose blood on a regular basis. Iron has no specific mechanism for excretion and it is generally only lost through blood loss, the breakdown of red blood cells, although most of that iron is reclaimed and recycled, and the sloughing of the cells lining the gut.[105] High intake of iron can rapidly cause toxicity and although iron poisoning in adults is rare, it can occur in children, usually as a result of a child accessing a parent's food supplements and believing them to be sweets.[106]

ZINC

This essential trace element is part of hundreds of enzymes that have roles in thousands of catalytic, structural, and regulatory functions within the body. The complexity and sheer number of processes that zinc is involved with means that how and why zinc does what it does in multiple biochemical pathways and interactions is still not fully understood. However, what is clear is that, because of its multiplicity of function, zinc deficiency, or even insufficiency, has a negative impact across the immune system. Dietary sources of zinc can be found in the nutrient cheat sheets in the last section of the book.

Zinc is central to maintaining the integrity of all epithelial tissues, from the gut to the airways, to the skin.[107,108,109] In fact around 6% of total body zinc is found in epithelial tissues where it helps to maintain the integrity of barrier function.[110] It regulates and maintains the tight junctions between cells so essential for the integrity of our membranes.[68] It is central in the development, differentiation, and function of cells in both the innate and acquired immune systems. Virtually all immune cell activity is regulated at some level by zinc signalling enzymes and pathways, and it is involved in the expression of hundreds of genes across all immune cells.[111] Zinc is also essential in the management of inflammation, the production of both pro- and anti-inflammatory cytokines and the modulation of inflammatory processes.[112]

Low zinc levels reduce the production and function of monocytes, macrophages, and NK cells, as well as reducing the function of the thymus gland, which in turn reduces the number of mature T cells and skews the proportions of T-helper cells.[113] Zinc insufficiency increases levels of ROS, putting pressure on antioxidant systems, and escalating the generation of inflammatory chemicals.[114]

Like iron, zinc is also used by invading pathogens; they use it for reproduction which enables them to establish a strong foothold within a host.[115] And like iron, our immune system sequesters zinc through nutritional immunity.[104] Plasma levels of zinc fall during infections as neutrophils synthesise calprotectin, an antimicrobial protein that binds zinc, thereby making it less available for use by pathogens.[116]

Zinc also appears to have specific antiviral properties and there is evidence that zinc supplementation can reduce the severity and duration of the common cold, herpes simplex outbreaks, and viral warts, and may even increase the CD4 T-cell count in HIV infection.[117] The precise mechanisms by which zinc does this are still being explored, however, some possibilities include the stimulation of increased production of antiviral proteins such as metallothioneins, creating a physical coating on a virus and interfering with a virus's ability to synthesise proteins.[117,118,119]

Although severe zinc deficiency in UK populations is rare, insufficiency is becoming increasingly common. Zinc intakes have fallen over the last two decades, and a significant proportion of UK citizens have intakes of zinc below the LRNI.[43] If taking zinc as a supplement, they should always be consumed with food as zinc on an empty stomach can cause nausea and GI cramping.

SELENIUM

Selenium is an essential trace element that is needed in microscopic amounts to maintain health. However, it cannot be used directly by the body, instead it is incorporated into the amino acid selenocysteine which in turn forms part of selenoproteins.[120] There are 25 selenoproteins and their functions range from cell maintenance to thyroid hormone metabolism, from forming part of several antioxidant enzyme families to protein synthesis, and from inflammatory modulation to immune cell activation.[121] Dietary sources of selenium can be found in the nutrient cheat sheets in the last section of the book.

The glutathione peroxidase and thioredoxin reductase antioxidant enzymes are highly active within the immune system, protecting immune cells from oxidation.[122] Selenium and vitamin E work together to protect and "reset" the glutathione enzymes through redox reactions and deficiency or insufficiency of either selenium or vitamin E are often interconnected.[123,124]

Although outright selenium deficiency is rare in the UK, low selenium status has been linked with poor immune function, increased susceptibility to viral diseases, and an increased risk of cardiovascular disease and some cancers, particularly those associated with inflammation.[125] Selenium insufficiency impairs the proliferation and function of almost all immune cells from both the innate and the acquired immune systems.[126] If selenium levels are boosted from inadequate to adequate through supplementation, there is an almost immediate increase in proliferation of T cells, NK cell activity and overall innate immune function.[127]

Whilst plants manufacture their own vitamins and other chemicals such as flavonoids, carotenoids, anthocyanins and polyphenols, minerals must be absorbed from the soil in which plants are grown. Soil levels of selenium across the UK are low and as a result the plants that grow in the UK, and the animals that eat them, also have low levels of selenium.[128] Selenium intakes in the UK have been falling for nearly 40 years and nearly 30% of the population have selenium intakes below the LRNI.[43,129,130] The impact of this on the long-term overall health of the nation is concerning.

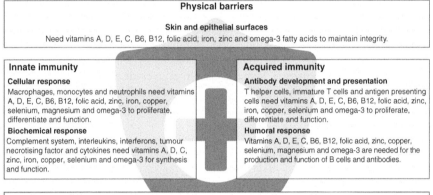

Physical barriers
Skin and epithelial surfaces
Need vitamins A, D, E, C, B6, B12, folic acid, iron, zinc and omega-3 fatty acids to maintain integrity.

Innate immunity	Acquired immunity
Cellular response	**Antibody development and presentation**
Macrophages, monocytes and neutrophils need vitamins A, D, E, C, B6, B12, folic acid, zinc, iron, copper, selenium, magnesium and omega-3 to proliferate, differentiate and function.	T helper cells, immature T cells and antigen presenting cells need vitamins A, D, E, C, B6, B12, folic acid, zinc, iron, copper, selenium and omega-3 to proliferate, differentiate and function.
Biochemical response	**Humoral response**
Complement system, interleukins, interferons, tumour necrotising factor and cytokines need vitamins A, D, C, zinc, iron, copper, selenium and omega-3 for synthesis and function.	Vitamins A, D, E, C, B6, B12, folic acid, zinc, copper, selenium, magnesium and omega-3 are needed for the production and function of B cells and antibodies.

Inflammatory response
Regulation of inflammation
Vitamins A, C, E, B6, zinc, iron, copper, selenium, magnesium and omega-3 fatty acids are needed to modulate inflammatory responses.
Antioxidant response
Immune cells use vitamin C and E, iron, zinc, copper, selenium and magnesium act as weapons, creating oxidative bursts to destroy pathogens. Also used as antioxidants to protect immune cells and wider tissues against inflammation.

Nutrients needed for effective immune system functioning.

Calcium

Immune responses are largely dependent on the ability of the different cells and chemicals of our immune system to communicate with each other and calcium forms part of that communication. It is used by B cells and mast cells in cell signalling, but recent evidence suggests that its key role is the regulation of the production of T cells, signalling to either ramp up production in response to pathogen invasion or damp down production once an infection has been dealt with.[131,132] Calcium also enables T cells to access the glucose needed to fund the energy demands of an immune response.[133]

Calcium's support in immunity does not stop there. It helps to protect the gut, a key battleground for the immune system. Calcium not only inhibits an over-proliferation of colonic cells, but it also supports the epithelial barrier, helping to maintain tight junctions and reduce inflammation in the gut.[134]

Calcium intakes have fallen over the last two decades.[43] Most women in the UK have intakes below the RNI, and an increasing number of both men and women have intakes that fall below the LRNI.[46] As with other vitamins and minerals discussed in this chapter, sources of calcium can be found in the nutrient cheat sheets at the end of this book.

OTHER FACTORS

β-GLUCANS

β-glucans are polysaccharides, long, indigestible, carbohydrate chains that form part of the cell walls in yeasts, grains, and fungi. There are many different forms of β-glucans. Some, found in grains, particularly oats and barley, reduce insulin resistance, improve dyslipidaemia, may help to reduce obesity and hypertension and actively reduce inflammation.[135,136] Others, found in fungi, particularly oyster, reishi, maitake, and shiitake mushrooms and yeasts, modulate the function of the immune system.[137]

Mushroom and yeast β-glucans have a direct effect on the epithelium, supporting the integrity of our barrier protection, particularly in the gut.[138] They appear to stimulate the migration of keratinocytes and fibroblasts to wound sites, where they accelerate tissue granulation and collagen deposition in scar formation.[139] And macrophages exposed to β-glucans carry long-term memory which allows them to recruit specific immune cells to deal with a pathogen that we have previously encountered.[140]

β-glucans impact on the immune system seems to be through the activation of immune cells. The β-glucans found in yeasts and fungi are identified by pattern recognition receptors on macrophages, monocytes, and dendritic cells in the gut.[141] These cells consume the β-glucans, chop them up and prime the fragments to trigger antimicrobial responses in other immune cells.[141] They are then incorporated into T cells, B cells, and NK cells where they enhance their functions and activity.[141]

β-glucans appear to have some anti-metastatic action, possibly as a result of the stimulation of NK cell activity and modulation of the balance between different types of T cells.[142] They also improve the anticancer effects of treatment and improve quality of life in cancer patients.[143]

β-glucans are available to purchase as food supplements from good health food shops.

FLAVONOIDS AND POLYPHENOLS

Actually, flavonoids are polyphenols; both are chemicals which act as antioxidants in plants. There are lots of different types of flavonoids, and they are found in all plant foods. Detailed dietary sources of flavonoids can be found in the nutrient cheat sheets in the last section of the book.

There are six different types of flavonoids; isoflavonoids, flavanones, flavanols, flavonols, flavones, and anthocyanidins. They each have different chemical structures and can influence our health in different ways. Over 5,000 have been identified thus far, and there are certainly more to discover.[144]

The mechanisms of action of flavonoids within the immune system are still being studied.[145] However, they go far beyond "simple" antioxidant effects; they are anti-inflammatory, they can reduce the risk of developing cardiovascular disease, help reduce blood pressure and prevent blood clots, and may reduce the risk of developing some dementias.[146] Some may even reduce the risk of developing some cancers, partially because of their potent antioxidant effects, but also because they induce programmed cell death and suppress cancer cell proliferation.[147]

Flavonoids are ubiquitous in plant foods because they are essential in so many aspects of plant life; they regulate development, ensure pigmentation which in turn provides UV protection, and are used in defence and signalling, within plants, between plants, and between plants and microorganisms.[148] All anyone needs to do to get a healthy dose of flavonoids is to consume fruit, vegetables, grains, nuts and seeds, roots, flowers, tea, coffee, chocolate, and wine.

THE MICROBIOME AND GALT

The gut microbiome comes up repeatedly in this book because it influences so many different aspects of our health and wellbeing. The relationship between the digestive system and immune function is discussed in more detail in Chapter 3.

Because the GI tract is exposed to more pathogenic threats than any other area of the body, it is a key training ground for our immune system which learns how to distinguish between the harmless and the pathogenic within the vast and constantly changing ecosystem of the microbiome.[149] The GI tract is also home to one of the largest immune organs in the body, gut-associated lymphoid tissue or GALT, and the microbiome is critical in maintaining both its structure and function.[150]

The interaction of the microbiome with the immune system is complex, involving multiple players including bacterial species, viruses, metabolic by-products of host, microbiome and pathogens, and a multitude of other factors. It is still being explored, however, what is becoming increasingly clear is that a well-balanced microbiome is critical in maintaining and supporting a strong immune system.[151] And to keep the microbiome happy you need to eat lots of plant foods because these contain the fibre which supports the microbiome.

Of course, there are many other factors which can have an impact on immunity – both positive and negative. Age, gender, genetics, how much sleep we have, our state of mind, our infection history, our exposure to environmental toxins, and a range of lifestyle factors can all affect how our immune system responds to challenges.

But underpinning everything else is nutrition. Micronutrients are essential for health and wellbeing throughout our lives and the general paucity of the UK diet means that almost everyone will have low intakes of at least some nutrients. As a basic health insurance measure healthcare professionals would be well advised to suggest patients eat lots of fruit and vegetables and take food supplements; a multivitamin, a multi-mineral, and an omega-3 fatty acid.

REFERENCES

1 Childs, C.E., Calder, P.C., & Miles, E.A. (2019). Diet and immune function. *Nutrients*, 11(8) 1933 doi: 10.3390/nu11081933

2 Alberts, B., Johnson, A., & Lewis, J. (2002). Molecular Biology of the Cell. 4th edition. New York: Garland Science. Chapter 25, Innate Immunity. Available from: https://www.ncbi.nlm.nih.gov/books/NBK26846/

3 Alberts, B., Johnson, A., & Lewis, J. (2002). Molecular Biology of the Cell. 4th edition. New York: Garland Science. Chapter 24, The Adaptive Immune System. Available from: https://www.ncbi.nlm.nih.gov/books/NBK21070/

4 Ratajczak, W., Niedźwiedzka-Rystwej, P., Tokarz-Deptuła, B., & Deptuła, W. (2018). Immunological memory cells. *Central-European Journal of Immunology*, *43*(2), 194–203. https://doi.org/10.5114/ceji.2018.77390

5 Killick, J., Morisse, G., Sieger, D., & Astier, A.L. (2018). Complement as a regulator of adaptive immunity. *Seminars in Immunopathology*, *40*(1), 37–48. https://doi.org/10.1007/s00281-017-0644-y

6 Zhang, J. M., & An, J. (2007). Cytokines, inflammation, and pain. *International Anesthesiology Clinics*, *45*(2), 27–37. https://doi.org/10.1097/AIA.0b013e318034194e

7 Gombart, A.F., Pierre, A., & Maggini, S. (2020). A review of micronutrients and the immune system – Working in harmony to reduce the risk of infection. *Nutrients*, 12(1), 236. https://doi.org/10.3390/nu12010236

8 Calder, P.C., Carr, A.C., Gombart, A.F., & Eggersdorfer, M. (2020). Optimal nutritional status for a well-functioning immune system is an important factor to protect against viral infections. *Nutrients,* 12(4): 1181 https://doi.org/10.3390/nu12041181

9 Wang, A., Luan, H.H., & Medzhitov, R. (2019). An evolutionary perspective on immunometabolism. *Science*, 363(6423), eaar3932. https://doi.org/10.1126/science.aar3932

10 Baracos, V. E., Whitmore, W. T., & Gale, R. (1987). The metabolic cost of fever. *Canadian Journal of Physiology and Pharmacology*, 65(6), 1248–1254. https://doi.org/10.1139/y87-199

11 Firth, J., Gangwisch, J.E., Borisini, A., Wootton, R.E., & Mayer, E.A. (2020). Food and mood: how do diet and nutrition affect mental wellbeing?. *BMJ*, *369*, m2382. https://doi.org/10.1136/bmj.m2382

12 Lee, C.H., & Giuliani, F. (2019). The role of inflammation in depression and fatigue. *Frontiers in Immunology*, *10*, 1696. https://doi.org/10.3389/fimmu.2019.01696

13 Barak, Y. (2006). The immune system and happiness. *Autoimmunity Reviews*, 5(8), 523–527. https://doi.org/10.1016/j.autrev.2006.02.010

14 de Carvalho, C., & Caramujo, M.J. (2018). The various roles of fatty acids. *Molecules,* 23(10), 2583. https://doi.org/10.3390/molecules23102583

15 Erasmus, U. (1999). Fats that Heal Fats that Kill (8th print). *Alive Books* Canada

16 Simopoulos, A.P. (2011). Evolutionary aspects of diet: The omega-6/omega-3 ratio and the Brain. *Molecular Neurobiology*, 44, 203–215. https://doi.org/10.1007/s12035-010-8162-0

17 Simopoulos, A.P. (2002). The importance of the ratio of omega-6/omega-3 essential fatty acids. *Biomedicine & Pharmacotherapy*, *56*(8), 365–379. https://doi.org/10.1016/s0753-3322(02)00253-6

18 Guitérrez, S., Svahn, S.L., & Johansson, M.E. (2019). Effects of omega-3 fatty acids on immune cells. *International Journal of Molecular Science*, 20(20), 5028. https://doi.org/10.3390/ijms20205028

19 Djuricic, I., & Calder, P.C. (2021). Beneficial outcomes of omega-6 and omega-3 polyunsaturated fatty acids on human health: An update for 2021. *Nutrients*, *13*(7), 2421. https://doi.org/10.3390/nu13072421

20 Greupner, T., Kutzner, L., Nolte, F., Strangmann, A., Kohrs, H., Hahn, A., Schebb, N.H., & Schuchardt, J. P. (2018). Effects of a 12-week high-α-linolenic acid intervention on EPA and DHA concentrations in red blood cells and plasma oxylipin pattern in subjects with a low EPA and DHA status. *Food & Function, 9*(3), 1587–1600. https://doi.org/10.1039/c7fo01809f

21 Derbyshire, E. (2019). Oily fish and omega-3s across the life stages: A focus on intakes and future directions. *Frontiers in Nutrition, 6,* 165. https://doi.org/10.3389/fnut.2019.00165

22 Alagawany, M., Elnesr, S.S., Farag, M.R., Abd El-Hack, M.E., Khafaga, A.F., Taha, A.E., Tiwari, R., Yatoo, M.I., Bhatt, P., Khurana, S.K., & Dhama, K. (2019). Omega-3 and omega-6 fatty acids in poultry nutrition: Effect on production performance and health. *Animals, 9*(8), 573. https://doi.org/10.3390/ani9080573

23 British Egg Industry Council; industry data. https://www.egginfo.co.uk/egg-facts-and-figures/industry-information/data

24 Dennis, E.A, & Norris, P.C. (2015). Eicosanoid storm in infection and inflammation. *Nature Reviews: Immunology*; 15(8), 511–523 https://doi.org/10.1038/nri3859

25 Ricciotti, E., & FitzGerald, G.A. (2011). Prostaglandins and inflammation. *Arteriosclerosis, Thrombosis and Vascular Biology*; 31(5), 986–1000 https://doi.org/10.1161/ATVBAHA.110.207449

26 Peters-Golden, M., Canetti, C., Mancuso, P., & Coffey, M.J. (2005). Leukotrienes: underappreciated mediators of innate immune responses. *Journal of Immunology, 174*(2), 589–594. https://doi.org/10.4049/jimmunol.174.2.589

27 Simonetto, M., Infante, M., Sacco, R.L., Rundek, T., & Della-Morte, D. (2019). A novel anti-inflammatory role of omega-3 PUFAs in prevention and treatment of atherosclerosis and vascular cognitive impairment and dementia. *Nutrients, 11*(10), 2279. https://doi.org/10.3390/nu11102279

28 Rucker, D., & Dhamoon, A.S. (2022). Physiology, Thromboxane A2. In: StatPearls [Internet]. Treasure Island (FL): StatPearls Publishing; Available from: https://www.ncbi.nlm.nih.gov/books/NBK539817/

29 Tang, S., Wan, M., Huang, W., Stanton, R.C., & Xu, Y. (2018). Maresins: Specialized proresolving lipid mediators and their potential role in inflammatory-related diseases. *Mediators of Inflammation*; 2380319. https://doi.org/10.1155/2018/2380319

30 Duvall, M.G., & Levy, B.D. (2016). DHA- and EPA- derived resolvins, protectins, and maresins in airway inflammation. *European Journal of Pharmacology*; 785,144–155. https://doi.org/10.1016/j.ejphar.2015.11.001

31 Seki, H., Sasaki, T., Ueda, T., & Arita, M. (2010). Resolvins as regulators of the immune system. *The Scientific World Journal, 10,* 818–831. https://doi.org/10.1100/tsw.2010.72

32 Farré, R., Fiorani, M., Abdu Rahiman, S., & Matteoli, G. (2020). Intestinal Permeability, inflammation and the role of nutrients. *Nutrients, 12*(4), 1185. https://doi.org/10.3390/nu12041185

33 Huang, Z., Lui Y., Qi G., Brand, D., & Zheng, S.G. (2018). Role of Vitamin A in the Immune System. *Journal of Clinical Medicine*; 7(9): 258 https://doi.org/10.3390/jcm7090258

34 Stephensen, C.B. Vitamin, A, infection, and immune function (2001). *Annual Review of Nutrition,* 21, 167–192. https://doi.org/10.1146/annurev.nutr.21.1.167

35 Beijer, M.R., Kraal G., & den Haan, J.M. (2014). Vitamin A and dendritic cell differentiation. *Immunology, 142*(1), 39–45. https://doi.org/10.1111/imm.12228

36 Mora, J.R., Iwata, M., von Andrian, U.H. (2008). Vitamin effects on the immune system: vitamins A and D take center stage. *Nature Reviews: Immunology,* 8(9), 685–698 https://doi.org/10.1038/nri2378

37 Trottier, C., Chabot, S., Mann, K.K., Colombo, M., Chatterjee, A., Miller, W.H., & Ward, B.J. (2008). Retinoids inhibit measles virus in vitro via nuclear retinoid receptor

signaling pathways. *Antiviral Research*, 80(1), 45–53 https://doi.org/10.1016/j.antiviral. 2008.04.003

38 World Health Organisation (2019). Fact Sheets. Measles. https://www.who.int/news-room/fact-sheets/detail/measles

39 D'Souza, R.M., & D'Souza, R. (2002). Vitamin A for the treatment of children with measles--a systematic review. *Journal of Tropical Pediatrics*, 48(6), 323–327. https://doi.org/10.1093/tropej/48.6.323

40 Soye, K.J., Trottier, C., Di Lenardo, T. Z., Restori, K.H., Reichman, L., Miller, W.H., & Ward, B.J. (2013). In vitro inhibition of mumps virus by retinoids. *Virology Journal*, 10, 337. DOI: https://doi.org/10.1186/1743-422X-10-337

41 Imdad, A., Mayo-Wilson E., Herzer, K., & Bhutta, Z.A. (2017). Vitamin A supplementation for preventing morbidity and mortality in children from six months to five years of age. *The Cochrane database of systematic reviews*, 3(3), CD008524. https://doi.org/10.1002/14651858.CD008524.pub3

42 Feskanich, D., Singh V., Willett W.C., & Colditz, G.A. (2002). Vitamin A intake and hip fractures among postmenopausal women. *JAMA*, 287(1), 47–54. https://doi.org/10.1001/jama.287.1.47

43 Derbyshire, E. (2019). UK dietary changes over the last two decades: A focus on vitamin and mineral intakes. *Journal of Vitamins and Minerals*, 2(2), 104. https://www.gavinpublishers.com/articles/research-article/Journal-of-Vitamins-Minerals/uk-dietary-changes-over-the-last-two-decades-a-focus-on-vitamin-mineral-intakes

44 Scientific Advisory Committee on Nutrition. (2005). Review of Dietary Advice on Vitamin A. https://assets.publishing.service.gov.uk/government/uploads/system/uploads/attachment_data/file/338853/SACN_Review_of_Dietary_Advice_on_Vitamin_A.pdf

45 Penniston, K.L., & Tanumihardjo, S.A. (2006). The acute and chronic toxic effects of vitamin A, *The American Journal of Clinical Nutrition*, 83(2), 191–201. https://doi.org/10.1093/ajcn/83.2.191

46 Derbyshire, E. (2018). Micronutrient intakes of British adults across mid-life: A secondary analysis of the UK national diet and nutrition survey. *Frontiers in Nutrition*, 5, 55. https://doi.org/10.3389/fnut.2018.00055

47 Haskell, M.J. (2012). The challenge to reach nutritional adequacy for vitamin A: β-carotene bioavailability and conversion—evidence in humans, *The American Journal of Clinical Nutrition*, 96(5), 1193S–1203 S. https://doi.org/10.3945/ajcn.112.034

48 Siddiqui, M., Manansala, J.S., Abdulrahman, H.A., Nasrallah, G.K., Smatti, M.K., Younes, N., Althani, A.A., & Yassine, H.M. (2020). Immune modulatory effects of vitamin D on viral infections. *Nutrients*, 12(9), 2879. https://doi.org/10.3390/nu12092879

49 Sassi, F., Tamone C., & D'Amelio, P. (2018). Vitamin D: Nutrient, hormone and immunomodulator. *Nutrients*, 10(11), 1656. https://doi.org/10.3390/nu10111656

50 Ao, T., Kikuta J., & Ishii, M. (2021). The effects of vitamin D on immune system and inflammatory diseases. *Biomolecules*, 11(11), 1624. https://doi.org/10.3390/biom11111624

51 Greulich, T., Regner, W., Branscheidt, M., Herr, C., Koczulla, A.R., Vogelmeier, C.F., & Bals, R. (2017). Altered blood levels of vitamin D, cathelicidin and parathyroid hormone in patients with sepsis-a pilot study. *Anaesthesia and Intensive Care*, 45(1), 36–45. https://doi.org/10.1177

52 Scheenstra, M.R., van Harten, R.M., Veldhuizen, E., Haagsman, H.P., & Coorens, M. (2020). Cathelicidins Modulate TLR-Activation and Inflammation. *Frontiers in Immunology*, 11, 1137. https://doi.org/10.3389/fimmu.2020.01137

53 Gombart, A.F., Bhan, I., Borregaard, N., Tamez, H., Camargo, C.A., Jr, Koeffler, H.P., & Thadhani, R. (2009). Low plasma level of cathelicidin antimicrobial peptide (hCAP18) predicts increased infectious disease mortality in patients undergoing hemodialysis. *Clinical Infectious Diseases*, 48(4), 418–424. https://doi.org/10.1086/596314

54 Cantorna, M.T., Snyder, L., & Arora, J. (2019). Vitamin A and vitamin D regulate the microbial complexity, barrier function, and the mucosal immune responses to ensure intestinal homeostasis. *Critical Reviews in Biochemistry and Molecular Biology*, *54*(2), 184–192. https://doi.org/10.1080/10409238.2019.1611734

55 Yamamoto, E.A., Jørgensen, T.N. (2020). Relationships Between Vitamin D, Gut Microbiome, and Systemic Autoimmunity. *Frontiers in Immunology*; 10: 3141. https://doi.org/10.3389/fimmu.2019.03141

56 Sutherland, J.P., Zhou, A., Leach, M.J., & Hyppönen, E. (2021). Differences and determinants of vitamin D deficiency among UK biobank participants: A cross-ethnic and socioeconomic study. *Clinical Nutrition, 40*(5), 3436–3447. https://doi.org/10.1016/j.clnu.2020.11.019

57 NHS (2020). Vitamin D. https://www.nhs.uk/conditions/vitamins-and-minerals/vitamin-d/

58 Sempos, C.T., Heijboer, A.C., Bikle, D.D., Bollerslev, J., Bouillon, R., Brannon, P.M., DeLuca, H.F., Jones, G., Munns, C.F., Bilezikian, J.P., Giustina, A., & Binkley, N. (2018). Vitamin D assays and the definition of hypovitaminosis D: results from the First International Conference on Controversies in Vitamin D. *British Journal of Clinical Pharmacology*, *84*(10), 2194–2207. https://doi.org/10.1111/bcp.13652

59 Lee, G.A., Han, S.N. (2018). The Role of Vitamin E in Immunity. *Nutrients*; 10(11):1614 https://doi.org/10.3390/nu10111614

60 Meydani, S.N., Lewis, E.D., & Wu, D. (2018). Perspective: Should Vitamin E recommendations for older adults be increased?, *Advances in Nutrition*, *9*(5), 533–543. https://doi.org/10.1093/advances/nmy035

61 Moriguchi, S., & Muraga, M. (2000). Vitamin E and immunity. *Vitamins and Hormones*, *59*, 305–336. https://doi.org/10.1016/s0083–6729(00)59011-6

62 Lewis, E.D., Meydani, S.N., & Wu, D. (2019). Regulatory Role of vitamin E in the immune system and inflammation. *IUBMB Life*, *71*(4), S 487–494. https://doi.org/10.1002/iub.1976

63 Singh, U., Devaraj, S., & Jialal, I. (2005). Vitamin E, oxidative stress, and inflammation. *Annual Review of Nutrition*, 25, 151–174. https://doi.org/10.1146/annurev.nutr.24.012003.132446

64 Anogeianaki, A., Castellani, M. L., Tripodi, D., Toniato, E., De Lutiis, M.A., Conti, F., Felaco, P., Fulcheri, M., Theoharides, T.C., Galzio, R., Caraffa, A., Antinolfi, P., Cuccurullo, C., Ciampoli, C., Felaco, M., Cerulli, G., Pandolfi, F., Sabatino, G., Neri, G., & Shaik-Dasthagirisaheb, Y. B. (2010). Vitamins and mast cells. *International Journal of Immunopathology and Pharmacology*. 2010;23(4):991-996. doi:10.1177/039463201002300403

65 Noaman, E., Zahran, A.M., Kamal, A.M., & Omran, M.F. (2002). Vitamin E and selenium administration as a modulator of antioxidant defense system: biochemical assessment and modification. *Biological Trace Element Research*, *86*(1), 55–64. https://doi.org/10.1385/BTER:86:1:55

66 Droge, W., & Breitkreutz, R. (2000). Glutathione and immune function. *Proceedings of the Nutrition Society*, 59, 595–600. https://doi.org/10.1017/S0029665100000847

67 Straub, R.H. (2017). The brain and immune system prompt energy shortage in chronic inflammation and ageing. *Nature reviews. Rheumatology*, *13*(12), 743–751. https://doi.org/10.1038/nrrheum.2017.172

68 Maggini, S., Pierre, A., & Calder, P.C. (2018). Immune function and micronutrient requirements change over the life course. *Nutrients*, *10*(10), 1531. https://doi.org/10.3390/nu10101531

69 Elmadfa, I., & Meyer, A.L. (2019). The role of the status of selected micronutrients in shaping the immune function. *Endocrine, Metabolic & Immune Disorders – Drug Targets*, *19*(8), 1100–1115. https://doi.org/10.2174/1871530319666190529101816

70 Stach, K., Stach, W., & Augoff, K. (2021). Vitamin B6 in health and disease. *Nutrients*, *13*(9), 3229. https://doi.org/10.3390/nu13093229

71 Yoshii, K., Hosomi K., Sawane K., & Kunisawa, J. (2019). Metabolism of dietary and microbial Vitamin B family in the regulation of host immunity. *Frontiers in Nutrition*, *6*, 48. https://doi.org/10.3389/fnut.2019.00048

72 Wintergerst, E.S, Maggini, S, & Hornig, D.H. (2007). Contribution of selected vitamins and trace elements to immune function. *Annals of Nutrition and Metabolism*, *51*(4), 301–323. https://doi.org/10.1159/000107673

73 Tourkochristou, E., Triantos C., & Mouzaki, A. (2021). The influence of nutritional factors on immunological outcomes. *Frontiers in Immunology*, *12*, 665968. https://doi.org/10.3389/fimmu.2021.665968

74 Tamura, J., Kubota, K., Murakami, H., Sawamura, M., Matsushima, T., Tamura, T., Saitoh, T., Kurabayshi, H., & Naruse, T. (1999). Immunomodulation by vitamin B12: augmentation of CD8+ T lymphocytes and natural killer (NK) cell activity in vitamin B12-deficient patients by methyl-B12 treatment. *Clinical and Experimental Immunology*, *116*(1), 28–32. https://doi.org/10.1046/j.1365-2249.1999.00870.x

75 Saeed, F., Nadeem, M., Ahmed, R.S., Nadeem, M.T., Arshad, M.S., & Ullah, A. (2016). Studying the impact of nutritional immunology underlying the modulation of immune responses by nutritional compounds – a review, *Food and Agricultural Immunology*, *27*(2), 205–229. https://doi.org/10.1080/09540105.2015.1079600

76 Yuan, S., Mason, A.M., Carter, P., Burgess, S., & Larsson, S.C. (2021). Homocysteine, B vitamins, and cardiovascular disease: a Mendelian randomization study. *BMC Medicine*, *19*(1), 97. https://doi.org/10.1186/s12916-021-01977-8

77 Li, T., Chen, Y., Li, J., Yang, X., Zhang, H., Qin, X., Hu, Y., & Mo, Z. (2015). Serum homocysteine concentration is significantly associated with inflammatory/immune factors. *PloS One*, *10*(9), e0138099. https://doi.org/10.1186/s12916-021-01977-8

78 McCully, K.S. (2017). Hyperhomocysteinemia, suppressed immunity, and altered oxidative metabolism caused by pathogenic microbes in atherosclerosis and dementia. *Frontiers in Aging Neuroscience*, *9*, 324. https://doi.org/10.3389/fnagi.2017.00324

79 Gilsing, A.M., Crowe, F.L., Lloyd-Wright, Z., Sanders, T.A., Appleby, P.N., Allen, N.E., & Key, T.J. (2010). Serum concentrations of vitamin B12 and folate in British male omnivores, vegetarians and vegans: results from a cross-sectional analysis of the EPIC-Oxford cohort study. *European Journal of Clinical Nutrition*, *64*(9), 933–939. https://doi.org/10.1038/ejcn.2010.142

80 Derbyshire, E. (2017). Associations between red meat intakes and the micronutrient Intake and status of UK females: A secondary analysis of the UK national diet and nutrition survey. *Nutrients*, *9*(7), 768. https://doi.org/10.3390/nu9070768

81 Drouin, G., Godin, J.R., & Pagé, B. (2011). The genetics of Vitamin C loss in vertebrates. *Current Genomics*, *12*(5), 371-378. doi: 10.2174/138920211796429736

82 Linus Pauling Institute. (2018). Vitamin C. *Micronutrient Information Center; Oregon State University*. https://lpi.oregonstate.edu/mic/vitamins/vitamin-C

83 Telang, P.S. (2013) Vitamin C in dermatology. *Indian Dermatology Online Journal*, *4*(2), 143–146. https://doi.org/10.4103/2229-5178.110593

84 Peterkofsky, B. (1991). Ascorbate requirement for hydroxylation and secretion of procollagen: relationship to inhibition of collagen synthesis in scurvy. *The American Journal of Clinical Nutrition*, *54*(6 Suppl), 1135S–1140 S. https://doi.org/10.1093/ajcn/54.6.1135s

85 Moores, J. (2013). Vitamin C: a wound healing perspective. *British Journal of Community Nursing*, *Suppl*, S6–S11. https://doi.org/10.12968/bjcn.2013.18.sup12.s6

86 Blass, S.C., Goost, H., Tolba, R.H., Stoffel-Wagner, B., Kabir, K., Burger, C., Stehle, P., & Ellinger, S. (2012). Time to wound closure in trauma patients with disorders in wound healing is shortened by supplements containing antioxidant

micronutrients and glutamine: A PRCT. *Clinical Nutrition*, 31(4), 469–475. https://doi.org/10.1016/j.clnu.2012.01.002

87 Evans, R.M., Currie, L., & Campbell, A. (1982). The distribution of ascorbic acid between various cellular components of blood, in normal individuals, and its relation to the plasma concentration. *The British Journal of Nutrition*, 47(3), 473–482. https://doi.org/10.1079/bjn19820059

88 Carr, A.C., & Maggini, S. (2017). Vitamin C and immune function. *Nutrients*, 9(11), 1211. https://doi.org/10.3390/nu9111211

89 Wintergerst, E.S., Maggini, S., & Hornig, D.H. (2006). Vitamin C and Zinc and effect on clinical conditions. *Annals of Nutrition and Metabolism*, 50(2), 85–94. https://doi.org/10.1159/000090495

90 Van Gorkom, G.N.Y., Wolterink, R.G.J.K., Van Elssen, C.H.M.J., Wieten, L., Germeraad, W.T.V., & Bos, G.M.J. (2018). Influence of vitamin C on lymphocytes: An overview. *Antioxidants*, 7(3), 41. https://doi.org/10.3390/antiox7030041

91 The Food Foundation (2021). Veg Facts 2021. *The Food Foundation* https://foodfoundation.org.uk/sites/default/files/2021-09/Peas-Please-Veg-Facts-2021.pdf

92 National Diet and Nutrition Survey (2019). Years 1 to 9 of the Rolling Programme (2008/2009 – 2016/2017): Time trend and income analyses. *Public Health England and the Food Standards Agency*. https://assets.publishing.service.gov.uk/government/uploads/system/uploads/attachment_data/file/772434/NDNS_UK_Y1-9_report.pdf.

93 NHS Digita.l (2021). Admissions for scurvy, rickets and malnutrition https://nhs-prod.global.ssl.fastly.net/binaries/content/assets/website-assets/supplementary-information/supplementary-info-2021/10977_scurvy_rickets_malnutrition_update_oct2021.xlsx

94 Department of Health (1991). Dietary Reference Values: A Guide. https://assets.publishing.service.gov.uk/government/uploads/system/uploads/attachment_data/file/743790/Dietary_Reference_Values_-_A_Guide__1991_.pdf

95 Linus Pauling Institute (2016). Iron. *Micronutrient Information Center; Oregon State University*. https://lpi.oregonstate.edu/mic/minerals/iron

96 Ganz, T. (2012). Macrophages and Systemic Iron Homeostasis. *Journal of Innate Immunity*, 4(5-6), 446–453. https://doi.org/10.1159/000336423

97 Sukhbaatar, N., & Weichhart, T. (2018). Iron regulation: Macrophages in control, *Pharmaceuticals;* 11(4), 137. https://doi.org/10.3390/ph11040137

98 Cronin, S., Woolf, C.J., Weiss, G., & Penninger, J.M. (2019). The role of iron regulation in immunometabolism and immune-related disease. *Frontiers in Molecular Biosciences*, 6, 116. https://doi.org/10.3389/fmolb.2019.00116

99 Aratani, Y. (2018). Myeloperoxidase: Its role for host defence, inflammation and neutrophil function. *Archives of Biochemistry and Biophysics*; 640, 47–52. https://doi.org/10.1016/j.abb.2018.01.004

100 Ni, S., Yuan, Y., Kuang, Y., & Li, X. (2022). Iron metabolism and immune regulation. *Frontiers in Immunology*, 13, 816282. https://doi.org/10.3389/fimmu.2022.816282

101 Frost, J.N., Tan, T.K., Abbas, M., Wideman, S.K., Bonadonna, M., Stoffel, N.U., Wray, K., Kronsteiner, B., Smits, G., Campagna, D.R., Duarte, T.L., Lopes, J.M., Shah, A., Armitage, A.E., Arezes, J., Lim, P.J., Preston, A.E., Ahern, D., Teh, M., Naylor, C., & Drakesmith, H. (2021). Hepcidin-mediated hypoferremia disrupts immune responses to vaccination and infection. *Med*, 2(2), 164–179.e12. https://doi.org/10.1016/j.medj.2020.10.004

102 Fraenkel, P.G. (2017). Anemia of inflammation: A review. *The Medical Clinics of North America*, 101(2), 285–296. https://doi.org/10.1016/j.mcna.2016.09.005

103 Ganz, T. (2009). Iron in innate immunity: starve the invaders. *Current Opinion in Immunology*, 21(1), 63–67. https://doi.org/10.1016/j.coi.2009.01.011

104 Hennigar, S.R., & McClung, J.P. (2016). Nutritional immunity: Starving pathogens of trace minerals. *American Journal of Lifestyle Medicine*, *10*(3), 170–173. https://doi.org/ 10.1177/1559827616629117

105 Gulec, S., Anderson, G.J., & Collins, J.F. (2014). Mechanistic and regulatory aspects of intestinal iron absorption. *American Journal of Physiology. Gastrointestinal and Liver Physiology*, *307*(4), G397–G409. https://doi.org/10.1152/ajpgi.00348.2013

106 Yuen, HW, & Becker, W. (2022). Iron Toxicity. In: StatPearls [Internet]. Treasure Island (FL): StatPearls Publishing; Available from: https://www.ncbi.nlm.nih.gov/ books/NBK459224/

107 Ohashi, W., & Fukada, T. (2019). Contribution of Zinc and Zinc transporters in the pathogenesis of inflammatory bowel diseases. *Journal of Immunology Research*, *2019*, 8396878. https://doi.org/10.1155/2019/8396878

108 Roscioli, E., Jersmann, H.P., Lester, S., Badiei, A., Fon, A., Zalewski, P., & Hodge, S. (2017). Zinc deficiency as a codeterminant for airway epithelial barrier dysfunction in an ex vivo model of COPD. *International Journal of Chronic Obstructive Pulmonary Disease*, *12*, 3503–3510. https://doi.org/10.2147/COPD.S149589

109 Ogawa, Y., Kinoshita, M., Shimada, S., & Kawamura, T. (2018). Zinc and skin disorders. *Nutrients*, *10*(2), 199. https://doi.org/10.3390/nu10020199

110 Gupta, M., Mahajan, V.K., Mehta, K.S., & Chauhan, P.S. (2014). Zinc therapy in dermatology: a review. *Dermatology Research and Practice*, *2014*, 709152. https://doi.org/ 10.1155/2014/709152

111 Haase, H., & Rink, L. (2014). Multiple impacts of zinc on immune function. *Metallomics*, *6*(7), 1175–1180. https://doi.org/10.1039/c3mt00353a

112 Gammoh, N.Z., & Rink, L. (2017). Zinc in infection and inflammation. *Nutrients*, *9*(6), 624. https://doi.org/10.3390/nu9060624

113 Wessels, I., Maywald, M., & Rink, L. (2017). Zinc as a gatekeeper of immune function. *Nutrients*, *9*(12), 1286. https://doi.org/10.3390/nu9121286

114 Prasad, A.S. (2008). Zinc in human health: Effect of zinc on immune cells. *Molecular Medicine*, *14*(5–6), 353–357. https://doi.org/10.2119/2008-00033.Prasad

115 Wang, S., Cheng, J., Niu, Y., Li, P., Zhang, X., & Lin, J. (2021). Strategies for zinc uptake in *Pseudomonas aeruginosa* at the host-pathogen interface. *Frontiers in Microbiology*, *12*, 741873. https://doi.org/10.3389/fmicb.2021.741873

116 Becker, K.W., & Skaar, E.P. (2014). Metal limitation and toxicity at the interface between host and pathogen. *FEMS Microbiology Reviews*, *38*(6), 1235–1249. https://doi.org/10.1111/1574-6976.12087

117 Read, S.A., Obeid, S., Ahlenstiel, C., & Ahlenstiel, G. (2019). The role of zinc in antiviral immunity. *Advances in Nutrition*, *10*(4), 696–710. https://doi.org/10.1093/ advances/nmz013

118 Mahajan, B.B., Dhawan, M., & Singh, R. (2013). Herpes genitalis - Topical zinc sulfate: An alternative therapeutic and modality. *Indian Journal of Sexually Transmitted Diseases and AIDS*, *34*(1), 32–34. https://doi.org/10.4103/0253-7184.112867

119 Lanke, K., Krenn, B. M., Melchers, W., Seipelt, J., & van Kuppeveld, F. (2007). PDTC inhibits picornavirus polyprotein processing and RNA replication by transporting zinc ions into cells. *The Journal of General Virology*, *88*(Pt 4), 1206–1217. https://doi.org/ 10.1099/vir.0.82634-0

120 Reeves, M.A., & Hoffmann, P.R. (2009). The human selenoproteome: recent insights into functions and regulation. *Cellular and Molecular Life Sciences*, *66*(15), 2457–2478. https://doi.org/10.1007/s00018-009-0032-4

121 Labunskyy, V.M., Hatfield, D.L., & Gladyshev, V.N. (2014). Selenoproteins: molecular pathways and physiological roles. *Physiological Reviews*, *94*(3), 739–777. https://doi.org/ 10.1152/physrev.00039.2013

122 Huang, Z., Rose, A.H., & Hoffmann, P.R. (2012). The role of selenium in inflammation and immunity: from molecular mechanisms to therapeutic opportunities. *Antioxidants & Redox Signalling, 16*(7), 705–743. https://doi.org/10.1089/ars.2011.4145

123 Van Haaften, R.I.M., Haenen, G.R.M.M., Evelo, C.T.A, & Bast, A. (2003). Effect of Vitamin E on glutathione-dependent enzymes. *Drug Metabolism Reviews, 35*(2–3), 215–253. https://doi.org/10.1081/DMR-120024086

124 Arthur, J.R., McKenzie, R.C., & Beckett, G.J. (2003). Selenium in the immune system, *The Journal of Nutrition, 133*(5), 1457S–1459 S. https://doi.org/10.1093/jn/133.5.1457S

125 Bae, M., & Kim, H. (2020). Mini-review on the roles of Vitamin C, Vitamin D, and selenium in the immune system against COVID-19. *Molecules), 25*(22), 5346. https://doi.org/10.3390/molecules25225346

126 Mehdi, Y., Hornick, J. L., Istasse, L., & Dufranse, I. (2013). Selenium in the environment, metabolism and involvement in body functions. *Molecules, 18*(3),3292–3311. https://doi.org/10.3390/molecules18033292

127 Avery, J.C., & Hoffman, P.R. (2018). Selenium, selenoproteins, and immunity. *Nutrients, 10*(9), 1203. https://doi.org/10.3390/nu10091203

128 Gill, H., & Walker, G. (2008). Selenium, immune function and resistance to viral infections. *Nutrition and Dietetics; Journal of Dietitians Australia, 65*(S3), S41–S47. https://doi.org/10.1111/j.1747-0080.2008.00260.x

129 Jackson, M.J., Broome, C.S., McArdle, F. (2003). Marginal dietary selenium intakes in the UK: Are there functional consequences?, *The Journal of Nutrition, 133*(5), 1557S–1559 S. https://doi.org/10.1093/jn/133.5.1557S

130 Stoffaneller, R., & Morse, N.L. (2015). A review of dietary selenium intake and selenium status in Europe and the Middle East. *Nutrients, 7*(3), 1494–1537. https://doi.org/10.3390/nu7031494

131 Zhu, Y., Yao, S., & Chen, L. (2011). Cell surface signaling molecules in the control of immune responses: A tide model. *Immunity, 34*(4), 466–478. https://doi.org/10.1016/j.immuni.2011.04.008

132 Vaeth, M., Eckstein, M., Shaw, P. J., Kozhaya, L., Yang, J., Berberich-Siebelt F., Clancy, R., Unutmaz, D., & Feske, S. (2016). Store-operated Ca(2+) entry in follicular T cells controls humoral immune responses and autoimmunity. *Immunity, 44*(6), 1350–1364. https://doi.org/10.1016/j.immuni.2016.04.013

133 Trebak, M., & Kinet, J.P. Calcium signalling in T cells (2019). *Nature Reviews: Immunology, 19,* 154–169. https://doi.org/10.1038/s41577-018-0110-7

134 Dimitrov, V., & White, J.H. (2016). Calcium, vitamin D, and immunity in the colon. *The American Journal of Clinical Nutrition, 103*(5), 1195–1196. https://doi.org/10.3945/ajcn.116.134247

135 El Khoury, D., Cuda, C., Luhovyy, B.L., & Anderson, G.H. (2012). Beta glucan: health benefits in obesity and metabolic syndrome. *Journal of Nutrition and Metabolism, 2012,* 851362. https://doi.org/10.1155/2012/851362

136 Żyła, E., Dziendzikowska, K., Kamola, D., Wilczak, J., Sapierzyński, R., Harasym, J., & Gromadzka-Ostrowska, J. (2021). Anti-inflammatory activity of oat beta-Glucans in a Crohn's disease model: Time- and molar mass-dependent effects. *International Journal of Molecular Sciences, 22*(9), 4485. https://doi.org/10.3390/ijms22094485

137 Kim, H.S., Hong, J.T., Kim, Y., & Han, S.B. (2011). Stimulatory effect of β-glucans on immune cells. *Immune Network, 11*(4), 191–195. https://doi.org/10.4110/in.2011.11.4.191

138 Ganda Mall, J.P., Casado-Bedmar, M., Winberg, M.E., Brummer, R.J., Schoultz, I., & Keita, Å.V. (2017). A β-Glucan-based dietary fiber reduces mast cell-induced hyperpermeability in ileum from patients with Crohn's disease and control subjects. *Inflammatory Bowel Diseases, 24*(1), 166–178. https://doi.org/10.1093/ibd/izx002

139 Majtan, J., & Jesenak, M. (2018). B-Glucans: Multi-functional modulator of wound healing. *Molecules, 23*(4), 806. https://doi.org/10.3390/molecules23040806

140 Stothers, C.L., Burelbach, K.R., Owen, A.M., Patil, N.K., McBride, M.A., Bohannon, J.K., Luan, L., Hernandez, A., Patil, T.K., Williams, D.L., & Sherwood E.R. (2021). β-Glucan induces distinct and protective innate immune memory in differentiated macrophages. *Journal of Immunology, 207*(11), 2785–2798. https://doi.org/10.4049/jimmunol.2100107

141 De Marco Castro, E., Calder, P.C., & Roche, H.M. (2021). β-1,3/1,6-Glucans and immunity: State of the art and future directions. *Molecular Nutrition & Food Research, 65*(1), e1901071. https://doi.org/10.1002/mnfr.201901071

142 Hetland, G., Tangen, J.M., Mahmood, F., Mirlashari, M.R., Nissen-Meyer, L., Nentwich, I., Therkelsen, S.P., Tjønnfjord, G.E., & Johnson, E. (2020). Antitumor, anti-inflammatory and antiallergic effects of *Agaricus blazei* mushroom extract and the related medicinal basidiomycetes mushrooms, *Hericium erinaceus* and *Grifolafrondosa*: A review of preclinical and clinical studies. *Nutrients, 12*(5), 1339. https://doi.org/10.3390/nu12051339

143 Vetvicka, V., Teplyakova, T.V., Shintyapina, A.B., & Korolenko, T.A. (2021). Effects of medicinal fungi-derived β-glucan on tumor progression. *Journal of Fungi, 7*(4), 250. https://doi.org/10.3390/jof7040250

144 Linus Pauling Institute Micronutrient Information Center (2016). Flavonoids. *Oregon State University* https://lpi.oregonstate.edu/mic/dietary-factors/phytochemicals/flavonoids

145 Pérez-Cano, F.J., & Castell, M. (2016). Flavonoids, inflammation and immune system. *Nutrients, 8*(10), 659. https://doi.org/10.3390/nu8100659

146 Panche, A.N., Diwan, A.D., & Chandra, S.R. (2016). Flavonoids: an overview. *Journal of Nutritional Science, 5*, e47. https://doi.org/10.1017/jns.2016.41

147 Kopustinskiene, D.M., Jakstas, V., Savickas, A., & Bernatoniene, J. (2020). Flavonoids as anticancer agents. *Nutrients, 12*(2), 457. https://doi.org/10.3390/nu12020457

148 Mathesius, U. (2018). Flavonoid functions in plants and their interactions with other organisms. *Plants, 7*(2), 30. https://doi.org/10.3390/plants7020030

149 Mowat, A.M. (2018). To respond or not to respond - a personal perspective of intestinal tolerance. *Nature Reviews. Immunology, 18*(6), 405–415. https://doi.org/10.1038/s41577-018-0002-x

150 Jiao, Y., Wu, L., Huntington, N.D., & Zhang, X. (2020). Crosstalk between Gut microbiota and innate immunity and its implication in autoimmune diseases. *Frontiers in Immunology, 11*, 282. https://doi.org/10.3389/fimmu.2020.00282

151 Lazar, V., Ditu, L.M., Pircalabioru, G.G., Gheorghe, I., Curutiu, C., Holban, A.M., Picu, A., Petcu, L., & Chifiriuc, M.C. (2018). Aspects of gut microbiota and immune system interactions in infectious diseases, immunopathology, and cancer. *Frontiers in Immunology, 9*, 1830. https://doi.org/10.3389/fimmu.2018.01830

6 Vitamin D

The importance of vitamin D cannot be understated, and research is starting to find out just how deep its influence runs.[1]

The substance we call vitamin D is not really a vitamin at all. Vitamins are nutrients derived from foods, but vitamin D is different. Although we do get some vitamin D from food, we also synthesise it from 7-dehydrocholesterol (a form of cholesterol) when our skin is exposed to the ultraviolet B (UVB) wavelength of light in sunlight.[2] Vitamin D is actually a type of steroid, a secosteroid that is converted into different steroid hormones in the body.[3] However, it is convenient to continue to use the terms "vitamin D", 25-hydroxyvitamin D (25(OH)D) and 1-α-25-dihydroxyvitamin D (1α,25(OH)$_2$D).

Once vitamin D has been ingested in food, or synthesised in the skin, it is transported to the liver where hydroxylase enzymes convert it into 25-hydroxyvitamin D (25(OH)D). This is transported to the kidneys where more hydroxylase enzymes further convert it to the biologically active form of 1-α-25-dihyroxyvitamin D (1α,25(OH)$_2$D).[4]

When blood levels of vitamin D are measured it is the inactive form, 25(OH)D, that is tested for. Measurements in the UK are shown in nanomoles per litre (nmol/L); however, in many countries, measurements are shown in nanograms per millilitre (ng/mL). To convert ng/mL to nmol/L, multiply the ng/mL by 2.5.

The active form, 1α,25(OH)$_2$D attaches to vitamin D receptors (VDRs). There are VDRs on almost every cell in the body, and the functions of vitamin D seem to be as diverse as the cells on which its receptors are found.[5] However, research is still working out what all of the receptors do.

VITAMIN D FROM FOOD

- If vitamin D is classified as a food, it is measured in micrograms (μg).
- If vitamin D is classified as a medicine, it is measured in International Units (IU).
- 400 IU is equivalent to 10 μg.
- There is some variability in national recommendations for vitamin D intake levels.
- In 2010, the American Institute of Medicine set the Dietary Reference Intake (DRI – the amount needed to be ingested per day to maintain health) for vitamin D at 15 μg/d, rising to 20 μg/d for those aged 70+.[6]
- In 2016, the European Food Safety Authority (EFSA) set the Dietary Reference Value (DRV – the amount needed to be ingested per day to maintain health) at 15 μg/d.[7]

DOI: 10.1201/b22900-7

- In 2016, the UK government's Scientific Advisory Committee on Nutrition (SACN) published a report amending the Reference Nutrient Intake (RNI, the amount most people need to maintain health) from 5 to 10 µg/d.[8]
- Intakes of vitamin D in the UK have consistently fallen over the last few decades and are currently only around 2.7 µg/d, far below even the previously recommended 5 µg.[9]

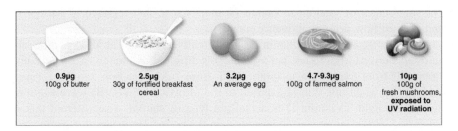

Vitamin D is only available in a limited number of foods.

Although the difference between 10, 15, and 20 µg may not seem much, vitamin D is not widely found in many foods. The richest sources of Vitamin D are oily fish, eggs, liver, fortified breakfast cereals, and mushrooms that have been exposed to UVB. But even these are not particularly rich sources. One hundred grams of farmed salmon, the most widely consumed oily fish in the UK, contains around 6.8 µg whilst an average egg contains around 3.2 µg. Mushrooms exposed to UVB are one of the richest sources, but few mushrooms sold in the UK are exposed to light.[10] Levels of vitamin D can vary, depending on how the food is cooked.[11]

Fish consumption in the UK is generally low, and intake of oily fish is even lower.[12] Egg consumption is rising, but one would need to eat three eggs a day, every day, to consume 10 µg of vitamin D, something that could be considered challenging.[13]

Vitamin D is fat soluble. It is only found in the fat content of food and can only be absorbed in the presence of dietary fat. The promotion of low-fat diets, and the prevalence of low-fat foods may be having a negative impact on vitamin D status as far less vitamin D is absorbed from food in a low-fat environment.[14]

VITAMIN D FROM SUNLIGHT

UVB in sunlight stimulates the synthesis of vitamin D in our skin. But in order for UVB to penetrate the Earth's atmosphere, the angle of the Sun in the sky needs to be at least 45°, or greater.[15] Thanks to the northerly latitude of this country, in the south of the UK from approximately the level of Cambridge down to the south coast, the Sun reaches 45° and above for a limited time each day for six months of the year, from mid-April to early September.[16] North of Cambridge, the Sun only reaches 45° and above from mid-May to the end of August, reducing vitamin D synthesis time to four months of the year.[17]

When *Homo sapiens* began migrating out of Africa, they met Neanderthal populations that had been living in northerly latitudes for several hundred thousand years. Through a mixture of interbreeding and genetic shift, *H. sapiens* moving north adapted and evolved a paler skin to allow more effective synthesis of vitamin D from less powerful sunlight.[18]

Because of the relatively low intensity of sunlight in northern latitudes and the protective effects of melanin, individuals with darker skins need longer sun exposure here in the north, to stimulate vitamin D production.[19] In our modern globalised world, people with pale skin moving to latitudes where sunlight has high intensity, have been told for decades to protect themselves against the sun.[20] But those with darker skins, moving to latitudes where the intensity of sunlight is less effective in stimulating vitamin D synthesis, have not been advised to increase their sun exposure in order to support their vitamin D levels. Perhaps it is time to start suggesting this.

How much sun exposure is needed to stimulate the synthesis of sufficient vitamin D depends on the latitude, the season, the time of day and an individual's sensitivity to sunburn. If you stand in the garden at midday on 25 December, your skin will not make a nanogram of vitamin D. So the same thing at midday on 25 June and you will make plenty. Our skin can synthesise vitamin D from sunlight when our shadow is shorter than we are.[21] For Caucasians, between 10 and 30 minutes of strong sun exposure on face, arms, hands and legs, without sunscreen, three times a week, should be enough; those with darker skins need about double that.[22]

Skin synthesises vitamin D from sunlight when your shadow is shorter than you are.

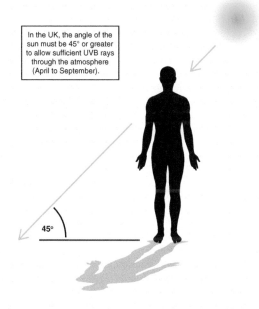

In the UK, the angle of the sun must be 45° or greater to allow sufficient UVB rays through the atmosphere (April to September).

45°

Vitamin D synthesis takes place when the sun is above a 45° angle in the sky and your shadow is shorter than you are.

SAFETY

There have been no recorded incidents of toxicity caused by excessive vitamin D production from sunlight.

Current understanding is 100 µg of supplemental vitamin D, in addition to any dietary intake, is safe over the long term.[6,23]

There are some medicines that can interact with vitamin D, some effect its absorption and some effect its metabolism.[24] Lipase inhibitors reduce fat absorption, and this can have a negative impact on the absorption of dietary vitamin D.[25] However, some statins appear to increase vitamin D levels and therefore it may be advisable to monitor levels in patients taking statins.[26]

SITUATION IN THE UK

The UK is deep in a vitamin D crisis. Rickets, a disease that should have vanished along with small boys being sent up chimneys, is re-emerging, particularly in ethnic South Asian, African and Afro-Caribbean populations.[27] At the opposite end of the age spectrum osteoporosis is on the increase with an estimated 500,000 fragility fractures in the UK every year.[28] Osteoporosis and the risk of fracture increases in women over 55 and men over 65.

For many years UK policy makers took the view that increasing the RNI (set in 1999) for vitamin D was unnecessary. It was assumed that enough would be synthesised during the summer months to cover the rest of the year. However, by 2010 it had become clear that vitamin D deficiency was a serious public health issue and SACN were asked to evaluate current evidence and make recommendations. In 2016 SACN made the following recommendations:

- A daily dietary intake of 10 µg for the UK general population aged over four years.
- Insufficient data to set RNIs for infants and children aged under four years therefore a "safe range" of 8.5–10 µg dietary intake per day for age 0–1 and 10 µg dietary intake per day for age 1–4 was set.
  - Babies under 1 year should have a daily 8.5–10 µg supplement but infants and young children receiving 500 mL or more of infant formula a day should not need any supplemental vitamin D as the formula is fortified with vitamin D.
- Children aged 1–4 years should have a daily 10 µg vitamin D supplement.

SACN advised these intakes applied throughout the year, regardless of sun exposure during the summer months and noted that obtaining 10 µg of vitamin D every day from natural food sources is difficult. They recommended that the government consider strategies to ensure all UK populations obtained sufficient daily vitamin D.

Public Health England (PHE) issued extremely unenthusiastic advice that people "should consider" taking a daily supplement containing 10 µg of vitamin D in autumn and winter.[29] PHE also suggested that individuals with little or no exposure to the sun, and ethnic minorities with darker skins, may not manage to get enough vitamin D from sunlight in the summer and "should consider" taking a supplement all year round.

The word "consider" means "to think carefully about something". UK government advice for general supplementation is not a call-to-arms for the UK population to take action to support their own health. It is a damp squib suggesting that the UK population might like to think about possibly taking action. It they can be bothered.

This advice has since been updated to be marginally more forceful.[30] However, virtually no public health messaging or promotion of the vitamin D message has been undertaken by any health authorities in the UK.

VITAMIN D DEFICIENCY RATES IN THE UK

Recent estimates suggest that severe Vitamin D deficiency in the UK's South Asian population could be as high as 82% in the summer, rising to 94% in the winter.[19] Vitamin D blood tests, taken at the end of summer when Vitamin D levels should be at their highest, found 25% of Afro-Caribbean adults to be severely deficient.[31] And even the Caucasian population is at risk, with12% of adults deficient in Vitamin D.[32]

Average intake of vitamin D is only 2.4 µg/d, less than a quarter of the recommended amount.[9] Fifteen percent of the total UK population are severely deficient and more than half have insufficient blood levels of vitamin D to maintain health.[33]

But what does vitamin D do exactly?

BONES

In relation to bone, vitamin D is both essential and potentially life changing. In 2009 the parents of a four-month-old were accused of murder by shaken baby syndrome. They were eventually cleared when tests revealed that their child had severe infantile rickets. The mother was so dangerously vitamin D deficient that the baby's bones crumbled whenever he was touched, which ultimately led to his death.[34]

The cells that build bone, osteoblasts, osteoclasts, and osteocytes, are packed with VDR, but vitamin D's function in bone goes further than that. It is linked with parathyroid hormone (PTH), manufactured by the parathyroid gland; calcitonin, manufactured by the thyroid gland; and fibroblast growth factor-23 (FGF23), a protein produced by osteoblasts and osteocytes. These elements regulate not only the absorption and excretion of calcium and phosphorus, but also each other.[35]

When calcium levels are high, calcitonin is released which reduces PTH synthesis, preventing resorption (the release of calcium from bone). Low PTH also inhibits the conversion of vitamin D in the kidneys from inactive 25(OH)D to active $1\alpha,25(OH)_2D$. This in turn reduces intestinal absorption of calcium and increases calcium loss through urine.

But when calcium levels are low, the flow of calcitonin is reduced which increases PTH secretion and stimulates greater conversion of 25(OH)D to $1\alpha,25(OH)_2D$. Higher PTH also increases the absorption of calcium from the gut, stimulates the release of calcium from bone, and prevents calcium loss through urine.[36]

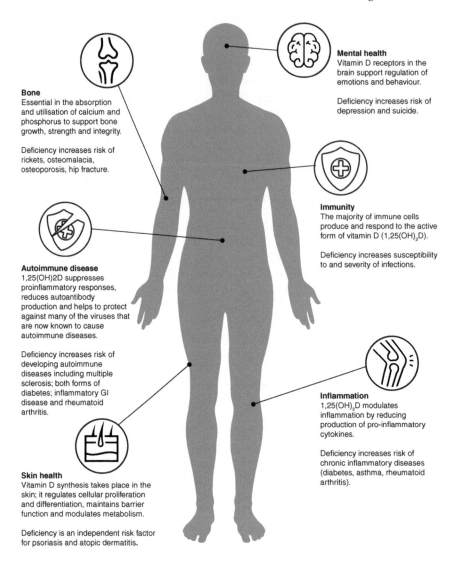

Mental health
Vitamin D receptors in the
brain support regulation of
emotions and behaviour.

Deficiency increases risk of
depression and suicide.

Bone
Essential in the absorption
and utilisation of calcium and
phosphorus to support bone
growth, strength and integrity.

Deficiency increases risk of
rickets, osteomalacia,
osteoporosis, hip fracture.

Immunity
The majority of immune cells
produce and respond to the active
form of vitamin D (1,25(OH)$_2$D).

Deficiency increases susceptibility
to and severity of infections.

Autoimmune disease
1,25(OH)2D suppresses
proinflammatory responses,
reduces autoantibody
production and helps to protect
against many of the viruses that
are now known to cause
autoimmune diseases.

Deficiency increases risk of
developing autoimmune
diseases including multiple
sclerosis; both forms of
diabetes; inflammatory GI
disease and rheumatoid
arthritis.

Inflammation
1,25(OH)$_2$D modulates
inflammation by reducing
production of pro-inflammatory
cytokines.

Deficiency increases risk of
chronic inflammatory diseases
(diabetes, asthma, rheumatoid
arthritis).

Skin health
Vitamin D synthesis takes place in the
skin; it regulates cellular proliferation
and differentiation, maintains barrier
function and modulates metabolism.

Deficiency is an independent risk factor
for psoriasis and atopic dermatitis.

Vitamin D's impact goes far beyond bone.

FGF23 is secreted by bone cells if high levels of calcitonin are detected. FGF23 and PTH act together in the kidneys, preventing phosphate from being absorbed, but increasing the absorption of calcium. So phosphate is excreted via urine whilst circulating calcium levels increase, thereby triggering the release of calcitonin. FGF23 also suppresses the conversion of 25(OH)D to 1α,25(OH)$_2$D meaning there is less circulating active vitamin D to ensure the laying down of mineral in bone.[37]

This carefully choreographed balancing act means that minerals in bone are subject to perpetual turn-over, constantly forming and breaking down to ensure that sufficient calcium and phosphorus are in circulation to fulfil the physiological roles they have beyond bone health. If insufficient calcium and or phosphorus are being absorbed from the diet to fulfil these biochemical requirements, then they are released from bone.[38]

The first areas of bone subject to resorption are the cores of vertebral bones and the ends of long bones like the femur. The loss of minerals in these bones is a key indicator of risk for osteoporotic fractures.[39] Vitamin D deficiency in older populations increases the risk of osteoporosis, particularly osteoporotic hip fractures. Every year in the UK there are around 76,000 hip fractures which cost the NHS and social care budgets around £2 billion annually.[40] On average, hospital costs alone for hip fracture are £13,000 per patient, however, because of pre-existing health inequalities, these costs increase by around £1,100 for patients living in deprived areas.[41]

MENTAL HEALTH

The brain is one of the few organs in the body, other than the kidneys, where 25(OH)D is converted into $1\alpha,25(OH)_2D$.[42] There are VDRs throughout the brain and they are particularly dense in the amygdala which regulates emotion, behaviour, and development.[43] Vitamin D also modulates the synthesis of neurotrophic proteins that support the development, survival, and function of neurons.[44]

There are strong associations between low maternal levels of vitamin D and impaired cognitive and neuro development in children.[45] Low maternal levels of vitamin D have also been linked with cognitive dysfunction disorders such as ADHD, disorders on the autistic spectrum and schizophrenia, particularly where this is combined with an additional lifetime of inadequacy.[46] In later life, vitamin D insufficiency increases the risk of developing neurodegenerative diseases including vascular dementia, Alzheimer's, and Parkinson's diseases.[47]

Patients with psychiatric disorders are often found to be deficient in vitamin D.[48] There is increasing evidence of a relationship between mild-to-moderate depression and low levels of vitamin D.[49] However, supplementation is only effective in reducing depression scores if baseline vitamin D shows deficiency or insufficiency; if an individual is vitamin D replete, adding more vitamin D is not going to help.[50] Having said that, depressed individuals often have low vitamin D status, possibly because they tend to spend less time out of doors and may have poor diets.[51] It's a bit of a negative feedback loop.

Although suicide is a multifactorial issue, depression is acknowledged as a significant risk factor.[52] And it seems that an independent risk factor for suicidal thoughts and behaviours is vitamin D deficiency.[53] Individuals with the lowest vitamin D status appear to be at the greatest risk for suicide.[54] It would certainly be worth including vitamin D in any suicide prevention programme or treatment protocol for depression, it costs very little, has no adverse effects, and could save lives.[55]

IMMUNITY

Although the role of vitamin D in immunity is discussed in the chapter on immunity, this section looks at the specific actions of vitamin D in relation to immune cells. It also notes the plethora of research which has come out about vitamin D and immunity since early 2020 and the start of the Covid-19 pandemic.

Vitamin D in immune function has gained a lot of interest over the last few years. Most of the cells of the immune system, particularly T cells, B cells, monocytes, macrophages and dendritic cells, carry VDR.[56] In a clear indication of exactly how important vitamin D is to our immune function, some of these cells can even convert the inactive 25(OH)D to the active 1α,25(OH)$_2$D because they express the enzyme 25-hydroxyvitamin D$_3$-1α-hydroxylase.[57]

Vitamin D increases the activity of monocytes, macrophages, and dendritic cells, and stimulates the production of antimicrobial cathelicidin peptides which destabilise pathogen cellular membranes.[56,57] It suppresses the maturation of dendritic cells, slowing their ability to present antigens to T cells.[58] This might not sound helpful, but when T cells become overstimulated, their ability to seek out and destroy specific threats becomes exhausted and they become less effective. In addition, many T cells are pro-inflammatory and the downregulation of T cell production also reduces inflammation.[59] When T cells become activated the number of VDR they carry increases; inactivated B cells do not have any VDR, these only develop once they have been activated.[60]

Vitamin D supplementation in individuals who are insufficient or deficient reduces the incidence of colds and flu.[61] This may be linked to the conversion of 25(OH)D into 1α,25(OH)$_2$D by the epithelial cells inside the lungs.[62] As a result of the global pandemic, research has ramped up significantly over the last few years. A simple PubMed search of the terms "vitamin D" and "Covid-19" turns up over 700 open access peer-review studies, many of which note that vitamin D deficiency, or even insufficiency, is associated with greater morbidity and mortality from respiratory tract infections, and Covid-19 in particular.

AUTOIMMUNE DISEASE

Inflammation which starts and ends swiftly is part of a normal immune response. But prolonged inflammation is not. It creates damage to tissues and organs and this damage can generate the self-perpetuating inflammatory cycle that often typifies autoimmune disease.[63] Vitamin D deficiency, or even insufficiency, is strongly associated with increased inflammation because of vitamin D's influence on inflammatory cells and processes.[64]

People living in more northerly latitudes (where the amount of time to synthesise vitamin D is limited), have a greater risk of developing autoimmune diseases.[2] And this correlation goes even further. Those born at a high latitude in the northern hemisphere in April (and therefore likely to be subject to low maternal vitamin D because gestation occurred over autumn and winter when vitamin D is lower), generally have the highest risk of developing autoimmune diseases, whilst those born in October and November (and therefore less likely to be subject to low maternal vitamin D), having a far lower risk.[65] Inadequate or deficient levels of vitamin D have been noted in multiple autoimmune diseases, including type II diabetes, multiple sclerosis, inflammatory bowel diseases, arthritic and rheumatic diseases, skin conditions such as psoriasis, and thyroid disease.[66]

Conventional management of autoimmune disease involves pharmaceutical anti-inflammatories, corticosteroids, pain management, and possibly even immunosuppressing drugs. But vitamin D can modulate inflammatory pathways.[67] It stimulates anti-inflammatory functions in regulatory T cells, inhibits the production of pro-inflammatory cytokines, promotes the production of anti-inflammatory cytokines, and strengthens the integrity of mucosal barriers throughout the body.[68,69] A daily supplement of 50 μg vitamin D can reduce the incidence of autoimmune disease by 39%.[70]

Several autoimmune conditions where there is good evidence to suggest a strong link with vitamin D are discussed next.

MULTIPLE SCLEROSIS

Living at latitudes further from the equator, both north and south, increases the risk of developing multiple sclerosis (MS).[71] The further one is from the equator, the less intense the sunlight, and the shorter the amount of time there is in the year to synthesise vitamin D. Some genetic variations also reduce the ability to synthesise vitamin D from sunlight, and these variations have been linked to an increased risk of developing MS.[72] Maternal levels of vitamin D are also a factor. The child of a vitamin D deficient mother is 90% more likely to develop MS than the child of a vitamin D replete mother, possibly because the child of a vitamin D deficient mother is also likely to be deficient, whereas the child of a vitamin D replete mother is likely to have a sufficiency of vitamin D.[73]

Vitamin D plays a role in myelination, protecting existing myelin, repairing damaged myelin, and even stimulating remyelination.[74] And vitamin D insufficiency may increase the autoimmune impact of the Epstein-Barr virus, a pathogen thought to be one of the key triggers of MS, however higher levels of vitamin D seem to be protective against this.[75]

There are few well-designed studies of supplementation with vitamin D in the management of MS. However two studies have found that supplementing with high-dose (just over 7,000 and 14,000 IU/d) vitamin D as an add-on to interferon-β may reduce the relapse rate in MS sufferers, slow disability progression, and may protect against the development of new lesions.[76,77]

DIABETES

Higher blood levels of vitamin D correlate with improved insulin resistance, whereas low blood levels are linked to impaired glucose tolerance, insulin resistance, and diabetes.[78] Vitamin D insufficiency increases the risk of developing both type II diabetes and gestational diabetes.[79,80] And, although evidence is inconclusive for low vitamin D levels being linked to an increased risk of type I diabetes, VDRs have been identified in the insulin-producing β cells in the pancreas, and newly diagnosed type I diabetes patients have lower plasma levels of vitamin D than age and gender-matched controls.[81,82]

There is a high prevalence of vitamin D deficiency in obesity, a factor which increases the risk of diabetes. As a fat-soluble substance, vitamin D is sequestered in fat deposits in the body meaning there is less available circulating serum $1\alpha,25(OH)_2D$.[83] Obesity, and vitamin D deficiency, are also strongly related to metabolic disorders, particularly insulin resistance and diabetes.[84]

Diabetes is an inflammatory disease and obesity promotes inflammation, stimulating the release of the inflammatory cytokines tumour necrosis factor (TNF) and interleukin 6 (IL6).[85] Vitamin D has a powerful role in regulating inflammatory processes and high-dose supplementation (up to 50,000IU) with vitamin D inhibits the production of both TNF and IL6.[86,87]

And vitamin D is also involved with the microbiome. A healthy and diverse microbiome helps to reduce inflammation and supports insulin management.[88] Whilst obesity has been found to reduce diversity in the gut microbiome, vitamin D supplementation actively increases diversity.[89,90]

INFLAMMATORY GI DISEASES

Vitamin D deficiency is prevalent across the spectrum of inflammatory GI disease, although it is not clear whether this is because of absorption issues, or a manifestation of widespread general vitamin D deficiency.[91] It is a bit chicken and egg; is the inflammatory disease state a result of a lack of vitamin D? Or is the lack of vitamin D the result of inflammatory disease?[92] Regardless, vitamin D improves gut integrity by strengthening the tight junctions in the epithelial barrier and modulates inflammatory responses.[93,94] And vitamin D sufficiency reduces disease severity and improves quality of life.[95]

Inflammatory GI conditions frequently result in absorptive issues and the absorption of fat-soluble vitamins is not simple (this is discussed in Chapter 3, on digestion). However, vitamin D is well absorbed through the buccal surfaces inside the mouth and sublingual drops and sprays have been found to reverse deficiency.[96]

SYSTEMIC LUPUS ERYTHEMATOSUS (SLE) AND RHEUMATOID ARTHRITIS (RA)

SLE is sometimes confused with RA in the early stages of the diseases because they have some similar symptoms, particularly inflammation in joints, tiredness and fatigue, and occasional low-grade fever.

Sun exposure can trigger flares of SLE, and many RA medications can increase photosensitivity.[97,98] As a result both cohorts are advised to avoid sun exposure, and it is therefore no surprise that vitamin D deficiency is widely prevalent among SLE and RA sufferers.[99,100] Although there is some debate about whether that deficiency is a cause, or an effect of acute inflammatory responses, vitamin D's effect on inflammation, and its modulation of the immune response, should really make it a frontline adjunct to pharmaceutical anti-inflammatories and corticosteroids.[101,102]

There is a growing body of evidence to support the benefit of vitamin D in the management of rheumatic diseases generally and optimum levels for health seem to range between 100 and 150 nmol/L.[103] Certainly higher serum levels of vitamin D are associated with reduced inflammation and disease activity in both SLE and RA.[99,104]

SOME CANCERS

Although cancer is not considered to be an autoimmune disease there is a strong association between autoimmunity and cancer.[105] And evidence is mounting for vitamin D's role in preventing, and mitigating, many forms of cancer.

In 1941 the first edition of Cancer Research published an evaluation of the relationship between sunlight and cancer mortality in North America.[106] Since then thousands of studies have supported the link between high vitamin D status and reduced risk of the development and progression of a range of cancers.[107] Many more studies have shown that vitamin D deficiency is associated with an increased risk of multiple cancers.[108] Indeed, in deficient individuals, the risk of cancer mortality decreases by 2% for every increase of 20 nmol/L of vitamin D.[109]

There appear to be several different mechanisms by which vitamin D protects against the development of cancers. These go beyond its actions in modulating inflammation and regulating immune function. Immune cells grow extremely fast and vitamin D forms part of the control of cellular proliferation, differentiation, and apoptosis.[110] Vitamin D inhibits tumour-derived cell proliferation by impacting protein production and gene expressions.[111] And at the same time, vitamin D stimulates apoptosis in cancer cells by upregulating tumour-suppressing mechanisms and downregulating anti-apoptotic proteins.[112]

Unfortunately, many of the clinical trials evaluating the impact of vitamin D in cancer are poorly designed, with no established baseline for vitamin D sufficiency or deficiency, and no evidence of where, on this non-existent continuum, their cohort may sit. Dosage of supplemental vitamin D also varies widely from huge bolus doses to relatively modest daily intakes. And genetic variability in responses to vitamin D are rarely taken into account.[113] As a consequence, there are no conclusive answers. However, given the potential for reduced risk of cancer morbidity and mortality, it could be worthwhile ensuring vitamin D adequacy (blood levels above 75 nmol/L) in the patient cohort.

SKIN HEALTH

Skin provides a waterproof barrier which helps to maintain water balance, protects against invasion by pathogens and damage from physical injury, helps to regulate temperature, and acts as a sensory organ. It takes between 40 and 60 days for skin cells to move through the skin, from the deepest layer, the stratum basale, up through the stratum spinosum and the granular layer, all the way to the top, the stratum corneum. On the way up, they differentiate and, if exposed to UVB, synthesise vitamin D.[114] But all those dermal cells, and the health and integrity of the skin are also dependent on vitamin D.

Vitamin D regulates the proliferation and differentiation of skin cells. Low levels of vitamin D stimulates an increased production of the type of cells that synthesise vitamin D; high levels of vitamin D slows this production down.[115] It regulates the synthesis of ceramides, chemicals that support the skin's barrier and selective permeability functions.[115] And it plays an important role in the synthesis of the antimicrobial peptide cathelicidin which is expressed by skin cells.[116]

Atopic dermatitis and psoriasis are two skin conditions linked with vitamin D and there is a strong association with vitamin D insufficiency and increased disease severity in both conditions.[117,118] In addition, the action of sunlight on skin is beneficial to both atopic dermatitis and psoriasis, although it is not clear whether this is the result of increased synthesis of vitamin D or another/additional effect of sunlight itself.[119]

Many of the studies looking at whether oral vitamin D supplements in psoriasis are effective have provided extremely low levels of vitamin D supplementation, ranging from 0.25 to 2 μg/d.[120] With such low doses it is not surprising that few have found any significant benefit. However, a few studies using high-dose vitamin D (750 μg/d to 1.5 mg/d) for a limited period and then reducing to a lower maintenance dose (250 μg/d), have shown clear benefits.[121,122] There are many studies on oral vitamin D supplementation in atopic dermatitis and there seems to be a general consensus that supplementation, in doses ranging between 40 and 125 μg/d is clinically useful, both on its own and as an adjuvant therapy.[123,124,125]

TO TEST OR NOT TO TEST

Testing for vitamin D deficiency (evaluating the inactive form of serum 25(OH)D levels) has increased significantly over the last decade. An evaluation of 6.41 million tests, undertaken between 2005 and 2015 found one-third of UK adults were deficient in vitamin D.[126]

The incidence of deficiency is unlikely to have improved in the intervening years, but the cost of testing is not insignificant. Although each individual test may not cost much, multiplying this by hundreds of thousands across the country adds a substantial cost burden to the NHS. In 2014 NICE estimated that the cost of vitamin D deficiency testing averaged out at approximately £17 per test and costs will have increased since then.[127] A 2017 audit of testing for vitamin D deficiency in Northumberland found that testing was not always warranted and calculated that a 70% national reduction in testing would give an annual cost saving of £1.9 million.[128] In addition, there is a lack of standardisation in the laboratory measurement of serum vitamin D which can create significant variability in results.[129]

If vitamin D deficiency is suspected, before ordering tests it may be advisable to recommend patients take vitamin D supplements of 50 μg a day for a month to see if symptoms improve.

SUPPLEMENTING TO PROTECT

Apart from the specific conditions outlined above, frequent infections; tiredness and fatigue; bone and joint pain; back pain; slow wound healing; muscle pain, low mood and depression are associated with vitamin D insufficiency, and are improved by vitamin D sufficiency.[130] One of the best pieces of advice any healthcare practitioner can give to a patient is to take a daily vitamin D supplement all year round.

But what dose to supplement at very much depends on how deficiency or sufficiency are classified. In the UK, official government policy states that anything above serum levels of 25(OH)D 25 nmol/L is sufficient. This level was set in 1998 by the Committee on Medical Aspects of Food and Nutrition Policy (COMA) and has not been reviewed since.[131] The 2016 SACN review claimed there was insufficient evidence of any health benefit, musculoskeletal or otherwise, for serum concentrations above 25 nmol/L and that this level represent a "population protective concentration".[8] The RNI was set at 10 μg/d because this is just enough to maintain a serum level of 25 nmol/L in individuals whose levels are not already below that point.[132]

RNIs are set at a level that is enough, or more than enough, to prevent deficiency in 97.5% of people within a group. But the UK "sufficiency" level of 25 nmol/L is the lowest anywhere in the world. Although there is ongoing international discussion on the most effective marker to determine vitamin D status, there is general scientific consensus that plasma levels below 50 nmol/L are deficient and that levels below 30 nmol/L are severely deficient.[130,133] By this globally accepted definition, practically the entire population of the UK is severely deficient in vitamin D, as a matter of government policy![134] It should be noted here that the NHS works to the global consensus level, defining 50 nmol/L as adequate in all assays.

As discussed above, serum levels of vitamin D are dependent on sun exposure and dietary intake. Living in an island nation famous for its cloud cover and rain, sun exposure in the UK cannot be guaranteed. Nor, given our indoor lifestyle and widespread predilection for covering up, can sun exposure be relied upon to generate sufficient vitamin D for the needs of most of the population.

Although a one-off loading dose of vitamin D can kick start the reversal of deficiency, bolus doses with monthly or even weekly intervals may not the best way to ensure sufficiency for everyone in the long term.[135] But one size does not fit all; different cohorts need different dietary intake levels to maintain vitamin D serum levels of 50nmol/L, the minimum needed to support health,[130] because the amount synthesised by sunlight is so variable.

Vitamin D Dosing for a Range of Cohorts to Maintain Serum Levels at 50 nmol/L[136,132]

Cohort	Caucasian	When	Those with Darker Skin	When
Age 0–12 months	10 μg/d	Year round	25 μg/d	Year round
Age 1–18 years	15–25 μg/d	September–April	25 μg/d	Year round
Age 18–60 years	30–50 μg/d	September–April	75 μg/d	Year round
Women 18–50 years	30–50 μg/d	September–April; throughout pregnancy & lactation	75 μg/d	Year round
Age 60+ years	30–50 μg/d	Year round	75 μg/d	Year round

Of course, many individuals may initially need higher intakes of vitamin D, because they start from a position of deficiency. It may be tempting, in these cases, to provide very high bolus or loading doses for a short period. Whilst this does significantly increase vitamin D levels, the effect is short term.[135] Advising individuals to supplement daily with 150 μg/d for a month, and then reduce to a daily intake of either 50 or 75 μg is likely to be more effective in the long term.

Vitamin D food supplements are widely available from high street chemists, health food stores, and even supermarkets. They are not overly expensive and come in a range of doses, from 10 μg (400IU) up to 100 μg (4,000 IU). In 2014 NICE noted the cost to the NHS of treating vitamin D deficiency was £50 for three months.[127] But it looks as if the NHS is being seriously overcharged. In April 2022, the cost to a consumer of 90 25 μg (1,000 IU) own-brand tablets (a three-month supply) from one high street retailer was only £4.99.

Nothing is single factorial, and that includes the plethora of health issues impacting across UK populations today. Whilst most of the health issues will not fall solely at the door of vitamin D insufficiency, many could be substantially improved by vitamin D sufficiency. This is something that should concern all health care practitioners, and which those same practitioners should seek to address. As the ideas of self-care and patients taking more responsibility for their own health and wellbeing grow, and as pressure on the NHS increases, it may be worth simply advising all patients to take a daily vitamin D supplement of between 50 and 75 μg throughout the year.

REFERENCES

1 Umar, M., Sastry, K.S., & Chouchane, A.I. (2018). Role of vitamin D beyond the skeletal function: A review of the molecular and clinical studies. *International Journal of Molecular Sciences, 19*(6), 1618. https://doi.org/10.3390/ijms19061618

2 Holick, M.F. (2008). Vitamin D: A D-Lightful health perspective. *Nutrition Reviews, 66*(10 Suppl 2), S182–S194. https://doi.org/10.1111/j.1753-4887.2008.00104.x

3 Demer, L.L., Hsu, J.J., & Tintut, Y. (2018). Steroid hormone vitamin D: Implications for cardiovascular disease. *Circulation Research, 122*(11), 1576–1585. https://doi.org/10.1161/CIRCRESAHA.118.311585

4 Bikle, D.D. (2020). Vitamin D: Newer concepts of its metabolism and function at the basic and clinical level. *Journal of the Endocrine Society, 4*(2), bvz038. https://doi.org/10.1210/jendso/bvz038

5 Bikle, D.D. (2016). Extraskeletal actions of vitamin D. *Annals of the New York Academy of Sciences, 1376*(1), 29–52. https://doi.org/10.1111/nyas.13219

6 Ross, C.A., Taylor, C.L., Yaktine, A.L., & Del Valle, H.B. (2010). DRI Dietary reference intakes Calcium Vitamin D. *The National Academies Press.* https://www.nap.edu/read/13050/chapter/1

7 EFSA. (2016). Dietary Reference Values for Vitamin D. *EFSA Journal.* http://www.efsa.europa.eu/en/efsajournal/pub/4547

8 Scientific Advisory Committee on Nutrition. (2016). Vitamin D and Health. https://assets.publishing.service.gov.uk/government/uploads/system/uploads/attachment_data/file/537616/SACN_Vitamin_D_and_Health_report.pdf

9 Derbyshire, E. (2019). UK dietary changes over the last two decades: A focus on vitamin & mineral intakes. *Journal of Vitamins and Minerals, 2*, 104. https://www.gavinpublishers.com/articles/research-article/Journal-of-Vitamins-Minerals/uk-dietary-changes-over-the-last-two-decades-a-focus-on-vitamin-mineral-intakes

10 Cardwell, G., Bornman, J.F., James, A.P., & Black, L.J. (2018). A review of mushrooms as a potential source of dietary vitamin D. *Nutrients*, *10*(10), 1498. https://doi.org/10.3390/nu10101498

11 McCance and Widdowson's Composition of Foods Integrated Dataset. (CoFID). https://www.gov.uk/government/publications/composition-of-foods-integrated-dataset-cofid

12 Derbyshire, E. (2019). Oily fish and omega-3s across the life stages: A focus on intakes and future directions. *Frontiers in Nutrition*, *6*, 165. https://doi.org/10.3389/fnut.2019.00165

13 British Egg Industry Council. (2020). https://www.egginfo.co.uk/egg-facts-and-figures/industry-information/data

14 Raimundo, F.V., Faulhaber, G.A., Menegatti, P.K., Marques, L., & Furlanetto, T.W. (2011). Effect of high- versus low-fat meal on serum 25-hydroxyvitamin D levels after a single oral dose of vitamin D: A single-blind, parallel, randomized trial. *International Journal of Endocrinology*, *2011*, 809069. https://doi.org/10.1155/2011/809069

15 Harinarayan, C.V., Holick, M.F., Prasad, U.V., Vani, P.S., & Himabindu, G. (2013). Vitamin D status and sun exposure in India. *Dermato-Endocrinology*, *5*(1), 130–141. https://doi.org/10.4161/derm.23873

16 US National Oceanic & Atmospheric Administration NOAA Solar Calculator https://gml.noaa.gov/grad/solcalc/

17 Holick, M.F. (1994). McCollum Award Lecture 1994: Vitamin D – new horizons for the 21st century. *American Journal of Clinical Nutrition, 60*, 619–630. https://doi.org/10.1093/ajcn/60.4.619

18 Deng, L., & Xu, S. (2017). Adaptation of human skin color in various populations. *Hereditas*, *155*, 1. https://doi.org/10.1186/s41065-017-0036-2

19 Lowe, N.M., & Bhojani I., (2017). Special considerations for vitamin D in the South Asian population in the UK. *Therapeutic Advances in Musculoskeletal Disease, 9*(6), 137–144. https://doi.org/10.1177/1759720×17704430

20 Voo, V., Stankovich, J., O'Brien, T. J., Butzkueven, H., & Monif, M. (2020). Vitamin D status in an Australian patient population: A large retrospective case series focusing on factors associated with variations in serum 25(OH)D. *BMJ Open*, *10*(3), e032567. https://doi.org/10.1136/bmjopen-2019-032567

21 Leal, A., Corrêa, M.P., Holick, M.F., Melo, E.V., & Lazaretti-Castro, M. (2021). Sun-induced production of vitamin D_3 throughout 1 year in tropical and subtropical regions: Relationship with latitude, cloudiness, UV-B exposure and solar zenith angle. *Photochemical & Photobiological Sciences*, *20*(2), 265–274. https://doi.org/10.1007/s43630-021-00015-z

22 Holick, M.F., (2002). Sunlight and vitamin D: both good for cardiovascular health. *Journal of General Internal Medicine, 17*(9), 733–735. https://doi.org/10.1046/j.1525-1497.2002.20731.x

23 EFSA Panel on Dietetic Products Nutrition and Allergies. (2012). Scientific opinion on the tolerable upper intake level of vitamin D. *EFSA Journal*, *10*(7), 2813. https://efsa.onlinelibrary.wiley.com/doi/pdf/10.2903/j.efsa.2012.2813

24 Kupisz-Urbańska, M., Płudowski, P., & Marcinowska-Suchowierska, E. (2021). Vitamin D deficiency in older patients-problems of sarcopenia, drug interactions, management in deficiency. *Nutrients*, *13*(4), 1247. https://doi.org/10.3390/nu13041247

25 Maurya, V.K., & Aggarwal, M. (2017). Factors influencing the absorption of vitamin D in GIT: An overview. *Journal of Food Science and Technology*, *54*(12), 3753–3765. https://doi.org/10.1007/s13197-017-2840-0

26 Riche, K.D., Arnall, J., Rieser, K., East, H.E., & Riche, D.M. (2016). Impact of vitamin D status on statin-induced myopathy. *Journal of Clinical & Translational Endocrinology*, *6*, 56–59. https://doi.org/10.1016/j.jcte.2016.11.002

27 Callaghan, A.L., Moy, R.J.D., Booth, I.W., Debelle, G. & Shaw, N.J. (2006). Incidence of symptomatic vitamin D deficiency. *Archives of Disease in Childhood, 91,* 606–607. http://dx.doi.org/10.1136/adc.2006.095075

28 Royal Osteoporosis Society Annual Impact Report. (2017). https://strwebstgmedia.blob. core.windows.net/media/dqab05ky/impact-report-2017.pdf

29 Public Health England. (2016). PHE publishes new advice on vitamin D. https://www. gov.uk/government/news/phe-publishes-new-advice-on-vitamin-d

30 Public Health England. (2020). Statement from PHE and NICE on vitamin D supplementation during winter. https://www.gov.uk/government/publications/vitamin-d-supplementation-during-winter-phe-and-nice-statement/statement-from-phe-and-nice-on-vitamin-d-supplementation-during-winter

31 Ford, L., Graham, V., Wall, A., & Berg, J., (2006). Vitamin D concentrations in an UK inner-city multicultural outpatient population. *Annals of Clinical Biochemistry, 43*(Pt 6), 468–473. https://doi.org/10.1258/000456306778904614

32 Lin, L.Y., Smeeth, L., Langan, S., & Warren-Gash, C. (2021). Distribution of vitamin D status in the UK: A cross-sectional analysis of UK Biobank. *BMJ Open, 11*(1), e038503. https://doi.org/10.1136/bmjopen-2020-038503

33 Calame, W., Street, L., & Hulshof, T. (2020). Vitamin D serum levels in the UK population, including a mathematical approach to evaluate the impact of vitamin D fortified ready-to-eat breakfast cereals: Application of the NDNS database. *Nutrients, 12*(6), 1868. https://doi.org/10.3390/nu12061868

34 Press Association. (2011, December 9). Couple cleared of killing son after doctors failed to diagnose rickets. *The Guardian.* https://www.theguardian.com/uk/2011/dec/09/couple-cleared-killing-baby-son

35 Shaker, J.L., & Deftos, L. (2018) Calcium and phosphate homeostasis. In: Feingold KR, Anawalt B, Boyce A, et al., editors. Endotext [Internet]. South Dartmouth (MA): MDText.com, Inc. Available from: https://www.ncbi.nlm.nih.gov/books/NBK279023/

36 Sun, M., Wu, X., Yu, Y., Wang, L., Xie, D., Zhang, Z., Chen, L., Lu, A., Zhang, G., & Li, F. (2020). Disorders of calcium and phosphorus metabolism and the proteomics/metabolomics-based research. *Frontiers in Cell and Developmental Biology, 8,* 576110. https://doi.org/10.3389/fcell.2020.576110

37 Erben, R.G. (2018). Physiological actions of fibroblast growth factor-23. *Frontiers in Endocrinology, 9,* 267. https://doi.org/10.3389/fendo.2018.00267

38 Zarei, A., Morovat, A., Javaid, K., & Brown, C.P. (2016). Vitamin D receptor expression in human bone tissue and dose-dependent activation in resorbing osteoclasts. *Bone Research, 4,* 16030. https://doi.org/10.1038/boneres.2016.30

39 Baldock, P.A., Thomas, G.P., Hodge, J.M., Baker, S.U., Dressel, U., O'Loughlin, P.D., Nicholson, G.C., Briffa, K.H., Eisman, J.A., & Gardiner, E.M. (2006). Vitamin D action and regulation of bone remodeling: Suppression of osteoclastogenesis by the mature osteoblast. *Journal of Bone Mineral Research, 21,* 1618–1626. https://doi.org/10.1359/jbmr.060714

40 Healthcare Quality Improvement Partnership. (2021). National Hip Fracture Database Annual Report 2020. https://data.gov.uk/dataset/fa2c8bc9-4230-4b8d-8ba9-1d6fc4affb68/national-hip-fracture-database-annual-report-2020

41 Glynn, J., Hollingworth, W., Bhimjiyani, A., Ben-Shlomo, Y., & Gregson, C.L. (2020). How does deprivation influence secondary care costs after hip fracture?. *Osteoporosis International, 31*(8), 1573–1585. https://doi.org/10.1007/s00198-020-05404-1

42 Holick, M.F. (2015). Vitamin D and brain health: The need for vitamin D supplementation and sensible sun exposure. *Journal of Internal Medicine, 277*(1), 90–93. https://doi.org/10.1111/joim.12308

43 Eyles, D.W. (2020). Vitamin D: Brain and behavior. *JBMR Plus, 5*(1), e10419. https://doi.org/10.1002/jbm4.10419

44 Anjum, I., Jaffery, S.S., Fayyaz, M., Samoo, Z., & Anjum, S. (2018). The role of vitamin D in brain health: A mini literature review. *Cureus, 10*(7), e2960. https://doi.org/10.7759/cureus.2960

45 García-Serna, A.M., & Morales, E. (2020). Neurodevelopmental effects of prenatal vitamin D in humans: Systematic review and meta-analysis. *Molecular Psychiatry, 25*(10), 2468–2481. https://doi.org/10.1038/s41380-019-0357-9

46 Gáll, Z., & Székely, O. (2021). Role of vitamin D in cognitive dysfunction: New molecular concepts and discrepancies between animal and human findings. *Nutrients, 13*(11), 3672. https://doi.org/10.3390/nu13113672

47 Łukaszyk, E., Bień-Barkowska, K., & Bień, B. (2018). Cognitive functioning of geriatric patients: Is hypovitaminosis D the next marker of cognitive dysfunction and dementia? *Nutrients, 10*(8), 1104. https://doi.org/10.3390/nu10081104

48 Cuomo, A., Maina, G., Bolognesi, S., Rosso, G., Beccarini Crescenzi, B., Zanobini, F., Goracci, A., Facchi, E., Favaretto, E., Baldini, I., Santucci, A., & Fagiolini, A. (2019). Prevalence and correlates of vitamin D deficiency in a sample of 290 inpatients with mental illness. *Frontiers in Psychiatry, 10*, 167. https://doi.org/10.3389/fpsyt.2019.00167

49 Kaviani, M., Nikooyeh, B., Zand, H., Yaghmaei, P., & Neyestani, T.R. (2020). Effects of vitamin D supplementation on depression and some involved neurotransmitters. *Journal of Affective Disorders, 269*, 28–35. https://doi.org/10.1016/j.jad.2020.03.029

50 Di Gessa, G., Biddulph, J.P., Zaninotto, P., & de Oliveira, C. (2021). Changes in vitamin D levels and depressive symptoms in later life in England. *Scientific Reports, 11*(1), 7724. https://doi.org/10.1038/s41598-021-87432-3

51 Wong, S.K., Chin, K.Y., & Ima-Nirwana, S. (2018). Vitamin D and depression: The evidence from an indirect clue to treatment strategy. *Current Drug Targets, 19*(8), 888–897. https://doi.org/10.2174/1389450118666170913161030

52 Brådvik, L. (2018). Suicide risk and mental disorders. *International Journal of Environmental Research and Public Health, 15*(9), 2028. https://doi.org/10.3390/ijerph15092028

53 Kim, S.Y., Jeon, S.W., Lim, W.J., Oh, K.S., Shin, D.W., Cho, S.J., Park, J.H., Kim, Y. H., & Shin, Y.C. (2020). Vitamin D deficiency and suicidal ideation: A cross-sectional study of 157,211 healthy adults. *Journal of Psychosomatic Research, 134*, 110125. https://doi.org/10.1016/j.jpsychores.2020.110125

54 Umhau, J.C., George, D.T., Heaney, R.P., Lewis, M.D., Ursano, R.J., Heilig, M., Hibbeln, J.R., & Schwandt, M.L. (2013). Low vitamin D status and suicide: A case-control study of active duty military service members. *PloS One, 8*(1), e51543. https://doi.org/10.1371/journal.pone.0051543

55 Atik, D., Cander, B., Dogan, S., Bulut, B., Yazıcı, R., & Taslidere, B. (2020). Relationship between suicidal patients and vitamin D: A prospective case-control study. *Journal of Surgery and Medicine, 4*(9), 766–770. https://doi.org/10.28982/josam.727963

56 Sassi, F., Tamone, C., & D'Amelio, P. (2018). Vitamin D: Nutrient, hormone, and immunomodulator. *Nutrients, 10*(11), 1656. https://doi.org/10.3390/nu10111656

57 Charoenngam, N., & Holick, M.F. (2020). Immunologic effects of vitamin D on human health and disease. *Nutrients, 12*(7), 2097. https://doi.org/10.3390/nu12072097

58 Martens, P.J., Gysemans, C., Verstuyf, A., & Mathieu, A.C. (2020). Vitamin D's effect on immune function. *Nutrients, 12*(5), 1248. https://doi.org/10.3390/nu12051248

59 Konijeti, G.G., Arora, P., Boylan, M.R., Song, Y., Huang, S., Harrell, F., Newton-Cheh, C., O'Neill, D., Korzenik, J., Wang, T. J., & Chan, A.T. (2016). Vitamin D supplementation modulates T cell-mediated immunity in humans: Results from a randomized control trial. *The Journal of Clinical Endocrinology and Metabolism, 101*(2), 533–538. https://doi.org/10.1210/jc.2015-3599

60 Giannini, S., Giusti, A., Minisola, S., Napoli, N., Passeri, G., Rossini, M., & Sinigaglia, L. (2022). The immunologic profile of vitamin D and its role in different immune-mediated diseases: An expert opinion. *Nutrients*, *14*(3), 473. https://doi.org/10.3390/nu14030473

61 Martineau, A.R., Jolliffe, D.A., Hooper, R.L., Greenberg, L., Aloia, J.F., Bergman, P., Dubnov-Raz, G., Esposito, S., Ganmaa, D., Ginde, A.A., Goodall, E. C., Grant, C.C., Griffiths, C.J., Janssens, W., Laaksi, I., Manaseki-Holland, S., Mauger, D., Murdoch, D.R., Neale, R., Rees, J.R., & Camargo, C.A., Jr (2017). Vitamin D supplementation to prevent acute respiratory tract infections: Systematic review and meta-analysis of individual participant data. *BMJ*, *356*, i6583. https://doi.org/10.1136/bmj.i6583

62 Hansdottir, S., Monick, M.M., Hinde, S.L., Lovan, N., Look, D.C., & Hunninghake, G.W. (2008). Respiratory epithelial cells convert inactive vitamin D to its active form: Potential effects on host defense. *Journal of Immunology*, *181*(10), 7090–7099. https://doi.org/10.4049/jimmunol.181.10.7090

63 Rosenblum, M.D., Remedios, K.A., & Abbas, A.K. (2015). Mechanisms of human autoimmunity. *The Journal of Clinical Investigation*, *125*(6), 2228–2233. https://doi.org/10.1172/JCI78088

64 Mousa, A., Misso, M., Teede, H., Scragg, R., & de Courten, B. (2016). Effect of vitamin D supplementation on inflammation: Protocol for a systematic review. *BMJ Open*, *6*(4), e010804. https://doi.org/10.1136/bmjopen-2015-010804

65 Dankers W., Colin E.M., van Hamburg J.P., Lubberts E. (2017) Vitamin D in autoimmunity: Molecular mechanisms and therapeutic potential. *Frontiers in Immunology*, *7*, 697. https://doi.org/10.3389/fimmu.2016.00697

66 Murdaca, G., Tonacci, A., Negrini, S., Greco, M., Borro, M., Puppo, F., & Gangemi, S. (2019). Emerging role of vitamin D in autoimmune diseases: An update on evidence and therapeutic implications. *Autoimmunity Reviews*, *18*(9), 102350. https://doi.org/10.1016/j.autrev.2019.102350

67 Fisher, S.A., Rahimzadeh, M., Brierley, C., Gration, B., Doree, C., Kimber, C.E., Plaza Cajide, A., Lamikanra, A.A., & Roberts, D.J. (2019). The role of vitamin D in increasing circulating T regulatory cell numbers and modulating T regulatory cell phenotypes in patients with inflammatory disease or in healthy volunteers: A systematic review. *PloS One*, *14*(9), e0222313. https://doi.org/10.1371/journal.pone.0222313

68 Schrumpf, J.A., van der Does, A.M., & Hiemstra, P.S. (2020). Impact of the local inflammatory environment on mucosal vitamin D metabolism and signaling in chronic inflammatory lung diseases. *Frontiers in Immunology*, *11*, 1433. https://doi.org/10.3389/fimmu.2020.01433

69 DiGuilio, K.M., Rybakovsky, E., Abdavies, R., Chamoun, R., Flounders, C.A., Shepley-McTaggart, A., Harty, R.N., & Mullin, J.M. (2022). Micronutrient improvement of epithelial barrier function in various disease states: A case for adjuvant therapy. *International Journal of Molecular Sciences*, *23*(6), 2995. https://doi.org/10.3390/ijms23062995

70 Hahn, J., Cook, N.R., Alexander, E.K., Friedman, S., Walter, J., Bubes, V., Kotler, G., Lee, I.M., Manson, J.E., & Costenbader, K.H. (2022). Vitamin D and marine omega 3 fatty acid supplementation and incident autoimmune disease: VITAL randomized controlled trial. *BMJ*, *376*, e066452. https://doi.org/10.1136/bmj-2021-066452

71 Simon, K.C., Munger, K.L., & Ascherio, A. (2012). Vitamin D and multiple sclerosis: Epidemiology, immunology, and genetics. *Current Opinion in Neurology*, *25*(3), 246–251. https://doi.org/10.1097/WCO.0b013e3283533a7e

72 Mokry, L.E., Ross, S., Ahmad, O.S., Forgetta, V., Smith, G.D., Goltzman, D., Leong, A., Greenwood, C.M., Thanassoulis, G., & Richards, J.B. (2015). Vitamin D and risk of multiple sclerosis: A Mendelian randomization study. *PLoS Medicine*, *12*(8), e1001866. https://doi.org/10.1371/journal.pmed.1001866

73 Munger, K.L., Åivo, J., Hongell, K., Soilu-Hänninen, M., Surcel, H.M., & Ascherio, A. (2016). Vitamin D status during pregnancy and risk of multiple sclerosis in offspring of women in the Finnish Maternity Cohort. *JAMA Neurology*, *73*(5), 515–519. https://doi.org/10.1001/jamaneurol.2015.4800

74 Gomez-Pinedo, U., Cuevas, J.A., Benito-Martín, M.S., Moreno-Jiménez, L., Esteban-Garcia, N., Torre-Fuentes, L., Matías-Guiu, J.A., Pytel, V., Montero, P., & Matías-Guiu, J. (2020). Vitamin D increases remyelination by promoting oligodendrocyte lineage differentiation. *Brain and Behavior*, *10*(1), e01498. https://doi.org/10.1002/brb3.1498

75 Brütting, C., Stangl, G.I., & Staege, M.S. (2021). Vitamin D, Epstein-Barr virus, and endogenous retroviruses in multiple sclerosis – facts and hypotheses. *Journal of Integrative Neuroscience*, *20*(1), 233–238. https://doi.org/10.31083/j.jin.2021.01.392

76 Hupperts, R., Smolders, J., Vieth, R., Holmøy, T., Marhardt, K., Schluep, M., Killestein, J., Barkhof, F., Beelke, M., Grimaldi, L., & SOLAR Study Group. (2019). Randomized trial of daily high-dose vitamin D_3 in patients with RRMS receiving subcutaneous interferon β-1a. *Neurology*, *93*(20), e1906–e1916. https://doi.org/10.1212/WNL.0000000000008445

77 Camu, W., Lehert, P., Pierrot-Deseilligny, C., Hautecoeur, P., Besserve, A., Jean Deleglise, A.S., Payet, M., Thouvenot, E., & Souberbielle, J.C. (2019). Cholecalciferol in relapsing-remitting MS: A randomized clinical trial (CHOLINE). *Neurology, Neuroimmunology & Neuroinflammation*, *6*(5), e597. https://doi.org/10.1212/NXI.0000000000000597

78 Rafiq, S., & Jeppesen, P.B. (2021). Vitamin D deficiency is inversely associated with homeostatic model assessment of insulin resistance. *Nutrients*, *13*(12), 4358. https://doi.org/10.3390/nu13124358

79 Park, S.K., Garland, C.F., Gorham, E.D., BuDoff, L., & Barrett-Connor, E. (2018). Plasma 25-hydroxyvitamin D concentration and risk of type 2 diabetes and pre-diabetes: 12-year cohort study. *PloS One*, *13*(4), e0193070. https://doi.org/10.1371/journal.pone.0193070

80 Hu, L., Zhang, Y., Wang, X., You, L., Xu, P., Cui, X., Zhu, L., Ji, C., Guo, X., & Wen, J. (2018). Maternal vitamin D status and risk of gestational diabetes: A meta-analysis. *Cellular Physiology and Biochemistry*, *45*(1), 291–300. https://doi.org/10.1159/000486810

81 Takiishi T., Gysemans C., Bouillon R., & Mathieu C., (2012). Vitamin D and diabetes. *Rheumatic Disease Clinics,* *38*(1), 179–206. DOI: https://doi.org/10.1016/j.rdc.2012.03.015

82 Littorin, B., Blom, P., Schölin, A., Arnqvist, H.J., Blohmé, G., Bolinder, J., Ekbom-Schnell, A., Eriksson, J.W., Gudbjörnsdottir, S., Nyström, L., Ostman, J., & Sundkvist, G. (2006). Lower levels of plasma 25-hydroxyvitamin D among young adults at diagnosis of autoimmune type 1 diabetes compared with control subjects: Results from the nationwide Diabetes Incidence Study in Sweden (DISS). *Diabetologia*, *49*(12), 2847–2852. https://doi.org/10.1007/s00125-006-0426-x

83 Walsh, J.S., Bowles, S., & Evans, A.L. (2017). Vitamin D in obesity. *Current Opinion in Endocrinology, Diabetes, and Obesity*, *24*(6), 389–394. https://doi.org/10.1097/MED.0000000000000371

84 Vranić, L., Mikolašević, I., & Milić, S. (2019). Vitamin D deficiency: Consequence or cause of obesity? *Medicina*, *55*(9), 541. https://doi.org/10.3390/medicina55090541

85 Ellulu, M.S., Patimah, I., Khaza'ai, H., Rahmat, A., & Abed, Y. (2017). Obesity and inflammation: The linking mechanism and the complications. *Archives of Medical Science: AMS*, *13*(4), 851–863. https://doi.org/10.5114/aoms.2016.58928

86 Tsalamandris, S., Antonopoulos, A.S., Oikonomou, E., Papamikroulis, G.A., Vogiatzi, G., Papaioannou, S., Deftereos, S., & Tousoulis, D. (2019). The role of inflammation

in diabetes: Current concepts and future perspectives. *European Cardiology, 14*(1), 50–59. https://doi.org/10.15420/ecr.2018.33.1

87 Haddad Kashani, H., Seyed Hosseini, E., Nikzad, H., Soleimani, A., Soleimani, M., Tamadon, M.R., Keneshlou, F., & Asemi, Z. (2018). The effects of vitamin D supplementation on signaling pathway of inflammation and oxidative stress in diabetic hemodialysis: A randomized, double-blind, placebo-controlled trial. *Frontiers in Pharmacology, 9*, 50. https://doi.org/10.3389/fphar.2018.00050

88 Scheithauer, T., Rampanelli, E., Nieuwdorp, M., Vallance, B.A., Verchere, C.B., van Raalte, D.H., & Herrema, H. (2020). Gut microbiota as a trigger for metabolic inflammation in obesity and type 2 diabetes. *Frontiers in Immunology, 11*, 571731. https://doi.org/10.3389/fimmu.2020.571731

89 Wen, L., & Duffy, A. (2017). Factors influencing the gut microbiota, inflammation, and type 2 diabetes. *The Journal of Nutrition, 147*(7), 1468S–1475 S. https://doi.org/10.3945/jn.116.240754

90 Singh, P., Rawat, A., Alwakeel, M., Sharif, E., & Al Khodor, S. (2020). The potential role of vitamin D supplementation as a gut microbiota modifier in healthy individuals. *Scientific Reports, 10*(1), 21641. https://doi.org/10.1038/s41598-020-77806-4

91 Nielsen, O.H., Hansen, T.I., Gubatan, J.M., Jensen, K.B., & Rejnmark, L. (2019). Managing vitamin D deficiency in inflammatory bowel disease. *Frontline Gastroenterology, 10*(4), 394–400. https://doi.org/10.1136/flgastro-2018-101055

92 Fletcher, J., Cooper, S.C., Ghosh, S., & Hewison, M. (2019). The role of vitamin D in inflammatory bowel disease: Mechanism to management. *Nutrients, 11*(5), 1019. https://doi.org/10.3390/nu11051019

93 Lobo de Sá, F.D., Backert, S., Nattramilarasu, P.K., Mousavi, S., Sandle, G.I., Bereswill, S., Heimesaat, M.M., Schulzke, J.D., & Bücker, R. (2021). Vitamin D reverses disruption of gut epithelial barrier function caused by *Campylobacter jejuni*. *International Journal of Molecular Sciences, 22*(16), 8872. https://doi.org/10.3390/ijms22168872

94 Vernia, F., Valvano, M., Longo, S., Cesaro, N., Viscido, A., & Latella, G. (2022). Vitamin D in inflammatory bowel diseases. Mechanisms of action and therapeutic implications. *Nutrients, 14*(2), 269. https://doi.org/10.3390/nu14020269

95 Karimi, S., Tabataba-Vakili, S., Yari, Z., Alborzi, F., Hedayati, M., Ebrahimi-Daryani, N., & Hekmatdoost, A. (2019). The effects of two vitamin D regimens on ulcerative colitis activity index, quality of life and oxidant/anti-oxidant status. *Nutrition Journal, 18*(1), 16. https://doi.org/10.1186/s12937-019-0441-7

96 Faisal, S., & Mirza, F.S. (2020). Sublingual vitamin D3 effective in a patient resistant to conventional vitamin D supplementation. *AACE Clinical Case Reports, 6*(6), e342–e345. https://doi.org/10.4158/ACCR-2020-0282

97 Chiruvolu, N.V., Safarpour, Y., & Sandhu, V.K. (2021). Vitamin D and Lupus: Are we doing enough?. *Journal of Community Hospital Internal Medicine Perspectives, 11*(5), 624–628. https://doi.org/10.1080/20009666.2021.1956049

98 National Rheumatoid Arthritis Society. Photosensitivity. https://nras.org.uk/resource/photosensitivity/

99 Magro, R., Saliba, C., Camilleri, L., Scerri, C., & Borg, A.A. (2021). Vitamin D supplementation in systemic lupus erythematosus: Relationship to disease activity, fatigue and the interferon signature gene expression. *BMC Rheumatology, 5*(1), 53. https://doi.org/10.1186/s41927-021-00223-1

100 Meena, N., Singh Chawla, S.P., Garg, R., Batta, A., & Kaur, S. (2018). Assessment of vitamin D in rheumatoid arthritis and its correlation with disease activity. *Journal of Natural Science, Biology, and Medicine, 9*(1), 54–58. https://doi.org/10.4103/jnsbm.JNSBM_128_17

101 Reid, D., Toole, B.J., Knox, S., Talwar, D., Harten, J., O'Reilly, D.S., Blackwell, S., Kinsella, J., McMillan, D.C., & Wallace, A.M. (2011). The relation between acute changes in the systemic inflammatory response and plasma 25-hydroxyvitamin D concentrations after elective knee arthroplasty. *The American Journal of Clinical Nutrition, 93*(5), 1006–1011. https://doi.org/10.3945/ajcn.110.008490

102 Reynolds, J.A., & Bruce, I.N. (2017). Vitamin D treatment for connective tissue diseases: Hope beyond the hype?. *Rheumatology, 56*(2), 178–186. https://doi.org/10.1093/rheumatology/kew212

103 Charoenngam, N. (2021). Vitamin D and rheumatic diseases: A review of clinical evidence. *International Journal of Molecular Sciences, 22*(19), 10659. https://doi.org/10.3390/ijms221910659

104 Guan, Y., Hao, Y., Guan, Y., Bu, H., & Wang, H. (2020). The effect of vitamin D supplementation on rheumatoid arthritis patients: A systematic review and meta-analysis. *Frontiers in Medicine, 7*, 596007. https://doi.org/10.3389/fmed.2020.596007

105 Elkoshi Z. (2022). Cancer and autoimmune diseases: A tale of two immunological opposites?. *Frontiers in Immunology, 13*, 821598. https://doi.org/10.3389/fimmu.2022.821598

106 Apperly, F.L. (1941). The relation of solar radiation to cancer mortality in North America. *Cancer Res, 1*, 191. https://aacrjournals.org/cancerres/article/1/3/191/472224/The-Relation-of-Solar-Radiation-to-Cancer

107 Grant, W.B. (2018). A review of the Evidence Supporting the Vitamin D-Cancer Prevention Hypothesis in 2017. *Anticancer Research: International Journal of Cancer Research and Treatment, 38*(2), 1121–1136. https://doi.org/10.21873/anticanres.12331

108 Jeon, S., & Shin, E. (2018). Exploring vitamin D metabolism and function in cancer. *Experimental and Molecular Medicine, 50*, 20. https://doi.org/10.1038/s12276-018-0038-9

109 Han, J., Guo, X., Yu, X., Liu, S., Cui, X., Zhang, B., & Liang, H. (2019). 25-hydroxyvitamin D and total cancer incidence and mortality: A meta-analysis of prospective cohort studies. *Nutrients, 11*(10), 2295. https://doi.org/10.3390/nu11102295

110 Cortes, M., Chen, M.J., Stachura, D.L., Liu, S.Y., Kwan, W., Wright, F., Vo, L. T., Theodore, L.N., Esain, V., Frost, I.M., Schlaeger, T.M., Goessling, W., Daley, G. Q., & North, T.E. (2016). Developmental vitamin D availability impacts hematopoietic stem cell production. *Cell Reports, 17*(2), 458–468. https://doi.org/10.1016/j.celrep.2016.09.012

111 Fleet, J.C., DeSmet, M., Johnson, R., & Li, Y. (2012). Vitamin D and cancer: A review of molecular mechanisms. *The Biochemical Journal, 441*(1), 61–76. https://doi.org/10.1042/BJ20110744

112 Carlberg, C., & Muñoz, A. (2022). An update on vitamin D signaling and cancer. *Seminars in Cancer Biology, 79*, 217–230. https://doi.org/10.1016/j.semcancer.2020.05.018

113 Young, M., & Xiong, Y. (2018). Influence of vitamin D on cancer risk and treatment: Why the variability?. *Trends in Cancer Research, 13*, 43–53. https://www.ncbi.nlm.nih.gov/pmc/articles/PMC6201256/

114 Mostafa, W.Z., & Hegazy, R.A. (2015). Vitamin D and the skin: Focus on a complex relationship: A review. *Journal of Advanced Research, 6*(6), 793–804. https://doi.org/10.1016/j.jare.2014.01.011

115 Umar,M., Sastry, K.S., Al Ali, F., Al-Khulaifi, M., Wang, E., & Chouchane, A.I. (2018). Vitamin D and the pathophysiology of inflammatory skin diseases. *Skin Pharmacology and Physiology, 31*(2), 74–86. https://doi.org/10.1159/000485132

116 Roider, E., Ruzicka, T., & Schauber, J. (2013). Vitamin D, the cutaneous barrier, antimicrobial peptides and allergies: Is there a link?. *Allergy, Asthma & Immunology Research, 5*(3), 119–128. https://doi.org/10.4168/aair.2013.5.3.119

117 Cheng, H.M., Kim, S., Park, G.H., Chang, S.E., Bang, S., Won, C.H., Lee, M. W., Choi, J.H., & Moon, K.C. (2014). Low vitamin D levels are associated with atopic dermatitis, but not allergic rhinitis, asthma, or IgE sensitization, in the adult Korean population. *The Journal of Allergy and Clinical Immunology, 133*(4), 1048–1055. https://doi.org/10.1016/j.jaci.2013.10.055

118 Ricceri, F., Pescitelli, L., Tripo, L., & Prignano, F. (2013). Deficiency of serum concentration of 25-hydroxyvitamin D correlates with severity of disease in chronic plaque psoriasis. *Journal of the American Academy of Dermatology, 68*(3), 511–512. https://doi.org/10.1016/j.jaad.2012.10.051

119 Kemény L., Varga E., & Novak Z. (2019). Advances in phototherapy for psoriasis and atopic dermatitis. *Expert Review of Clinical Immunology, 15*(11), 1205–1214. https://doi.org/10.1080/1744666X.2020.1672537

120 Stanescu, A., Simionescu, A.A., & Diaconu, C.C. (2021). Oral vitamin D therapy in patients with psoriasis. *Nutrients, 13*(1), 163. https://doi.org/10.3390/nu13010163

121 Finamor, D.C., Sinigaglia-Coimbra, R., Neves, L.C., Gutierrez, M., Silva, J.J., Torres, L.D., Surano, F., Neto, D.J., Novo, N.F., Juliano, Y., Lopes, A.C., & Coimbra, C.G. (2013). A pilot study assessing the effect of prolonged administration of high daily doses of vitamin D on the clinical course of vitiligo and psoriasis. *Dermato-Endocrinology, 5*(1), 222–234. https://doi.org/10.4161/derm.24808

122 Mahtani, R., Nair, & P.M.K., (2022). Daily Oral vitamin D3 without concomitant therapy in the management of psoriasis: A case series. *Clinical Immunology Communications, 2*, 17–22. https://doi.org/10.1016/j.clicom.2022.01.001

123 Hattangdi-Haridas, S.R., Lanham-New, S.A., Wong, W., Ho, M., & Darling, A. L. (2019). Vitamin D deficiency and effects of vitamin D supplementation on disease severity in patients with atopic dermatitis: A systematic review and meta-analysis in adults and children. *Nutrients, 11*(8), 1854. https://doi.org/10.3390/nu11081854

124 Sánchez-Armendáriz, K., García-Gil, A., Romero, C.A., Contreras-Ruiz, J., Karam-Orante, M., Balcazar-Antonio, D., & Domínguez-Cherit, J. (2018). Oral vitamin D3 5000 IU/day as an adjuvant in the treatment of atopic dermatitis: A randomized control trial. *International Journal of Dermatology, 57*(12), 1516–1520. https://doi.org/10.1111/ijd.14220

125 Mansour, N.O., Mohamed, A.A., Hussein, M., Eldemiry, E., Daifalla, A., Hassanin, S., Nassar, N., Ghaith, D., & Mohamed Salah, E. (2020). The impact of vitamin D supplementation as an adjuvant therapy on clinical outcomes in patients with severe atopic dermatitis: A randomized controlled trial. *Pharmacology Research & Perspectives, 8*(6), e00679. https://doi.org/10.1002/prp2.679

126 Crowe, F.L., Jolly, K., MacArthur, C., Manaseki-Holland, S., Gittoes, N., Hewison, M., Scragg, R., & Nirantharakumar, K. (2019) Trends in the incidence of testing for vitamin D deficiency in primary care in the UK: A retrospective analysis of The Health Improvement Network (THIN), 2005–2015. *BMJ Open, 9*(6), e028355. https://doi.org/10.1136/bmjopen-2018-028355

127 York Health Economics Consortium. (2014). NICE: An Economic Evaluation of Interventions to Improve the Uptake of Vitamin D Supplements in England and Wales. *University of York.* https://www.nice.org.uk/guidance/ph56/evidence/economic-evaluation-final-69290605

128 Woodford, H.J., Barrett, S., & Pattman, S., (2018). Vitamin D: Too much testing and treating? *Clinical Medicine, 18*(3), 196–200. doi: 10.7861/clinmedicine.18-3-196

129 Pilz, S., Zittermann, A., Trummer, C., Theiler-Schwetz, V., Lerchbaum, E., Keppel, M.H., Grübler, M.R., März, W., & Pandis, M. (2019). Vitamin D testing and treatment: A narrative review of current evidence. *Endocrine Connections, 8*(2), R27–R43. https://doi.org/10.1530/EC-18-0432

130 Amrein, K., Scherkl, M., Hoffmann, M., Neuwersch-Sommeregger, S., Köstenberger, M., Tmava Berisha, A., Martucci, G., Pilz, S., & Malle, O. (2020). Vitamin D deficiency 2.0: An update on the current status worldwide. *European Journal of Clinical Nutrition, 74*(11), 1498–1513. https://doi.org/10.1038/s41430-020-0558-y

131 Nutrition and bone health: with particular reference to calcium and vitamin D. Report of the Subgroup on Bone Health, Working Group on the Nutritional Status of the Population of the Committee on Medical Aspects of the Food Nutrition Policy. (1998). *Reports on health and social subjects, 49,* iii–24. https://assets.publishing.service.gov. uk/government/uploads/system/uploads/attachment_data/file/743523/Nutrition_and_ Bone_Health_-_with_particular_reference_to_calcium_and_vitamin_D__1998_.pdf

132 Hall, L.M., Kimlin, M.G., Aronov, P.A., Hammock, B.D., Slusser, J.R., Woodhouse, L.R., & Stephensen, C.B. (2010). Vitamin D intake needed to maintain target serum 25-hydroxyvitamin D concentrations in participants with low sun exposure and dark skin pigmentation is substantially higher than current recommendations. *The Journal of Nutrition, 140*(3), 542–550. https://doi.org/10.3945/jn.109.115253

133 Cashman, K.D. (2018). Vitamin D requirements for the future-lessons learned and charting a path forward. *Nutrients, 10*(5), 533. https://doi.org/10.3390/nu10050533

134 Griffin, G., Hewison, M., Hopkin, J., Kenny, R.A., Quinton, R., Rhodes, J., Subramanian, S., & Thickett, D. (2021). Preventing vitamin D deficiency during the COVID-19 pandemic: UK definitions of vitamin D sufficiency and recommended supplement dose are set too low. *Clinical Medicine, 21*(1), e48–e51. https://doi.org/ 10.7861/clinmed.2020-0858

135 Mazess, R.B., Bischoff-Ferrari, H.A., & Dawson-Hughes, B. (2021). Vitamin D: Bolus is Bogus – A narrative review. *JBMR Plus, 5*(12), e10567. https://doi.org/10.1002/jbm4. 10567

136 Holick, M.F., Binkley, N.C., Bischoff-Ferrari, H.A., Gordon, C.M., Hanley, D.A., Heaney, R.P., Murad, M.H., Weaver, C.M., & Endocrine Society. (2011). Evaluation, treatment, and prevention of vitamin D deficiency: An Endocrine Society clinical practice guideline. *The Journal of Clinical Endocrinology and Metabolism, 96*(7), 1911–1930. https://doi.org/10.1210/jc.2011-0385

7 Conception, Pregnancy and Foetal Development

This chapter looks at three separate but interrelated issues, the relevance of nutrition to conception for both parents, the mother's nutritional requirements throughout pregnancy, and the nutrition requirements of the developing foetus. There are crossover nutrients in all three areas, for example zinc is essential in gene transcription, protein synthesis, and a range of antioxidant and pro-oxidant cellular processes.[1] Zinc contributes to strong, healthy, motile sperm as well as the growth and development of the embryo, foetus, and neonate.[2,3] It also seems to reduce the amount of time taken to fall pregnant, although the mechanisms for this are not yet clear.[4]

The nutritional demands for mother and baby are so tightly interlinked that the two are discussed concurrently next. There is a separate section for fathers because, whilst sperm is obviously essential in the reproductive process, once the original donation is made, from a nutrition perspective, the role of the father can take a back seat for 40 weeks – apart from going out for ice-cream (or similar) at 2 am.

Of course, it should be possible to obtain all the nutrients we need from a varied and balanced diet. But as previously discussed, the UK diet is generally poor, being high in ultra-processed foods and sugars, and low in fruit, vegetables, dietary fibre, and oily fish.[5,6] Poor diet, leading to either over-nutrition or under-nutrition, is not a good starting place to build a new person. It can impact the quality and viability of sperm and egg and can adversely affect both mother and baby. A lack of some micronutrients has been linked with poor neurodevelopment, issues with visual and motor development, and an increased risk of neuropsychiatric disorders in later life.[7] The consequences of poor nutrition can follow a baby through childhood, into adulthood and even continue to influence future generations.[8] On the other hand, good nutrition benefits parents, children, and the wider society, reducing the incidence of physical and mental ill health and decreasing the burden of cost on healthcare providers.

DOI: 10.1201/b22900-8

MUM AND BABY

Micronutrients needed for healthy foetal and infant development.

Nutrients in **bold** are known to have low intakes in the UK.

B VITAMINS
Riboflavin
Vitamin B6
Vitamin B12
Folic acid
Inositol
Choline
Betaine

FAT SOLUBLE
VITAMINS
Vitamin A
Vitamin D

OMEGA-3 FATTY ACIDS
Eicosapentaenoic acid (EPA) &
Docosahexaenoic Acid (DHA)

OMEGA-6 FATTY ACID
Arachidonic Acid (AA)

MINERALS
Calcium
Iodine
Iron

Human milk oligosaccharides

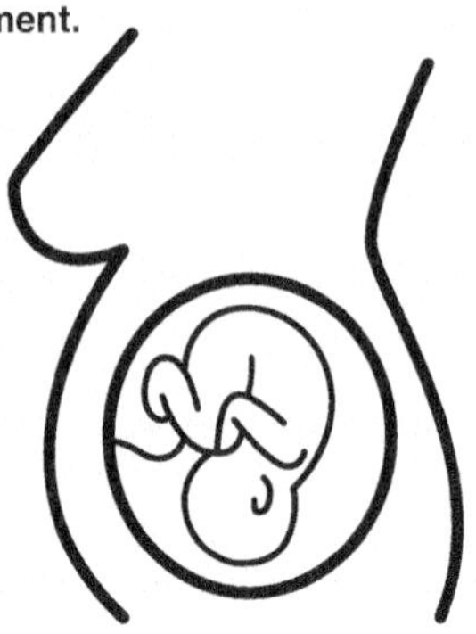

Micronutrients needed for healthy foetal and infant development.

FOLIC ACID

Since 1991, folic acid has been the most well recognised nutrient related to pre-conception and early pregnancy.[9] If taken in sufficient quantities (400 µg for at least three months prior to pregnancy and for the first three months of pregnancy) it protects against the development of neural tube defects (NTDs).

The neural tube is the structure within the embryo where the brain and spinal cord develop. It forms within the first few days of cell division following fertilisation and should fully close between the 18th and 28th day after conception. Failure to close creates a malformation of the brain and/or spine, known as a NTD.[10] NTDs range from spina bifida, which can result in a lifetime of disability and healthcare costs, through to anencephaly, where a brain does not form, leading to the death of the foetus.

In the UK, 90% of women of childbearing age have such low red blood cell folate levels that any unborn children are at increased risk of NTDs.[6] Between 1995 and 1998 the Health Education Authority ran a public health campaign to raise awareness of the importance of folic acid.[11] There has been no public health messaging around folic acid since that time.

Public health messages fade in public consciousness unless they continue to be effectively promoted. Whilst many prospective mothers may have heard of folic acid, most do not understand its relevance or the importance of timing in relation to pregnancy.[12] Women of ethnic minorities in the UK are even less likely to either know about, or take, folic acid.[13] And although women may "know" about folic acid, only around one-third of women supplement with folic acid when planning a pregnancy.[14] However, approximately 45% of pregnancies in the UK are unplanned, and many women may not be aware they are pregnant until between six and eight weeks gestation.[15] By which point any intervention with folic acid is far too late, as the neural tube will have already closed.[10]

Folic acid is part of the B complex which consists of eight vitamins and a couple of allied nutrients. These all work synergistically with each other in a range of functions, so it is not surprising that some B vitamins and allied nutrients are also involved in the formation of the neural tube. Low levels of vitamin B12 have been associated with an increased risk of NTDs.[16] As are low levels of inositol, a carbocyclic sugar which works with the B complex.[17] And sufficiency in vitamins B2, B6, choline, and betaine (more allied nutrients) may also reduce the risk of NTDs.[18]

OTHER BENEFITS OF B VITAMINS

B vitamins have a significant role to play, from pre-conception onwards. Placental development is dependent on sufficient vitamins B2, B3, B12, and folic acid.[19] Supplementing with vitamin B6 can increase the chance of conception and possibly reduce the risk of miscarriage in early pregnancy.[20] It can also reduce symptoms of nausea and vomiting.[21] And high levels of vitamins B2, B6, and folate pre-conception, and during the first and second trimesters, have been linked to a reduced risk of gestational diabetes.[22]

The B complex are vital in the metabolism of homocysteine, an amino acid produced in the body as part of the breakdown pathway of another amino acid, methionine. Methionine metabolism needs B2, B6, B12, folic acid, and betaine (synthesised from dietary choline) to ensure the pathway works properly.[23] Insufficient levels of these nutrients slows or even halts methionine breakdown which leads to an increased level of homocysteine.[24] High levels of circulating homocysteine have been linked to difficulty in conceiving and poor pregnancy outcomes, including an increased risk of preeclampsia and placental abruption.[25,26,27]

Serum levels of both vitamin B12 and folate are low in women of childbearing age in the UK, whilst homocysteine levels are high.[28] Although vitamin B12 intakes mostly meet recommended levels, requirements in pregnancy and lactation cannot be met by the current RNI of 1.5 µg.[29,30] Indeed, the European Food Safety Authority recommends increasing intakes of vitamin B12 to 4.5 µg from preconception to lactation.[31] Vegetarians and vegans are particularly at risk because vitamin B12 is primarily found in foods of animal origin, although fortified products such as breakfast cereals and nutritional yeast are available.[32]

One of the allied nutrients that works with the B complex is biotin, a key enzymatic cofactor in the metabolism of fats, amino acids, and sugars, as well as in gene regulation and cell signalling.[33] Biotin requirements increase in pregnancy and, although outright deficiency is rare, insufficiency has been linked to restricted foetal growth, birth defects, and preterm delivery.[34,35]

Another substance allied with the B complex is choline which is critical in foetal development.[36] During the final trimester it is essential for cell growth and division, particularly of the brain and spinal cord, as well as neurotransmitter synthesis.[37] Sufficient foetal supply of choline seems to impact on lifelong memory function, and choline continues to be important post birth, as neonates have three times the levels of choline in their blood that their mothers have.[38] Choline also seems to help the body make more efficient use of omega-3 fatty acids, particularly docosahexaenoic acid (DHA) which is key in foetal brain, cognition and visual development.[39] Although the UK has no recommended intake level, intakes among women of childbearing age is worryingly low.[40]

The B complex and associated substances (biotin, choline, betaine, and inositol) are extremely safe. Although most are widely available from a range of foods, intakes of folic acid, B12, biotin, and choline are potentially dangerously low. Added to which, many of the sources of B12, biotin, and choline are animal foods, which increases the risk of insufficiency among vegetarians and vegans. The calorie-dense, nutrient-poor UK diet simply does not provide all necessary micronutrients in sufficient amounts. Food supplements can be an extremely useful adjunct to support good nutrition, particularly during critical points in the life cycle such as pregnancy. B complex food supplements are safe in pregnancy, and the UK market provides a wide range of good quality and affordable products. Given the importance of these substances in supporting the health and wellbeing of the next generation, healthcare practitioners may wish to consider recommending all women of childbearing age, from teens to fifties should take a daily B complex food supplement as a form of health insurance.

FATS AND OILS

Fat is an essential part of our diets; the fat we eat allows us to absorb the fat-soluble vitamins (A, D, E, and K). Our bodies use it to create cell structures and membranes as well as a range of chemicals including neurotransmitters, hormones, and immune substances like cytokines and eicosanoids. We use it to generate energy and keep ourselves warm. And there are some fats which are key in healthy conception, gestation, and development for both mum and baby.

TRANS FATS

Of course, not all fats are beneficial, and trans fats are at the top of that list. Although they occur naturally in trace amounts in meat and dairy products, most are artificial, created by modern food-processing techniques. As discussed in chapter 4, these processes alter the molecular structure of fats, making them inflexible. Our bodies do not know what to do with these artificially created substances and so they tend to get pushed into cell membranes, at the expense of the fatty acids that should be placed there. Because trans-fats are inflexible, this makes cell membranes rigid, reducing permeability and disrupting cell signalling and metabolism (see infographic in chapter 4).[41]

Trans fats disrupt cholesterol balance, stimulate inappropriate inflammation, increase insulin resistance, and create endothelial dysfunction.[42] Consumption of trans fats also has a detrimental effect on female fertility, particularly ovarian functions.[43]

Ultra-processed food accounts for more than half of all dietary energy consumed in the UK.[44] The industrial nature of ultra-processed foods means that many contain hefty amounts of trans fats.[45,46] High intakes of trans reduce the likelihood of falling pregnant, possibly because of the impact of trans fats on cell membranes, including those of the sperm and egg.[47,48] Consuming as little as 4 g of trans fats a day can increase the risk of ovarian infertility by as much as 73%.[49] Trans fats also reduce overall gestation time, and high intakes are associated with an increased risk of preeclampsia.[50,51]

Trans fats can cross the placental barrier and have been found in foetal blood.[52] They disrupt lipid metabolism which can negatively impact foetal growth and development.[53] Children with higher levels of trans fats in umbilical blood have minor neurological dysfunction, and foetal exposure to trans fats can increase the risk of developing metabolic diseases later in life.[54,55]

Trans fats are found in foods such as margarine and anything containing hydrogenated vegetable oils such as commercially produced cakes and biscuits, ice cream, doughnuts, and "fast" foods. The advice on trans fats should be to avoid them at all costs. Unfortunately, this can be difficult to do as there is no legal requirement for trans fats to be listed on food labels. So avoiding any foods which are heavily processed is probably the best idea.

Omega Fats

On the flip side of fats and oils are the essential polyunsaturated fatty acids (PUFAs) omega-3 (n-3), and omega-6 (n-6). These are "essential" because they are needed for human survival, cannot be synthesised by the human body and must be obtained through the diet. Both n-3 and n-6 PUFAs can increase the chances of conceiving and provide health benefits to both mother and baby.

Both n-3 and n-6 PUFAs are major components of cell membranes where they enable fluidity and flexibility, facilitate permeability, and determine the functioning of cell-signalling pathways.[56] PUFAs are also used to manufacture eicosanoids, compounds that, among other things, regulate ovulation, fertilisation, implantation, embryo development, and childbirth.[56]

The n-3 fats eicosapentaenoic acid (EPA) and DHA and the n-6 fat arachidonic acid (AA) form cell membrane phospholipids and are used in the manufacture of both pro and anti-inflammatory eicosanoids. n-3 PUFAs are broadly anti-inflammatory whilst n-6 PUFAs are more pro-inflammatory, it is the balance between n-3 and n-6 that is key. The pro-inflammatory action of n-6 stimulates favourable conditions for embryo implantation, whilst the anti-inflammatory effects of n-3 support oocyte maturation.[57]

In in-vitro fertilisation (IVF), a higher n-6 linoleic acid (LA) to n-3 α-linolenic acid (ALA) ratio seems to increase the chance of embryo implantation, initiating pregnancy.[58] And overall high serum levels of the n-3 fats EPA and ALA in IVF are associated with successful pregnancy outcomes.[59]

Of course, extrapolations of studies of women undergoing IVF cannot necessarily be extended to the wider population. However supplementation with n-3 EPA and DHA does seem to improve fertility in normal weight young women, whilst consumption of a diet rich in n-3 fatty acids can improve egg quality and the health of ovarian reserves in older women.[60,61]

n-3 fatty acid supplementation, particularly in women with low food n-3 consumption, slightly increases the length of gestation, reducing the incidence of premature births.[62] Even the notoriously precautionary Cochrane review has acknowledged that supplementing with n-3 fatty acids during pregnancy reduces the risk of low-birthweight babies, and reduces the risk of perinatal death and neonatal care admissions to hospital.[63]

The n-3 fats EPA and DHA, and the n-6 fat AA are also crucial in foetal and infant development. The developing foetus can only gain these PUFAs through maternal consumption, and maternal stores fall rapidly following fertilisation unless they are continuously topped up.[64]

The brain and retina contain very high levels of DHA and AA in comparison to other tissues in the body. Both are needed for the growth and development of the foetal brain, nervous system, and eyes.[65] DHA requirements increase during the last trimester of pregnancy when the brain accumulates this PUFA at a faster rate than any other fatty acid.[66] This accumulation continues in the first two years of life when the brain and retinal membranes undergo substantial growth and development.[67] An insufficient supply of n-3 fatty acids during pregnancy is associated with poor developmental and behaviour scores in childhood and insufficiency during the first two years of infancy can lead to permanent abnormalities in mental and visual development and performance.[64,65,67]

The best source of n-3 fatty acids is seafood, particularly oily fish and some shellfish. The n-6 fatty acids are widely found in seed oils and animal products. The UK diet is low in oily fish but high in seed oils and animal products which tips the balance of PUFAs to higher n-6/lower n-3. The ideal ratio between n-3 and n-6 is 1:1, but the patterns in most Western diets, including the UK have skewed the ratio n-6 to n-3 to around 20:1.[68]

Consumption of any kind of fish in the UK is low with only 26% of UK consumers knowing that the recommended weekly intake of fish is two portions a week, one of which should be oily.[69] Only 15% eat the recommended 140 g portion of oily fish a week.[70] Adding a layer of difficulty to this, women who intend to become pregnant, or are pregnant, are advised to limit their intakes of most oily fish because of high levels of contaminants such as mercury, lead, cadmium, dioxins and polychlorinated biphenyls (PCBs) which can be found in it.[71]

Some nuts and seeds (flax, hemp and chia seeds, and walnuts) contain omega-3 in the form of ALA. Unfortunately human biochemistry is not great at converting ALA into EPA and DHA.[72] Therefore vegetarians and vegans can be at risk of omega-3 insufficiency, if not outright deficiency, and vegetarian and vegan women generally have lower levels of both EPA and DHA than omnivorous women.[73,74] There are some algal food supplements which have recently come on to the UK market that provide some EPA and DHA, although at lower levels than those found in fish oils.

There is a broad consensus among researchers that women of childbearing age who are vegetarian or vegan should be provided with nutritional guidance in planning a nutritionally balanced diet to avoid inadequate intakes and, if needed, should take food supplements to ensure sufficiency of these key nutrients.[75,76]

Although good nutrition should always be "food first", the low intakes of oily fish in the UK and the importance of the omega-3 fatty acids EPA and DHA mean that advising women of childbearing age to take a daily fish oil (or algal oil) food supplement is sensible advice. The fish oils used in supplements are filtered and processed to remove all of the contaminants found in oily fish and they are a convenient way of ensuring sufficient intakes of these essential nutrients.

Micronutrients needed before conception and during pregnancy
to ensure maternal health and the healthy development of the foetus.

Nutrients in **bold** are known to have low intakes in the UK.

B VITAMINS	**MINERALS**
Riboflavin	**Calcium**
Niacin	**Iodine**
Vitamin B6	**Iron**
Vitamin B12	**Zinc**
Folic acid	**Selenium**
Biotin	**Magnesium**
Choline	
	OMEGA-3 FATTY ACIDS
FAT SOLUBLE	**Eicosapentaenoic acid (EPA) &**
VITAMINS	**Docosahexaenoic Acid (DHA)**
Vitamin A	
Vitamin D	**Dietary fibre**

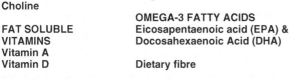

Micronutrients needed before conception and during pregnancy.

Vitamin A

In the context of pregnancy, vitamin A is considered to be a controversial nutrient.

There are two forms of vitamin A; the retinoids which are found in animal products, and β-carotene found in red- and orange-coloured fruit and vegetables. Excessive levels of the retinoid forms of vitamin A (retinols, retinoic acid, and retinyls) are teratogenic.[77] Certain defects, originating from malformation of the neural crest, including cleft palate; small or absent ears and auditory canals; extremely small, missing, or malformed eyes; and malformation of the cardiovascular system are collectively known as "foetal retinoid syndrome."[78]

High consumption of the β-carotene form of vitamin A is not teratogenic, and it may even have some protective effect against some genetic damage.[79]

In 1990, the UK Department of Health issued precautionary advice for the intake of retinoid forms of vitamin A in pregnancy. Women intending to become pregnant, or already pregnant, were warned not to take food supplements containing vitamin A unless advised to do so by their general practitioner, and not to eat liver or liver products such as paté.[80] In 1991 an agreement was reached between the Ministry of Agriculture, Fisheries and Food and the UK food supplements industry to include a warning statement on food supplements. Any product containing more than 800 μg (approximately 2,650 IU) of retinoid vitamin A should carry a warning statement on the label advising women not to take the product if they were pregnant or were intending to become pregnant. This advice remains extant to this day.[81]

But is it time that this was reviewed? Foetal retinoid syndrome seems to be pretty rare, occurring primarily as a result of maternal consumption within the first trimester of isotretinoin, a pharmaceutical prescribed for the treatment of chronic acne.[82] Advice on vitamin A provided to women across the world varies, but there is consistent evidence that excessive intake is most risky up to the 60th day of pregnancy, and that intakes below 3,000 µg (approximately 10,000 IU) per day of retinoids have been shown to be safe with no observed adverse effects (NOAEL).[83,84]

What makes vitamin A so very contentious is that, whilst excess is teratogenic, deficiency is also damaging to both mother and baby. Vitamin A requirements increase substantially during pregnancy because it is used in so many functions. Vitamin A is essential for iron metabolism, the need for which rises sharply during pregnancy.[85] Low levels of vitamin A are often associated with maternal anaemia and low haemoglobin levels in neonates.[86] It is needed for the formation of the foetal heart, liver and kidneys, ears (and inner ears), limbs, and immune system.[87] It is also essential in the development of the eyes and the maintenance of night vision.[88]

Vitamin A deficiency (VAD) in early pregnancy can result in abnormalities in foetal growth and development.[86] VAD later in pregnancy is linked with impaired neonatal immunity, increased susceptibility to infection for both mother and baby, and increased risk of maternal morbidity and mortality.[89] Vitamin A sufficiency in pregnancy reduces the risk of gestational diabetes, whilst foetal vitamin A sufficiency in-utero reduces the risk of developing diabetes in adulthood.[22,90]

It would be hoped that the Royal College of Obstetricians and Gynaecologists would be aware of developments in this area. However, a leaflet, published by them in October 2014, states that women should not take any supplement of vitamin A that contains more than 700 µg.[91] This is 100 µg below the UK acknowledged safe level for retinol, and a very long way from the internationally recognised NOAEL. In addition, the leaflet makes no mention of the β-carotene form of vitamin A. Intakes at such a low level could place both mother and baby at risk of insufficiency, if not outright deficiency. And there are no risks from high intakes of the β-carotene form of vitamin A, something that supposed experts in the field seem unaware of.

Vitamin A intakes in the UK have fallen slowly but consistently over the last two decades and government data shows that 13% of adults have intakes of vitamin A below the lower reference nutrient intake (LRNI, the level below which deficiency is likely to occur).[6] Given the benefits of vitamin A, supplementing with β-carotene, or even retinol (up to 800 µg) should be recommended throughout pregnancy.

Vitamin D

The importance of vitamin D to health is discussed in detail in chapter 6. This section will focus on vitamin D solely in relation to conception, pregnancy, and foetal development.

Vitamin D impacts female fertility in a multitude of ways. The ovaries, endometrium, placenta, and myometrium all carry vitamin D receptors (VDRs).[92] These tissues are some of the few that can actively metabolise the inactive 25(OH)D into the active (1,25-(OH)$_2$D), and this conversion appears to be optimised during pregnancy.[93]

Vitamin D's functions within the immune system influence conception and pregnancy.[94] Seminal fluid triggers a pro-inflammatory immune response which stimulates changes to the endometrium, facilitating implantation.[95] Following implantation, T cells exert an immuno-suppressant function, regulated by vitamin D, which is critical in both establishing pregnancy, and allowing it to continue.[96]

Throughout pregnancy, vitamin D regulates maternal immune tolerance. It inhibits pro-inflammatory Th1 cytokines which induce autoimmune responses and enhances anti-inflammatory Th2 interleukin cytokines.[97] This balance enables the mother's body to continue to recognise the growing foetus as "self" rather than "other", thereby reducing the risk of rejection and miscarriage.[98]

Vitamin D deficiency is very common among women of reproductive age and is particularly prevalent among infertile women.[99] It is associated with endometriosis and polycystic ovary disease, both of which are known obstacles to successful conception and pregnancy.[100] Low levels of vitamin D have also been linked to increased risk of preeclampsia and gestational diabetes.[101,102] And in IVF, vitamin D deficiency is associated with a decreased probability of live birth, whilst sufficiency (vitamin D serum levels above 75nmol/L) is associated with greater success of falling pregnant.[103,104]

As with all nutrients, vitamin D is only available to the growing foetus through maternal intake. It is critical to foetal development, enabling the growth and development of bone and muscle; the laying down of fat reserves; and the development of the immune system, the brain, and the lungs.[93,105] Yet despite this, most UK parents are unaware of advice around vitamin D supplementation in pregnancy or infancy and the quality of information provided is often poor.[106]

As discussed in detail in chapter 6, intakes of vitamin D in the UK are extremely concerning. The UK has, by far, the worst policy and supplementation programme of any European nation.[107] Infantile rickets is a growing concern, particularly within Black, Asian, and minority populations and there have been several instances where vitamin D deficiency and its attendant complications have resulted in infant deaths.[108,109]

Recently a group of senior academics published the view that UK definitions of sufficiency and deficiency require substantial revision, as does the recommended intake of 10 μg a day.[110] That intake is intended to maintain blood plasma levels of vitamin D at 25 nmol/L, the level which the UK defines as sufficiency. Yet this level of "sufficiency" is the lowest in the world; all other national or international organisations view this level as severe deficiency.[111]

Despite regular discussion of vitamin D in the press, the UK continues to suffer a public health crisis of vitamin D deficiency. There is a lack of knowledge about the health benefits of vitamin D and where it can be obtained.[112] Almost half of UK adults, and most UK healthcare practitioners are unaware of the UK government advice around the need for vitamin D supplementation.[113,114] Advice that itself is deeply inadequate.

Vitamin D's central role in the health of both mother and child means that all healthcare practitioners should be promoting the use of vitamin D food supplements. Recommended doses should be at least 25 μg of vitamin D in all women of childbearing age, increasing to at least 50 μg during pregnancy and lactation.

Calcium

Calcium is the most abundant mineral in the body. It provides structure and strength to bones and teeth; is used in the transmission of nerve signals and intercellular signalling; regulates muscle movement, including the contraction and expansion of the cardiovascular system; and is involved in the synthesis and secretion of some hormones.

Vitamin D is central to calcium absorption and utilisation and both mother and baby are dependent on a sufficiency of these nutrients.[115] The efficiency of intestinal calcium absorption increases during pregnancy, but insufficient dietary calcium results in it being removed from the mother's skeleton to compensate.[116] However, whilst bone health is certainly important, one of the less familiar functions of calcium may be the most relevant in pregnancy.

Calcium helps to regulate blood pressure through its function in the expansion and contraction of smooth muscle tissues throughout the body, including the gut, heart, and blood vessels.[117] Supplementation of between 1,000 and 1,500 mg of calcium significantly reduces the risk of gestational hypertension, preeclampsia, and eclampsia.[118] Even the Cochrane agrees, recommending a cautious 500 mg daily dose, however other research recommends a dose of 1,000 mg for optimal absorption and efficacy.[119,120]

Calcium is widely available from multiple food sources and yet, despite this, intakes in the UK have been falling slowly but steadily over the last two decades, with a significant proportion of women having intakes that put them at risk of deficiency.[6] An overall intake of calcium up to 1,500 mg is considered safe.[121] Its importance to both mother and baby means that daily supplementation of at least 1,000 mg is advisable throughout pregnancy.

Iodine

Iodine may be one of the most important nutrients most people have never heard of. Although some may know it as a disinfectant, or a yellow dye, many are not aware that it is a nutrient and have no idea what it does, or where it comes from.

It is an essential component of the thyroid hormones thyroxine (T4) and triiodothyronine (T3) which regulate multiple metabolic processes, including growth and development throughout life.[122] It is a key element in successful conception, and it is also critical in foetal neurodevelopment.[123]

It is not only the thyroid gland that absorbs iodine, the ovaries and endometrium also have high iodine requirements, but in iodine insufficiency, these organs lose out to the higher priority demands of metabolism.[124] A woman with low iodine levels has a reduced probability of falling pregnant and requires more time to become pregnant.[125] Low iodine is not just associated with reduced fertility, it also increases the risk of miscarriage.[126] And if pregnancy does occur (and continue) iodine insufficiency has negative impacts on both mother and baby.[127] Low levels of iodine are linked with poor foetal growth and a greater probability of stillbirth and neonatal mortality, as well as gestation-induced hypertension, preeclampsia, and preterm delivery.[128]

Maternal iodine requirements increase throughout pregnancy because the developing foetus is completely reliant on maternal intakes.[129] Initially maternal thyroid hormones supply the foetus, but at some point between 16 and 20 weeks, the foetal thyroid develops sufficiently to function independently and produce its own hormones.[130] However, the foetus still draws on maternal iodine because it has no other source.[131] At the same time, possibly because renal function generally increases during pregnancy, maternal urinary excretion of iodine rises by between 30% and 50%.[132]

Following birth, iodine requirements remain high because, although urinary excretion returns to normal levels, it is supplied in breast milk to the growing infant. Ideally iodine concentrations in breast milk should be around 150 μg/L.[133] However, more than half the women in the UK of childbearing age have iodine concentration levels far below what would be required to maintain this level.[6]

As with most nutrients, recommended intakes of iodine in the UK (140 μg/d) were set in 1991 and have not been reviewed since. There is no recommended increase for pregnancy or lactation. Yet the World Health Organisation recommends an intake of 150 μg per day for all adults, which rises to 250 μg per day in pregnancy.[134] Concerns have repeatedly been raised about the issue, however public health nutrition policy has not yet seen fit to review recommendations.[129,135,136]

Encouraging women intending to become pregnant, or who are pregnant, to eat fish and other seafood, which are rich sources of iodine, will help to support iodine levels. Women who do not habitually eat fish, or who are vegetarian or vegan should be encouraged to take a good quality food supplement which supplies at least 150 μg of iodine per day, increasing to 250 μg per day in the event of pregnancy.

Iron

Everyone knows about iron, right? Iron is so crucial in pregnancy that long before anyone knew that food contained substances essential to health, women would put an iron nail in into an apple and leave it overnight before consuming the apple. Nobody understood the science at the time; that acids in the apple oxidised the iron making it bioavailable when consumed. They just knew that pregnant women felt better if they did this. Of course, putting an iron nail into an apple is not something that should be practiced in the modern world. Iron nails are no longer pure iron and often contain other highly toxic metals including cadmium and nickel. But the issue of iron in pregnancy remains.

The two different forms of iron (haem from meat, and non-haem from plants) have different absorption pathways. Haem iron is easily absorbed because specific transport proteins allow it to pass directly through cell membranes and into the blood. Non-haem iron is less bioavailable because it must undergo a complex series of enzymatic reduction and oxidation processes, before being attached to transferrin, the glycoprotein which transports iron around the body.[137] Vitamin C increases the bioavailability of non-haem iron by up to four times; however phytate, a substance found in plants, significantly inhibits the absorption of iron, both haem and non-haem.[138] The absorption of non-haem iron is regulated by the protein hepcidin which blocks iron absorption channels, but hepcidin concentrations fall during pregnancy which means that more iron can be absorbed, so long as it is present in the diet.[139]

Iron requirements in pregnancy increase significantly because both placenta and foetus require iron to grow and develop, and the mother's blood volume expands significantly to ensure sufficient oxygen and nutrition can be delivered to her own organs and the growing baby.[139] Although the need for iron actually falls in the first trimester because blood is not being lost via menstruation, it then increases through the second and third trimester.[85] It peaks in the final few months when the infant builds stores to ensure that it has a sufficiency for the first six months of life, as human breast milk is very low in iron.[140]

Iron insufficiency not only leads to fatigue and reduced quality of life for the mother, it also affects the growing foetus. Iron is essential in foetal brain growth and development and maternal insufficiency can result in poor cognitive and behavioural outcomes in offspring that can last throughout life.[141] It increases the risk of low birth weight, preterm birth, and still birth.[142,143] Iron is also needed for thyroid function and deficiency disrupts thyroid metabolism which, as discussed above, impacts pregnancy and foetal development.[144] Iron deficiency also increases the overall risk of all cause maternal mortality.[145]

Despite the increase in requirements for iron in pregnancy, the UK does not recommend increased intake levels during this critical time. Government rationale for this lack of increase is that iron is not being lost through menstruation, but iron intakes in the UK are often inadequate. More than 40% of females aged 11–64 have iron intakes below the LRNI, putting them at risk of deficiency, even under "normal" circumstances.[146]

A note of caution should be sounded around iron. Whilst it is essential to health, too much iron is toxic because it is extremely pro-oxidative. The body regulates iron levels very tightly, conserving and reabsorbing much of the iron released from the breakdown of red blood cells. Whilst it is important to stay within safe parameters when considering iron supplementation, it is equally important to be aware of the implications of insufficiency, which may not necessarily present as outright deficiency. It is worth advising any women who are pregnant or who are intending to become pregnant to take a food supplement formulated for pregnancy, all of which will contain iron at safe levels.

Zinc

Zinc is more commonly associated with male fertility, but it equally essential to female fertility.

It is part of hundreds of enzymatic processes with roles in growth, development, and reproduction, and the synthesis of RNA and DNA. It is used in the production of hormones, including androgens, is involved in multiple antioxidant systems, regulates inflammatory processes, modulates glucose and lipid metabolism, and is a key element in thousands of human proteins.[147] The enzymes that enable ovulation, development of oocytes into viable eggs, placental development, the maintenance of a normal pregnancy, and foetal development are all zinc dependent.[4] And it is needed for the absorption and utilisation of folate and folic acid through its action on the methylene tetrahydrofolate reductase (MTHFR) enzyme which converts both folate and folic acid to the biologically active form 5-methyltetrahydrofolate.[148]

Women with low levels of zinc take longer to conceive than women with higher levels.[4] Low serum zinc also increases the risk of miscarriage, preterm delivery, placental disruption, poor neural development, restricted foetal growth, and low birth weight.[149] And outright zinc deficiency can result in defects in the formation of the neural tube because zinc deficiency disrupts cell proliferation.[150]

Zinc, in conjunction with vitamin D, calcium, and magnesium (all nutrients of concern among women of childbearing age in the UK, reduces the biomarkers of inflammation and oxidative stress associated with gestational diabetes.[151] This is not surprising as zinc is crucial in maintaining the redox balance through several antioxidant systems.[152] Zinc is also needed in the production and secretion of insulin and deficiency increases the risk of insulin resistance.[153]

Maternal requirements for zinc during the third trimester are around double those of non-pregnant women.[154] But, as with most micronutrients, the UK recommended intakes were set in 1991, have not been reviewed since, and make no allowance for any increased need in pregnancy. Yet 35% of females of childbearing age have intakes of zinc that fall below the LRNI.[146]

Considering the importance of this trace element, and the cohorts who have insufficient intakes, some health insurance in the form of a food supplement is likely to be a good idea.

Selenium

Like zinc, selenium is more commonly associated with masculine fertility and its role in female reproduction is still not well understood. However that is beginning to change, at least partially because of an increased understanding of the wide range of functions selenium has within the body and their relevance to conception and pregnancy.

Selenium cannot act on its own; in a unique process it combines with proteins to form the amino acid selenocysteine, which in turn combines with other amino acids to form selenoproteins.[155] There are 25 known selenoproteins which work in multiple different areas. Selenium-dependent antioxidant enzymes provide protection during follicle growth and maturation as well as protecting embryos and placental tissues.[156] There is a strong link between low selenium intakes and increased placental oxidative stress, which is associated with poor birth outcomes.[157]

Some selenium-dependent enzymes help to regulate thyroid function, converting thyroxine (T4) into the active form of triiodothyronine (T3).[158] Low selenium intake increases the risk of thyroid dysfunction and has a negative impact on foetal psychomotor and language development.[159]

Some selenoproteins modulate inflammatory and immune responses, both important factors in starting and maintaining a pregnancy.[160] And some work structurally, folding polypeptide chains into three-dimensional proteins, and in the synthesis of deoxynucleotides for DNA formation, key elements in cell proliferation and differentiation.[161]

Selenium inadequacy is linked with an increased risk of pregnancy-related hypertension, including preeclampsia, but supplementing with selenium throughout pregnancy can reduce the risk of preeclampsia.[162,163] Low levels are also linked with overall reduced fertility in women and a longer time to fall pregnant as well as an increased risk of miscarriage, autoimmune thyroid disease, small-for-gestational-age birth weight babies, and pre-term birth.[164,165]

Possibly because UK soil is particularly low in selenium, 100% of women in the UK have intakes below the RNI and more than 50% have intakes so low that they are at risk of deficiency.[29] Selenium requirements in pregnancy increase, and unless supplemented, levels fall with each trimester.[158] It is therefore somewhat concerning that most food supplement products formulated for pregnancy contain only 55 μg of selenium, below the UK RNI of 75 μg.

Magnesium

Magnesium is involved in hundreds of enzymes that work in energy production, in the synthesis of DNA, RNA, and proteins; in the transportation of ions across cell membranes, and the conduction of nerve impulses and cell signalling and cell migration. It is also a key structural component of bone, cell membranes, and chromosomes.[166] And it works on vascular smooth muscle, stimulating relaxation and reducing blood pressure.[167]

Low maternal magnesium increases the risk of insulin resistance and gestational diabetes; can restrict foetal growth and inhibit foetal development; and increase the risk of premature labour, pregnancy-induced hypertension, and preeclampsia.[168,169]

Magnesium has been used for many years in the suppression of premature labour and as the first-line therapy in the management of preeclampsia.[170] However, it would clearly be preferable to prevent the occurrence of these issues before they begin. Ongoing work suggests that supplementing with 300 mg/d magnesium throughout pregnancy reduces leg cramps and decreases the risk of preterm birth, low-birth-weight neonates, and the incidence of preeclampsia.[171]

The UK RNI and LRNI for magnesium varies between ages and genders, ranging from 270 to 300 mg/d and 150 to 190 mg/d, respectively. Over 60% of women of childbearing age have intakes that fall below the LRNI, putting them at risk of deficiency.[28] To make matters worse, magnesium is not particularly well absorbed.[172] Even if magnesium status is low, only around 75% of magnesium consumed is absorbed.[172]

Many food supplements designed to be consumed in pregnancy do not even contain magnesium and those that do contain it have levels below the LRNI. It may therefore be advisable to discuss diet with women who are pregnant or who intend to become pregnant, to ensure that they are consuming sufficient magnesium, or suggest additional supplementation.

THE MICROBIOME

Evidence is building about the importance of the microbiome throughout life, including in pregnancy and foetal development.[173]

Dietary fibre is central to the existence and function of the gut microbiome. There is a lot of detailed information about fibre in chapter 3; rather than repeat that, it is sufficient to note that fibre is a keystone to our overall health. For every 8 g increase in fibre consumed, the risk of all-cause mortality, cardiovascular disease, type II diabetes, and colorectal cancer falls by between 2% and 19%, depending on the amount and type of fibre consumed.[174] In pregnancy, dietary fibre reduces the risk of excessive weight gain, gestational diabetes, increased blood pressure, and preeclampsia.[175,176] Research is exploring whether this is the fibre itself, or its impact on the microbiome.

The hormonal, metabolic, and immunological changes in the mother's body during pregnancy stimulate significant changes in the microbiome.[177] Disruption in the microbiome (dysbiosis) is known to create inflammatory conditions. And dysbiosis has been linked with an increased risk of hyperemesis gravidarum, gestational diabetes, gestational hypertension, and preeclampsia.[178,179,180]

It is difficult to gain definitive evidence of specific influences that the maternal microbiome may have on the foetus. However, there is data that suggests that specific bacterial types may protect against future food allergies and that antibiotic use in pregnancy (which impacts the diversity of the microbiome) may increase the incidence of atopic dermatitis and asthma in offspring.[181,182] As if that were not enough, we now know that breast milk is full of bacteria that kick start the microbiome of the neonate.[183] More than 200 different types of FODMAP fibre are also present in human breast milk.[184] These fibres constitute the third largest solid component in human milk and are there solely for the purpose of feeding and developing the gut microbiome of the neonate.[185]

The UK recommendation for fibre intake in adults is 30 g/d however the average intake of dietary fibre among adults is only 19 g/d.[6] Without adequate fibre in the diet the microbiome cannot function effectively which may have potentially negative impacts on the long-term health of both mother and child.[173]

ENERGY INTAKES

Whilst the myth of "eating for two" has long been dispelled, energy restriction in pregnancy can lead to a decrease in birthweight.[186] Therefore it is not advisable to undertake any efforts towards weight loss during pregnancy, particularly as energy requirements increase significantly from about 10 weeks, funding the growth of foetal tissue.[16] Having said that, there are concerns that women with pre-existing diabetes, and who develop gestational diabetes may misreport their intake of foods, particularly foods which are higher in calories.[187]

Excessive energy intakes during pregnancy increase the risk of excessive gestational weight gain, gestational diabetes, high blood pressure and preeclampsia, and having a caesarean section.[188] And these in turn increase the risks of excessive birth weight which can continue throughout life, as well as an increased risk of metabolic and cardiovascular disease in adulthood.[189]

PROTEIN INTAKE

Good quality protein is essential in the growth and development of foetal structures as well as the synthesis of hormones and enzymes. Protein requirements, like energy requirements increase in the second and third trimesters, particularly of the nine "essential" amino acids.[190] Protein should constitute about 14% of total energy intake during the first trimester and about 17.5% of total energy intake during the second and third trimesters.[190]

Both very high and very low protein intakes have been linked with growth restriction and low-birth weight babies and a higher protein diet during pregnancy has been linked with lower gestational weight gain.[191,192] As high gestational weight gain is associated with negative pregnancy outcomes and negative long-term impacts on offspring, it may be worth suggesting to women who intend to become pregnant, or who are already pregnant, that they think about their protein intake.

FINALLY ... FOR MUM AND BABY

Although the constant repetition of the food supplement message in this chapter may have become tedious, given the inadequacy of the UK diet and the evidence of widespread insufficiency of multiple micronutrients, it is worth re-peating. All women of childbearing age in the UK should take a good quality multivitamin as well as a fish oil supplement to ensure sufficiency of omega-3 fatty acids, and an additional B complex supplement to ensure good levels of folate.

There are no guarantees about anything in life, but a good nutrition foundation is an excellent place to start for a healthy and successful pregnancy.

PRECONCEPTION FOR DAD

Micronutrients needed for healthy sperm development to support successful conception.

Nutrients in **bold** are known to have low intakes in the UK.

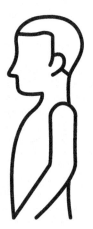

B VITAMINS & VITAMIN C
Folic acid
Vitamin B12
Vitamin C

FAT SOLUBLE VITAMINS
Beta-carotene
Vitamin E

MINERALS
Zinc
Selenium

OMEGA-3 FATTY ACIDS
Eicosapentaenoic acid (EPA) &
Docosahexaenoic Acid (DHA)

Micronutrients needed for healthy sperm development to support successful conception.

It takes two to tango and, whilst the heavy lifting in reproduction is done by mum, way back at the beginning when a baby is only a twinkle in two pairs of eyes, the quality of sperm is as important as the quality of egg. Globally, sperm counts are falling.[193] Whilst all the causative factors behind this are not yet fully understood, sperm quality and numbers do seem to reflect the effects of modern living, including exposure to environmental stressors.[194]

Although exposure to environmental toxins such as endocrine disrupting chemicals, pesticides and electromagnetic frequencies are not necessarily within the control of the individual, nutrition and diet are. The evidence that nutritional factors are vital in ensuring healthy fertility and reproduction is just as powerful in men as in women.

Making sperm is a complex multistage process that takes 74 days.[195] Making healthy sperm requires sufficient folate, vitamin B12, vitamin E, vitamin C, zinc, and selenium to be available throughout that process.[196] But government data shows that these nutrients have worryingly low intakes in the UK.[29]

As previously noted, the UK diet is not the healthiest, being high in ultra-processed foods and low in unprocessed nutrient-dense foods like fruit, vegetables, and oily fish. Ultra-processed food is high in sugar, salt, and processed fats; has a high glycaemic index; and has been found to impair sperm production, with a negative effect on both semen quality and quantity.[197,198]

A high glycaemic index also creates oxidative stress caused by reactive oxygen species (ROS), unstable molecules that can create damage in genetic material.[199] High levels of ROS can damage DNA in sperm, affecting motility and vitality in sperm and potentially causing foetal developmental abnormalities and even miscarriage.[200]

Unprocessed foods, particularly fruit and vegetables, contain antioxidant nutrients like vitamins C and E, β-carotene, folate, magnesium, zinc and selenium, as well as flavonoids and anthocyanins which give fruit and vegetables their bright colours. These nutrients protect sperm by actively removing ROS from seminal fluid and converting them to less damaging compounds.[201]

Folic acid may be just as important in the formation of healthy sperm as it is in the development of the foetus.[202] It is a key substance in the synthesis of S-adenosylmethionine which is essential in the metabolism of both DNA and RNA.[203] And higher paternal folate intakes before conception result in slightly longer gestation time, suggesting that paternal nutrition, prior to conception has an impact on the overall health of offspring.[204]

Vitamin D plays a significant role in male fertility. Male reproductive tissues, such as the prostate, testes and sperm, are just as packed with VDRs as the female reproductive system.[205] And, just as in the female reproductive system, there are enzymes present that metabolise the inactive 25(OH)D into the active (1,25-(OH)$_2$D).[206] Vitamin D also improves sperm motility, and low levels of serum vitamin D have been linked to lower pregnancy rates.[207] Vitamin D status in the UK is so poor that even the government has noticed the problem.

Omega-3 and omega-6 essential fatty acids also play significant roles in male fertility. Both are integral to cell membranes, allowing flexibility and permeability.[208] However, intakes in men are just as unbalanced as they are in women, and a higher n-6 to n-3 intake can reduce the quality of semen and lower concentrations of testosterone.[209] Omega-3 supplementation improves the quality, number, morphology, and motility of sperm in men with a low sperm count.[210] DHA seems to be particularly relevant as it is the predominant PUFA in human sperm, particularly in its head.[211] Even in healthy young men, fish oil supplements increase semen volume, total sperm count, and sperm motility.[212] Oily fish intakes in the UK are poor with an average intake of only 8 g/d.[70]

Zinc is found in high concentrations in the testes and seminal fluid where it supports normal sperm formation, healthy sperm count, and good motility.[213] Because of this, zinc deficiency is linked to reduced male fertility.[214] Zinc stabilises and protects chromatin, the mixture of DNA and proteins that form chromosomes; in zinc deficiency the DNA contained in sperm becomes fragmented, making the sperm less viable.[215] Zinc is also a potent antioxidant, it displaces the redox minerals iron and copper by competitive absorption, and it forms part of several antioxidant enzyme families. Its antioxidant functions help to reduce ROS by preventing their creation or by neutralising them.[216] Zinc is also involved in sperm motility which is probably why it is found in very high levels in the mitochondria and the tails of mature sperm.[217] Zinc intakes in around 12% of men in the UK falls below the LRNI, putting them at risk of deficiency.[29]

Selenium has a strong link with masculine sexual development. The motility and morphology of sperm are both enhanced by adequate selenium intakes.[218] It influences testicular development, and inadequate intakes have been linked to the late onset of puberty in boys (but not in girls).[219] Selenium is a cofactor in the glutathione peroxidase enzymes which protect immature sperm cells from oxidative stress.[220] Glutathione peroxidase 4 also has a structural role, forming over 50% of the mitochondrial capsule in mature sperm.[221] In the UK, 25% of men aged 19–64 have intakes below the LRNI.[29]

Not all of the nutrients mentioned here in relation to male fertility are necessarily of concern; however the UK diet is generally pretty dire and the recommended intakes for most nutrients have not been reevaluated since 1991. If a couple comes to a healthcare practitioner with concerns about fertility it may be worth considering diet and nutrition as a first line of action. And if IVF is on the cards, nutrition can be even more important. Recommending a good all-round multivitamin and mineral and a good quality fish oil capsule will improve overall nutrient status, is likely to have a beneficial impact on overall health and may even help in the creation of the next generation.

REFERENCES

1 Wessels, I., Maywald, M., & Rink, L. (2017). Zinc as a gatekeeper of immune function. *Nutrients*, *9*(12), 1286. https://doi.org/10.3390/nu9121286

2 Kerns, K., Zigo, M., & Sutovsky, P. (2018). Zinc: A necessary ion for mammalian sperm fertilization competency. *International Journal of Molecular Sciences*, *19*(12), 4097. https://doi.org/10.3390/ijms19124097

3 Terrin, G., Berni Canani, R., Di Chiara, M., Pietravalle, A., Aleandri, V., Conte, F., & De Curtis, M. (2015). Zinc in early life: A key element in the fetus and preterm neonate. *Nutrients*, *7*(12), 10427–10446. https://doi.org/10.3390/nu7125542

4 Grieger, J.A., Grzeskowiak, L.E., Wilson, R.L., Bianco-Miotto, T., Leemaqz, S.Y., Jankovic-Karasoulos, T., Perkins, A.V., Norman, R.J., Dekker, G.A., & Roberts, C.T. (2019). Maternal selenium, copper and zinc concentrations in early pregnancy, and the association with fertility. *Nutrients, 11*(7), 1609. https://doi.org/10.3390/nu11071609

5 Rauber, F., Louzada, M., Martinez Steele, E., Rezende, L., Millett, C., Monteiro, C.A., & Levy, R.B. (2019). Ultra-processed foods and excessive free sugar intake in the UK: A nationally representative cross-sectional study. *BMJ Open, 9*(10), e027546. https://doi.org/10.1136/bmjopen-2018-027546

6 Derbyshire, E. (2019). UK dietary changes over the last two decades: A focus on vitamin and mineral intakes. *Journal of Vitamins and Minerals, 2*(2), 104. https://www.gavinpublishers.com/articles/research-article/Journal-of-Vitamins-Minerals/uk-dietary-changes-over-the-last-two-decades-a-focus-on-vitamin-mineral-intakes

7 Cortés-Albornoz, M.C., García-Guáqueta, D.P., Velez-van-Meerbeke, A., & Talero-Gutiérrez, C. (2021). Maternal nutrition and neurodevelopment: A scoping review. *Nutrients, 13*(10), 3530. https://doi.org/10.3390/nu13103530

8 King, J.C. (2016). A summary of pathways or mechanisms linking preconception maternal nutrition with birth outcomes. *The Journal of Nutrition, 146*(7), 1437S–44 S. https://doi.org/10.3945/jn.115.223479

9 MRC Vitamin Study Research Group. (1991). Prevention of neural tube defects: Results of the Medical Research Council Vitamin Study. *The Lancet, 338*(8760), 131–137. https://doi.org/10.1016/0140–6736(91)90133-A

10 Cavalli, P. (2008). Prevention of neural tube defects and proper folate periconceptional supplementation. *Journal of Prenatal Medicine, 2*(4), 40–41. https://www.ncbi.nlm.nih.gov/pmc/articles/PMC3279093/

11 Raats, M., Thorpe, L., Hurren, C., & Elliott, K. (1998). Changing preconceptions (volume 2): The HEA folic acid campaign 1995–1998 (research report). http://citeseerx.ist.psu.edu/viewdoc/download?doi=10.1.1.692.8005&rep=rep1&type=pdf

12 Garcia, R., Ali, N., Griffiths, M., & Randhawa, G. (2018). Understanding the consumption of folic acid during preconception, among Pakistani, Bangladeshi and white British mothers in Luton, UK: A qualitative study. *BMC Pregnancy and Childbirth, 18*(1), 234. https://doi.org/10.1186/s12884-018-1884-0

13 Peake, J.N., Copp, A.J., & Shawe, J. (2013). Knowledge and periconceptional use of folic acid for the prevention of neural tube defects in ethnic communities in the United Kingdom: Systematic review and meta-analysis. *Birth Defects Research. Part A; Clinical and Molecular Teratology, 97*(7), 444–451. https://doi.org/10.1002/bdra.23154

14 McDougall, B., Kavanagh, K., Stephenson, J., Poston, L., Flynn, A.C., & White, S.L. (2021). Health behaviours in 131,182 UK women planning pregnancy. *BMC Pregnancy and Childbirth, 21*(1), 530. https://doi.org/10.1186/s12884-021-04007-w

15 Mann, S. (2018). Health matters: Reproductive health and pregnancy planning. *UK Health Security Agency.* https://ukhsa.blog.gov.uk/2018/06/26/health-matters-reproductive-health-and-pregnancy-planning/

16 Mousa, A., Naqash, A., & Lim, S. (2019). Macronutrient and micronutrient intake during pregnancy: An overview of recent evidence. *Nutrients, 11*(2), 443. https://doi.org/10.3390/nu11020443

17 Greene, N.D., Leung, K.Y., & Copp, A.J. (2017). Inositol, neural tube closure and the prevention of neural tube defects. *Birth Defects Research, 109*(2), 68–80. https://doi.org/10.1002/bdra.23533

18 Li, K., Wahlqvist, M.L., & Li, D. (2016). Nutrition, one-carbon metabolism and neural tube defects: A review. *Nutrients, 8*(11), 741. https://doi.org/10.3390/nu8110741

19 Fowles, E.R., Walker, L.O., Marti, C.N., Ruiz, R.J., Wommack, J., Bryant, M., Kim, S., & Timmerman, G.M. (2012). Relationships among maternal nutrient intake and placental biomarkers during the 1st trimester in low-income women. *Archives of Gynecology and Obstetrics*, *285*(4), 891–899. https://doi.org/10.1007/s00404-011-2213-2

20 Ronnenberg, A.G., Venners, S.A., Xu, X., Chen, C., Wang, L., Guang, W., Huang, A., & Wang, X. (2007). Preconception B-vitamin and homocysteine status, conception, and early pregnancy loss. *American Journal of Epidemiology*, *166*(3), 304–312. https://doi.org/10.1093/aje/kwm078

21 Sharifzadeh, F., Kashanian, M., Koohpayehzadeh, J., Rezaian, F., Sheikhansari, N., & Eshraghi, N. (2018). A comparison between the effects of ginger, pyridoxine (vitamin B6) and placebo for the treatment of the first trimester nausea and vomiting of pregnancy (NVP). *The Journal of Maternal-Fetal & Neonatal Medicine*, *31*(19), 2509–2514. https://doi.org/10.1080/14767058.2017.1344965

22 Chen, Q., Feng, Y., Yang, H., Wu, W., Zhang, P., Wang, K., Wang, Y., Ko, J., Shen, J., Guo, L., Zhao, F., Du, W., Ru, S., Wang, S., & Zhang, Y. (2019). A vitamin pattern diet is associated with decreased risk of gestational diabetes mellitus in Chinese women: Results from a Case Control Study in Taiyuan, China. *Journal of Diabetes Research*, *2019*, 5232308. https://doi.org/10.1155/2019/5232308

23 Lyon, P., Strippoli, V., Fang, B., & Cimmino, L. (2020). B Vitamins and one-carbon metabolism: Implications in human health and disease. *Nutrients*, *12*(9), 2867. https://doi.org/10.3390/nu12092867

24 Linus Pauling Institute (2022). High Homocysteine. *Micronutrient Information Center; Oregon State University* https://lpi.oregonstate.edu/mic/health-disease/high-homocysteine

25 Refsum, H., Nurk, E., Smith, A.D., Ueland, P.M., Gjesdal, C.G., Bjelland, I., Tverdal, A., Tell, G.S., Nygård, O., & Vollset, S.E. (2006). The Hordaland Homocysteine Study: A community-based study of homocysteine, its determinants, and associations with disease. *The Journal of Nutrition*, *136*(6 Suppl), 1731S–1740S. https://doi.org/10.1093/jn/136.6.1731S

26 Vujkovic, M., de Vries, J.H., Lindemans, J., Macklon, N.S., van der Spek, P.J., Steegers, E.A., & Steegers-Theunissen, R.P. (2010). The preconception Mediterranean dietary pattern in couples undergoing in vitro fertilization/intracytoplasmic sperm injection treatment increases the chance of pregnancy. *Fertility and Sterility*, *94*(6), 2096–2101. https://doi.org/10.1016/j.fertnstert.2009.12.079

27 Chaudhry, S.H., Taljaard, M., MacFarlane, A.J., Gaudet, L.M., Smith, G.N., Rodger, M., Rennicks White, R., Walker, M.C., & Wen, S.W. (2019). The role of maternal homocysteine concentration in placenta-mediated complications: findings from the Ottawa and Kingston birth cohort. *BMC Pregnancy and Childbirth*, *19*(1), 75. https://doi.org/10.1186/s12884-019-2219-5

28 Sukumar, N., Adaikalakoteswari, A., Venkataraman, H., Maheswaran, H., & Saravanan, P. (2016). Vitamin B12 status in women of childbearing age in the UK and its relationship with national nutrient intake guidelines: Results from two National Diet and Nutrition Surveys. *BMJ Open*, *6*(8), e011247. https://doi.org/10.1136/bmjopen-2016-011247

29 Derbyshire, E. (2018). Micronutrient intakes of British adults across mid-life: A secondary analysis of the UK National Diet and Nutrition Survey. *Frontiers in Nutrition*, *5*, 55. https://doi.org/10.3389/fnut.2018.00055

30 Obeid, R., Heil, S.G., Verhoeven, M., van den Heuvel, E., de Groot, L., & Eussen, S. (2019). Vitamin B12 intake from animal foods, biomarkers, and health aspects. *Frontiers in Nutrition*, *6*, 93. https://doi.org/10.3389/fnut.2019.00093

31 European Food Safety Authority (2017). Dietary Reference Values for Nutrients: Summary Report https://www.efsa.europa.eu/sites/default/files/2017_09_DRVs_summary_report.pdf

32 Rashid, S., Meier, V., & Patrick, H. (2021). Review of Vitamin B12 deficiency in pregnancy: A diagnosis not to miss as veganism and vegetarianism become more prevalent. *European Journal of Haematology, 106*(4), 450–455. https://doi.org/10.1111/ ejh.13571

33 Mock, D.M. (2017). Biotin: From nutrition to therapeutics. *The Journal of Nutrition, 147*(8), 1487–1492. https://doi.org/10.3945/jn.116.238956

34 Perry, C.A., West, A.A., Gayle, A., Lucas, L.K., Yan, J., Jiang, X., Malysheva, O., & Caudill, M.A. (2014). Pregnancy and lactation alter biomarkers of biotin metabolism in women consuming a controlled diet. *The Journal of Nutrition, 144*(12), 1977–1984. https://doi.org/10.3945/jn.114.194472

35 Ichihara, Y., Suga, K., Fukui, M., Yonetani, N., Shono, M., Nakagawa, R., & Kagami, S. (2020). Serum biotin level during pregnancy is associated with fetal growth and preterm delivery. *The Journal of Medical Investigation: JMI, 67*(1.2), 170–173. https://doi.org/10.2152/jmi.67.170

36 Zeisel, S.H. (2006). Choline: Critical role during fetal development and dietary requirements in adults. *Annual Review of Nutrition, 26,* 229–250. https://doi.org/10.1146/ annurev.nutr.26.061505.111156

37 Korsmo, H.W., Jiang, X., & Caudill, M.A. (2019). Choline: Exploring the growing science on its benefits for moms and babies. *Nutrients, 11*(8), 1823. https://doi.org/ 10.3390/nu11081823

38 Derbyshire, E. (2019). Could we be overlooking a potential choline crisis in the United Kingdom? *BMJ Nutrition, Prevention & Health, 2*(2), 86–89. https://doi.org/10.1136/ bmjnph-2019-000037

39 Klatt, K.C., McDougall, M.Q., Malysheva, O.V., Taesuwan, S., Loinard-González, A., Nevins, J., Beckman, K., Bhawal, R., Anderson, E., Zhang, S., Bender, E., Jackson, K.H., King, D.J., Dyer, R. A., Devapatla, S., Vidavalur, R., Brenna, J.T., & Caudill, M.A. (2022). Prenatal choline supplementation improves biomarkers of maternal docosahexaenoic acid status among pregnant participants consuming supplemental DHA: A randomized controlled trial. *The American Journal of Clinical Nutrition, 116*(3), 820–832. https://doi.org/10.1093/ajcn/nqac147

40 Derbyshire, E., Obeid, R., & Schön, C. (2021). Habitual choline intakes across the childbearing years: A review. *Nutrients, 13*(12), 4390. https://doi.org/10.3390/ nu13124390

41 Oteng, A.B., & Kersten, A. (2020). Mechanisms of action of *trans* fatty acids. *Advances in Nutrition, 11*(3), 697–708 https://doi.org/10.1093/advances/nmz125

42 Micha, R., & Mozaffarian, D. (2008). Trans fatty acids: Effects on cardiometabolic health and implications for policy. *Prostaglandins, Leukotrienes, and Essential Fatty Acids, 79*(3–5), 147–152. https://doi.org/10.1016/j.plefa.2008.09.008

43 Fontana, R., & Della Torre, S. (2016). The deep correlation between energy metabolism and reproduction: A view on the effects of nutrition for women fertility. *Nutrients, 8*(2), 87. https://doi.org/10.3390/nu8020087

44 Rauber, F., da Costa Louzada, M.L., Steele, E.M., Millett, C., Monteiro, C.A., & Levy, R.B. (2018). Ultra-Processed food consumption and chronic non-communicable diseases-related dietary nutrient profile in the UK (2008–2014). *Nutrients, 10*(5), 587. https://doi.org/10.3390/nu10050587

45 Cornwell, B., Villamor, E., Mora-Plazas, M., Marin, C., Monteiro, C.A., & Baylin, A. (2018). Processed and ultra-processed foods are associated with lower-quality nutrient profiles in children from Colombia. *Public Health Nutrition, 21*(1), 142–147. https://doi.org/10.1017/S1368980017000891

46 Poti, J.M., Braga, B., & Qin, B. (2017). Ultra-processed food intake and obesity: What really matters for health-processing or nutrient content? *Current Obesity Reports, 6*(4), 420–431. https://doi.org/10.1007/s13679-017-0285-4

47 Wise, L.A., Wesselink, A.K., Tucker, K.L., Saklani, S., Mikkelsen, E.M., Cueto, H., Riis, A.H., Trolle, E., McKinnon, C.J., Hahn, K.A., Rothman, K.J., Sørensen, H.T., & Hatch, E.E. (2018). Dietary fat intake and fecundability in 2 preconception cohort studies. *American Journal of Epidemiology, 187*(1), 60–74. https://doi.org/10.1093/aje/kwx204

48 Çekici, H., & Akdevelioğlu, Y. (2019). The association between trans fatty acids, infertility and fetal life: A review. *Human Fertility, 22*(3), 154–163. https://doi.org/10.1080/14647273.2018.1432078

49 Chavarro, J.E., Rich-Edwards, J.W., Rosner, B.A., & Willett, W.C. (2007). Dietary fatty acid intakes and the risk of ovulatory infertility. *The American Journal of Clinical Nutrition, 85*(1), 231–237. https://doi.org/10.1093/ajcn/85.1.231

50 Dhaka, V., Gulia, N., Ahlawat, K.S., & Khatkar, B.S. (2011). Trans fats-sources, health risks and alternative approach – A review. *Journal of Food Science and Technology, 48*(5), 534–541. https://doi.org/10.1007/s13197-010-0225-8

51 Arvizu M., Gaskins A., Stuart J., Rich-Edwards J., & Chavarro J.E. (2020). Intakes of major types of fat before pregnancy and hypertensive disorders of pregnancy. *Current Developments in Nutrition, 4*(S2), 936, https://doi.org/10.1093/cdn/nzaa054_008

52 Enke, U., Jaudszus, A., Schleussner, E., Seyfarth, L., Jahreis, G., & Kuhnt, K. (2011). Fatty acid distribution of cord and maternal blood in human pregnancy: Special focus on individual trans fatty acids and conjugated linoleic acids. *Lipids in Health and Disease, 10*, 247. https://doi.org/10.1186/1476-511X-10-247

53 Larqué, E., Zamora, S., & Gil, A. (2001). Dietary trans fatty acids in early life: A review. *Early Human Development, 65 Suppl*, S31–S41. https://doi.org/10.1016/s0378-3782(01)00201-8

54 Bouwstra, H., Dijck-Brouwer, J., Decsi, T., Boehm, G., Boersma, E.R., Muskiet, F.A., & Hadders-Algra, M. (2006). Neurologic condition of healthy term infants at 18 months: Positive association with venous umbilical DHA status and negative association with umbilical trans-fatty acids. *Pediatric Research, 60*(3), 334–339. https://doi.org/10.1203/01.pdr.0000233043.16674.1d

55 Mennitti, L.V., Oliveira, J.L., Morais, C.A., Estadella, D., Oyama, L.M., Oller do Nascimento, C.M., & Pisani, L.P. (2015). Type of fatty acids in maternal diets during pregnancy and/or lactation and metabolic consequences of the offspring. *The Journal of Nutritional Biochemistry, 26*(2), 99–111. https://doi.org/10.1016/j.jnutbio.2014.10.001

56 de Carvalho, C., & Caramujo, M.J. (2018). The various roles of fatty acids. *Molecules, 23*(10), 2583. https://doi.org/10.3390/molecules23102583

57 Chiu, Y.H., Karmon, A.E., Gaskins, A.J., Arvizu, M., Williams, P.L., Souter, I., Rueda, B.R., Hauser, R., Chavarro, J.E., & EARTH Study Team (2018). Serum omega-3 fatty acids and treatment outcomes among women undergoing assisted reproduction. *Human Reproduction, 33*(1), 156–165. https://doi.org/10.1093/humrep/dex335

58 Jungheim, ES., Frolova, A.I., Jiang, H., & Riley, J.K. (2013). Relationship between serum polyunsaturated fatty acids and pregnancy in women undergoing in vitro fertilization. *The Journal of Clinical Endocrinology and Metabolism, 98*(8), E1364–E1368. https://doi.org/10.1210/jc.2012-4115

59 Mirabi, P., Chaichi, M.J., Esmaeilzadeh, S., Ali Jorsaraei, S.G., Bijani, A., Ehsani, M., & Hashemi Karooee, S.F. (2017). The role of fatty acids on ICSI outcomes: A prospective cohort study. *Lipids in Health and Disease, 16*(1), 18. https://doi.org/10.1186/s12944-016-0396-z

60 Bauer, J.L., Kuhn, K., Bradford, A.P., Al-Safi, Z.A., Harris, M. A., Eckel, R.H., Robledo, C.Y., Malkhasyan, A., Johnson, J., Gee, N.R., & Polotsky, A.J. (2019). Reduction in FSH throughout the menstrual cycle after omega-3 fatty acid supplementation in young normal weight but not obese women. *Reproductive Sciences, 26*(8), 1025–1033. https://doi.org/10.1177/1933719119828099

61 Nehra, D., Le, H.D., Fallon, E.M., Carlson, S.J., Woods, D., White, Y.A., Pan, A.H., Guo, L., Rodig, S.J., Tilly, J.L., Rueda, B.R., & Puder, M. (2012). Prolonging the female reproductive lifespan and improving egg quality with dietary omega-3 fatty acids. *Aging Cell*, *11*(6), 1046–1054. https://doi.org/10.1111/acel.12006

62 Ciesielski, T.H., Bartlett, J., & Williams, S.M. (2019). Omega-3 polyunsaturated fatty acid intake norms and preterm birth rate: A cross-sectional analysis of 184 countries. *BMJ Open*, *9*(4), e027249. https://doi.org/10.1136/bmjopen-2018–027249

63 Middleton, P., Gomersall, J.C., Gould, J.F., Shepherd, E., Olsen, S.F., & Makrides, M. (2018). Omega-3 fatty acid addition during pregnancy. *The Cochrane Database of Systematic Reviews*, *11*(11), CD003402. https://doi.org/10.1002/14651858.CD003402. pub3

64 Coletta, J.M., Bell, S.J., & Roman, A.S. (2010). Omega-3 fatty acids and pregnancy. *Reviews in Obstetrics & Gynecology*, *3*(4), 163–171.

65 Nyaradi, A., Li, J., Hickling, S., Foster, J., & Oddy, W.H. (2013). The role of nutrition in children's neurocognitive development, from pregnancy through childhood. *Frontiers in Human Neuroscience*, *7*, 97. https://doi.org/10.3389/fnhum.2013.00097

66 Calder, P.C. (2016). Docosahexaenoic acid. *Annals of Nutrition & Metabolism*, *69 Suppl 1*, 7–21. https://doi.org/10.1159/000448262

67 Devarshi, P.P., Grant, R.W., Ikonte, C.J., & Hazels Mitmesser, S. (2019). Maternal omega-3 nutrition, placental transfer and fetal brain development in gestational diabetes and preeclampsia. *Nutrients*, *11*(5), 1107. https://doi.org/10.3390/nu11051107

68 Simopoulos, A.P. (2016). An increase in the omega-6/omega-3 fatty acid ratio increases the risk for obesity. *Nutrients*, *8*(3), 128. https://doi.org/10.3390/nu8030128

69 Seafish (2018). State of the Nation Research. https://www.seafish.org/document/?id= 8a28f065-aed3–472a-85b8–069613e5dd39

70 Derbyshire, E. (2019). Oily fish and omega-3s across the life stages: A focus on intakes and future directions. *Frontiers in Nutrition*, *6*, 165. https://doi.org/10.3389/fnut. 2019.00165

71 NHS Eat Well (2018). Fish and shellfish. https://www.nhs.uk/live-well/eat-well/fish-and-shellfish-nutrition/

72 Burns-Whitmore, B., Froyen, E., Heskey, C., Parker, T., & San Pablo, G. (2019). Alpha-linolenic and linoleic fatty acids in the vegan diet: Do they require dietary reference intake/adequate intake special consideration? *Nutrients*, *11*(10), 2365. https://doi.org/ 10.3390/nu11102365

73 Saunders, A.V., Davis, B.C., & Garg, M.L. (2013). Omega-3 polyunsaturated fatty acids and vegetarian diets. *The Medical Journal of Australia*, *199*(S4), S22–S26. https://pubmed.ncbi.nlm.nih.gov/25369925/

74 Burdge, G.C., Tan, S.Y., & Henry, C.J. (2017). Long-chain *n*-3 PUFA in vegetarian women: A metabolic perspective. *Journal of Nutritional Science*, *6*, e58. https://doi.org/ 10.1017/jns.2017.62

75 Elorinne, A.L., Alfthan, G., Erlund, I., Kivimäki, H., Paju, A., Salminen, I., Turpeinen, U., Voutilainen, S., & Laakso, J. (2016). Food and nutrient intake and nutritional status of Finnish vegans and non-vegetarians. *PloS One*, *11*(2), e0148235. https://doi.org/ 10.1371/journal.pone.0148235

76 Sebastiani, G., Herranz Barbero, A., Borrás-Novell, C., Alsina Casanova, M., Aldecoa-Bilbao, V., Andreu-Fernández, V., Pascual Tutusaus, M., Ferrero Martínez, S., Gómez Roig, M.D., & García-Algar, O. (2019). The effects of vegetarian and vegan diet during pregnancy on the health of mothers and offspring. *Nutrients*, *11*(3), 557. https://doi.org/10.3390/nu11030557

77 Rothman, K.J., Moore, L.L., Singer, M.R., Nguyen, U.S., Mannino, S., & Milunsky, A. (1995). Teratogenicity of high vitamin A intake. *The New England Journal of Medicine*, *333*(21), 1369–1373. https://doi.org/10.1056/NEJM199511233332101

78 National Organization for Rare Disorders (2019). Rare Diseases Database; Fetal Retinoid Syndrome. https://rarediseases.org/rare-diseases/fetal-retinoid-syndrome/

79 Mathews-Roth, M.M. (1988). Lack of genotoxicity with beta-carotene. *Toxicology Letters*, *41*(3), 185–191. https://doi.org/10.1016/0378–4274(88)90053-7

80 Scientific Advisory Committee on Nutrition (2005). Review of Dietary Advice on Vitamin A. *The Stationary Office, London*. https://assets.publishing.service.gov.uk/government/uploads/system/uploads/attachment_data/file/338853/SACN_Review_of_Dietary_Advice_on_Vitamin_A.pdf

81 Department of Health and Social Care (2011). Food supplements label advisory statements and suggested reformulations. https://assets.publishing.service.gov.uk/government/uploads/system/uploads/attachment_data/file/204323/Advisory_Statements_DH_FINAL.pdf

82 Mondal, D., R Shenoy, S., & Mishra, S. (2017). Retinoic acid embryopathy. *International Journal of Applied & Basic Medical Research*, *7*(4), 264–265. https://doi.org/10.4103/ijabmr.IJABMR_469_16

83 Scientific Committee on Food (2006). Tolerable Upper Intake Levels for Vitamins and Minerals. Opinion of the Scientific Committee On Food on the Tolerable Upper Intake Level of Preformed Vitamin A (Retinol and Retinyl Esters). http://www.efsa.europa.eu/sites/default/files/efsa_rep/blobserver_assets/ndatolerableuil.pdf

84 National Institutes of Health (2020). Office of Dietary Supplements; Vitamin A Fact Sheet for Health Professionals. https://ods.od.nih.gov/factsheets/VitaminA-HealthProfessional/

85 Fisher, A.L., & Nemeth, E. (2017). Iron homeostasis during pregnancy. *The American Journal of Clinical Nutrition*, *106*(Suppl 6), 1567S–1574 S. https://doi.org/10.3945/ajcn.117.155812

86 Bastos Maia, S., Rolland Souza, A.S., Costa Caminha, M.F., Lins da Silva, S., Callou Cruz, R., Carvalho Dos Santos, C., & Batista Filho, M. (2019). Vitamin A and pregnancy: A narrative review. *Nutrients*, *11*(3), 681. https://doi.org/10.3390/nu11030681

87 Spiegler, E., Kim, Y.K., Wassef, L., Shete, V., & Quadro, L. (2012). Maternal-fetal transfer and metabolism of vitamin A and its precursor β-carotene in the developing tissues. *Molecular and Cell Biology of Lipids*, *1821*(1), 88–98. https://doi.org/10.1016/j.bbalip.2011.05.003

88 Christian, P., West, K.P., Jr, Khatry, S.K., Kimbrough-Pradhan, E., LeClerq, S.C., Katz, J., Shrestha, S.R., Dali, S.M., & Sommer, A. (2000). Night blindness during pregnancy and subsequent mortality among women in Nepal: Effects of vitamin A and beta-carotene supplementation. *American Journal of Epidemiology*, *152*(6), 542–547. https://doi.org/10.1093/aje/152.6.542

89 West, K.P., Jr, Christian, P., Katz, J., Labrique, A., Klemm, R., & Sommer, A. (2010). Effect of vitamin A supplementation on maternal survival. *The Lancet*, *376*(9744), 873–874. https://doi.org/10.1016/S0140–6736(10)61411-0

90 Keller, A., Ängquist, L., Jacobsen, R., Vaag, A., & Heitmann, B.L. (2017). A retrospective analysis of a societal experiment among the Danish population suggests that exposure to extra doses of vitamin A during fetal development may lower type 2 diabetes mellitus (T2DM) risk later in life. *The British Journal of Nutrition*, *117*(5), 731–736. https://doi.org/10.1017/S000711451700037X

91 Royal College of Obstetricians and Gynaecologists (2014). Healthy eating and vitamin supplements in pregnancy. https://www.rcog.org.uk/globalassets/documents/patients/patient-information-leaflets/pregnancy/pi-healthy-eating-and-vitamin-supplements-in-pregnancy.pdf

92 Cermisoni, G.C., Alteri, A., Corti, L., Rabellotti, E., Papaleo, E., Viganò, P., & Sanchez, A.M. (2018). Vitamin D and endometrium: A systematic review of a neglected area of research. *International Journal of Molecular Sciences*, *19*(8), 2320. https://doi.org/10.3390/ijms19082320

93 Curtis E.M., Moon R.J., Harvey N.C., & Cooper C. (2018). Maternal vitamin D supplementation during pregnancy, *British Medical Bulletin*, *126*(1), 57–77, https://doi.org/10.1093/bmb/ldy010

94 Schröder-Heurich, B., Springer, C., & von Versen-Höynck, F. (2020). Vitamin D effects on the immune system from periconception through pregnancy. *Nutrients*, *12*(5), 1432. https://doi.org/10.3390/nu12051432

95 Miller, D.J. (2018). Review: The epic journey of sperm through the female reproductive tract. *Animal*, *12*(s1), s110–s120. https://doi.org/10.1017/S1751731118000526

96 Cyprian, F., Lefkou, E., Varoudi, K., & Girardi, G. (2019). Immunomodulatory effects of Vitamin D in pregnancy and beyond. *Frontiers in Immunology*, *10*, 2739. https://doi.org/10.3389/fimmu.2019.02739

97 Ikemoto, Y., Kuroda, K., Nakagawa, K., Ochiai, A., Ozaki, R., Murakami, K., Jinushi, M., Matsumoto, A., Sugiyama, R., & Takeda, S. (2018). Vitamin D regulates maternal T-Helper cytokine production in infertile women. *Nutrients*, *10*(7), 902. https://doi.org/10.3390/nu10070902

98 Berger, A. (2000). Th1 and Th2 responses: What are they? *BMJ*, *321*, 424. https://doi.org/10.1136/bmj.321.7258.424

99 Pilz, S., Zittermann, A., Obeid, R., Hahn, A., Pludowski, P., Trummer, C., Lerchbaum, E., Pérez-López, F.R., Karras, S.N., & März, W. (2018). The role of Vitamin D in fertility and during pregnancy and lactation: A review of clinical data. *International Journal of Environmental Research and Public Health*, *15*(10), 2241. https://doi.org/10.3390/ijerph15102241

100 Voulgaris, N., Papanastasiou, L., Piaditis, G., Angelousi, A., Kaltsas, G., Mastorakos, G., & Kassi, E. (2017). Vitamin D and aspects of female fertility. *Hormones*, *16*(1), 5–21. https://doi.org/10.14310/horm.2002.1715

101 Akbari, S., Khodadadi, B., Ahmadi, S., Abbaszadeh, S., & Shahsavar, F. (2018). Association of vitamin D level and vitamin D deficiency with risk of preeclampsia: A systematic review and updated meta-analysis. *Taiwanese Journal of Obstetrics & Gynecology*, *57*(2), 241–247. https://doi.org/10.1016/j.tjog.2018.02.013

102 Ojo, O., Weldon, S.M., Thompson, T., & Vargo, E.J. (2019). The effect of vitamin D supplementation on glycaemic control in women with gestational diabetes mellitus: A systematic review and meta-analysis of randomised controlled trials. *International Journal of Environmental Research and Public Health*, *16*(10), 1716. https://doi.org/10.3390/ijerph16101716

103 Zhao, J., Huang, X., Xu, B., Yan, Y., Zhang, Q., & Li, Y. (2018). Whether vitamin D was associated with clinical outcome after IVF/ICSI: A systematic review and meta-analysis. *Reproductive Biology and Endocrinology: RB&E*, *16*(1), 13. https://doi.org/10.1186/s12958-018-0324-3

104 Mumford, S.L., Garbose, R.A., Kim, K., Kissell, K., Kuhr, D.L., Omosigho, U.R., Perkins, N.J., Galai, N., Silver, R.M., Sjaarda, L.A., Plowden, T.C., & Schisterman, E.F. (2018). Association of preconception serum 25-hydroxyvitamin D concentrations with livebirth and pregnancy loss: A prospective cohort study. *The Lancet: Diabetes & Endocrinology*, *6*(9), 725–732. https://doi.org/10.1016/S2213–8587(18)30153-0

105 Hart, P.H., Lucas, R.M., Walsh, J.P., Zosky, G.R., Whitehouse, A.J., Zhu, K., Allen, K.L., Kusel, M.M., Anderson, D., & Mountain, J.A. (2015). Vitamin D in fetal development: Findings from a birth cohort study. *Pediatrics*, *135*(1), e167–e173. https://doi.org/10.1542/peds.2014–1860

106 Day, R.E., Krishnarao, R., Sahota, P., & Christian, M.S. (2019). We still don't know that our children need vitamin D daily: A study of parents' understanding of vitamin D requirements in children aged 0–2 years. *BMC Public Health*, *19*(1), 1119. https://doi.org/10.1186/s12889-019-7340-x

107 Uday, S., Kongjonaj, A., Aguiar, M., Tulchinsky, T., & Högler, W. (2017). Variations in infant and childhood vitamin D supplementation programmes across Europe and factors influencing adherence. *Endocrine Connections*, *6*(8), 667–675. https://doi.org/10.1530/EC-17-0193

108 Uday, S., Fratzl-Zelman, N., Roschger, P., Klaushofer, K., Chikermane, A., Saraff, V., Tulchinsky, T., Thacher, T.D., Marton, T., & Högler, W. (2018). Cardiac, bone and growth plate manifestations in hypocalcemic infants: Revealing the hidden body of the vitamin D deficiency iceberg. *BMC Pediatrics*, *18*(1), 183. https://doi.org/10.1186/s12887-018-1159-y

109 Uday, S., & Högler, W. (2017). Nutritional rickets and osteomalacia in the twenty-first century: Revised concepts, public health, and prevention strategies. *Current Osteoporosis Reports*, *15*(4), 293–302. https://doi.org/10.1007/s11914-017-0383-y

110 Griffin, G., Hewison, M., Hopkin, J., Kenny, R.A., Quinton, R., Rhodes, J., Subramanian, S., & Thickett, D. (2021). Preventing vitamin D deficiency during the COVID-19 pandemic: UK definitions of vitamin D sufficiency and recommended supplement dose are set too low. *Clinical Medicine*, *21*(1), e48–e51. https://doi.org/10.7861/clinmed.2020–0858

111 Cashman, K.D. (2018). Vitamin D requirements for the future-lessons learned and charting a path forward. *Nutrients*, *10*(5), 533. https://doi.org/10.3390/nu10050533

112 Kotta, S., Gadhvi, D., Jakeways, N., Saeed, M., Sohanpal, R., Hull, S., Famakin, O., Martineau, A., & Griffiths, C. (2015). "Test me and treat me" -- Attitudes to vitamin D deficiency and supplementation: A qualitative study. *BMJ Open*, *5*(7), e007401. https://doi.org/10.1136/bmjopen-2014–007401

113 British Nutrition Foundation (2021). BNF survey reveals 49% of adults unaware of UK government guidelines for vitamin D. https://www.nutrition.org.uk/news/2021/british-nutrition-foundation-survey-reveals-49-adults-unaware-of-uk-government-guidelines-for-vitamin-d/

114 Fallon, E., Lanham-New, S., Williams, P., & Ray, S. (2020). An investigation of the vitamin D Knowledge, Attitudes and Practice of UK practising doctors and nurses: The D-KAP study. *Proceedings of the Nutrition Society*, *79*(OCE1), E20. https://doi.org/10.1017/S0029665119001411

115 Mohammad-Alizadeh-Charandabi, S., Mirghafourvand, M., Mansouri, A., Najafi, M., & Khodabande, F. (2015). The effect of Vitamin D and calcium plus Vitamin D during pregnancy on pregnancy and birth outcomes: A randomized controlled trial. *Journal of Caring Sciences*, *4*(1), 35–44. https://doi.org/10.5681/jcs.2015.004

116 Kumar, A., & Kaur, S. (2017). Calcium: A nutrient in pregnancy. *Journal of Obstetrics and Gynaecology of India*, *67*(5), 313–318. https://doi.org/10.1007/s13224-017-1007-2

117 Hill-Eubanks, D.C., Werner, M.E., Heppner, T.J., & Nelson, M.T. (2011). Calcium signaling in smooth muscle. *Cold Spring Harbor Perspectives in Biology*, *3*(9), a004549. https://doi.org/10.1101/cshperspect.a004549

118 Chen, D., Wang, H., Xin, X., Zhang, L., Yu, A., Li, S., & He, R. (2022). Different doses of calcium supplementation to prevent gestational hypertension and pre-eclampsia: A systematic review and network meta-analysis. *Frontiers in Nutrition*, *8*, 795667. https://doi.org/10.3389/fnut.2021.795667

119 Hofmeyr, G.J., Lawrie, T.A., Atallah, Á.N., & Torloni, M.R. (2018). Calcium supplementation during pregnancy for preventing hypertensive disorders and related problems. *The Cochrane Database of Systematic Reviews*, *10*(10), CD001059. https://doi.org/10.1002/14651858.CD001059.pub5

120 Omotayo, M.O., Dickin, K.L., O'Brien, K.O., Neufeld, L.M., De Regil, L.M., & Stoltzfus, R.J. (2016). Calcium supplementation to prevent preeclampsia: Translating guidelines into practice in low-income countries. *Advances in Nutrition*, *7*(2), 275–278. https://doi.org/10.3945/an.115.010736

121 Expert Group on Vitamins and Minerals (2003). Safe upper levels for vitamins and minerals. https://cot.food.gov.uk/sites/default/files/vitmin2003.pdf

122 Zbigniew, S. (2017). Role of iodine in metabolism. *Recent Patents on Endocrine, Metabolic & Immune Drug Discovery*, *10*(2), 123–126. https://doi.org/10.2174/1872214 811666170119110618

123 Threapleton, D.E., Snart, C., Keeble, C., Waterman, A.H., Taylor, E., Mason, D., Reid, S., Azad, R., Hill, L., Meadows, S., McKillion, A., Alwan, N.A., Cade, J. E., Simpson, N., Stewart, P.M., Zimmermann, M., Wright, J., Waiblinger, D., Mon-Williams, M., Hardie, L.J., & Greenwood, D.C. (2021). Maternal iodine status in a multi-ethnic UK birth cohort: Associations with child cognitive and educational development. *Paediatric and Perinatal Epidemiology*, *35*(2), 236–246. https://doi.org/10.1111/ppe.12719

124 Bilal, M.Y., Dambaeva, S., Brownstein, D., Kwak-Kim, J., Gilman-Sachs, A., & Beaman, K.D. (2020). Iodide transporters in the endometrium: A potential diagnostic marker for women with recurrent pregnancy failures. *Medical Principles and Practice*, *29*(5), 412–421. https://doi.org/10.1159/000508309

125 Mills, J.L., Buck Louis, G.M., Kannan, K., Weck, J., Wan, Y., Maisog, J., Giannakou, A., Wu, Q., & Sundaram, R. (2018). Delayed conception in women with low-urinary iodine concentrations: A population-based prospective cohort study. *Human Reproduction*, *33*(3), 426–433. https://doi.org/10.1093/humrep/dex379

126 Mathews, D.M., Johnson, N.P., Sim, R.G., O'Sullivan, S., Peart, J.M., & Hofman, P.L. (2021). Iodine and fertility: Do we know enough?. *Human Reproduction*, *36*(2), 265–274. https://doi.org/10.1093/humrep/deaa312

127 Toloza, F., Motahari, H., & Maraka, S. (2020). Consequences of severe iodine deficiency in pregnancy: Evidence in humans. *Frontiers in Endocrinology*, *11*, 409. https://doi.org/10.3389/fendo.2020.00409

128 Abel, M.H., Caspersen, I.H., Sengpiel, V., Jacobsson, B., Meltzer, H.M., Magnus, P., Alexander, J., & Brantsæter, A.L. (2020). Insufficient maternal iodine intake is associated with subfecundity, reduced foetal growth, and adverse pregnancy outcomes in the Norwegian Mother, Father and Child Cohort Study. *BMC Medicine*, *18*(1), 211. https://doi.org/10.1186/s12916-020-01676-w

129 Snart, C., Keeble, C., Taylor, E., Cade, J.E., Stewart, P.M., Zimmermann, M., Reid, S., Threapleton, D.E., Poston, L., Myers, J. E., Simpson, N., Greenwood, D.C., & Hardie, L.J. (2019). Maternal Iodine Status and Associations with birth outcomes in three major cities in the United Kingdom. *Nutrients*, *11*(2), 441. https://doi.org/10.3390/nu11020441

130 Moog, N.K., Entringer, S., Heim, C., Wadhwa, P.D., Kathmann, N., & Buss, C. (2017). Influence of maternal thyroid hormones during gestation on fetal brain development. *Neuroscience*, *342*, 68–100. https://doi.org/10.1016/j.neuroscience.2015.09.070

131 Velasco, I., Bath, S.C., & Rayman, M.P. (2018). Iodine as essential nutrient during the first 1000 days of life. *Nutrients*, *10*(3), 290. https://doi.org/10.3390/nu10030290

132 Anderson S.L., & Laurberg P. (2016). Iodine supplementation in pregnancy and the dilemma of ambiguous recommendations. *European Thyroid Journal*, *5*(1), 35–43. https://doi.org/10.1159/000444254

133 Dror, D.K., & Allen, L.H. (2018). Iodine in human milk: A systematic review. *Advances in Nutrition*, *9*(suppl_1), 347S–357 S. https://doi.org/10.1093/advances/nmy020

134 Bouga, M., Lean, M., & Combet, E. (2018). Iodine and pregnancy-a qualitative study focusing on dietary guidance and information. *Nutrients*, *10*(4), 408. https://doi.org/ 10.3390/nu10040408

135 Bath, S.C., & Rayman, M.P. (2015). A review of the iodine status of UK pregnant women and its implications for the offspring. *Environmental Geochemistry and Health*, *37*(4), 619–629. https://doi.org/10.1007/s10653-015-9682-3

136 Bath, S.C., Walter, A., Taylor, A., Wright, J., & Rayman, M.P. (2014). Iodine deficiency in pregnant women living in the South East of the UK: The influence of diet

and nutritional supplements on iodine status. *The British Journal of Nutrition, 111*(9), 1622–1631. https://doi.org/10.1017/S0007114513004030

137 Young, I., Parker, H.M., Rangan, A., Prvan, T., Cook, R.L., Donges, C.E., Steinbeck, K.S., O'Dwyer, N.J., Cheng, H.L., Franklin, J.L., & O'Connor, H.T. (2018). Association between haem and non-haem iron intake and serum ferritin in healthy young women. *Nutrients, 10*(1), 81. https://doi.org/10.3390/nu10010081

138 Cook, J.D. & Reddy, M.B. (2001). Effects of ascorbic acid intake on nonheme-iron absorption from a complete diet. *American Journal of Clinical Nutrition, 73*(1), 93–98. https://doi.org/10.1093/ajcn/73.1.93

139 Georgieff, M.K., Krebs, N.F., & Cusick, S.E. (2019). The benefits and risks of iron supplementation in pregnancy and childhood. *Annual Review of Nutrition, 39*, 121–146. https://doi.org/10.1146/annurev-nutr-082018-124213

140 Brannon, P.M., & Taylor, C.L. (2017). Iron supplementation during pregnancy and infancy: Uncertainties and implications for research and policy. *Nutrients, 9*(12), 1327. https://doi.org/10.3390/nu9121327

141 Juul, S.E., Derman, R.J., & Auerbach, M. (2019). Perinatal iron deficiency: Implications for mothers and infants. *Neonatology, 115*(3), 269–274. https://doi.org/10.1159/0004 95978

142 Rahman, M.M., Abe, S.K., Rahman, M.S., Kanda, M., Narita, S., Bilano, V., Ota, E., Gilmour, S., & Shibuya, K. (2016). Maternal anemia and risk of adverse birth and health outcomes in low- and middle-income countries: Systematic review and meta-analysis. *The American Journal of Clinical Nutrition, 103*(2), 495–504. https://doi.org/10.3945/ ajcn.115.107896

143 Nair, M., Churchill, D., Robinson, S., Nelson-Piercy, C., Stanworth, S.J., & Knight, M. (2017). Association between maternal haemoglobin and stillbirth: A cohort study among a multi-ethnic population in England. *British Journal of Haematology, 179*(5), 829–837. https://doi.org/10.1111/bjh.14961

144 Luo, J., Wang, X., Yuan, L., & Guo, L. (2021). Iron deficiency, a risk factor of thyroid disorders in reproductive-age and pregnant women: A systematic review and meta-analysis. *Frontiers in Endocrinology, 12*, 629831. https://doi.org/10.3389/fendo.2021. 629831

145 Daru, J., Zamora, J., Fernández-Félix, B.M., Vogel, J., Oladapo, O.T., Morisaki, N., Tunçalp, Ö., Torloni, M.R., Mittal, S., Jayaratne, K., Lumbiganon, P., Togoobaatar, G., Thangaratinam, S., & Khan, K. S. (2018). Risk of maternal mortality in women with severe anaemia during pregnancy and post partum: A multilevel analysis. *The Lancet, 6*(5), e548–e554. https://doi.org/10.1016/S2214-109X(18)30078-0

146 Public Health England (2019). NDNS results from years 1–9: Report. https://assets. publishing.service.gov.uk/government/uploads/system/uploads/attachment_data/file/ 772434/NDNS_UK_Y1–9_report.pdf

147 Nasiadek, M., Stragierowicz, J., Klimczak, M., & Kilanowicz, A. (2020). The role of zinc in selected female reproductive system disorders. *Nutrients, 12*(8), 2464. https://doi.org/10.3390/nu12082464

148 Ebisch, I.M., Thomas, C.M., Peters, W.H., Braat, D.D., & Steegers-Theunissen, R.P. (2007). The importance of folate, zinc and antioxidants in the pathogenesis and prevention of subfertility. *Human Reproduction Update, 13*(2), 163–174. https://doi.org/10.1093/ humupd/dml054

149 Garner, T.B., Hester, J.M., Carothers, A., & Diaz, F.J. (2021). Role of zinc in female reproduction. *Biology of Reproduction, 104*(5), 976–994. https://doi.org/10.1093/biolre/ ioab023

150 Nuttall, J.R., Supasai, S., Kha, J., Vaeth, B.M., Mackenzie, G.G., Adamo, A.M., & Oteiza, P.I. (2015). Gestational marginal zinc deficiency impaired fetal neural progenitor cell proliferation by disrupting the ERK1/2 signaling pathway. *The Journal*

of Nutritional Biochemistry, *26*(11), 1116–1123. https://doi.org/10.1016/j.jnutbio.2015.05.007

151 Jamilian, M., Mirhosseini, N., Eslahi, M., Bahmani, F., Shokrpour, M., Chamani, M., & Asemi, Z. (2019). The effects of magnesium-zinc-calcium-vitamin D co-supplementation on biomarkers of inflammation, oxidative stress and pregnancy outcomes in gestational diabetes. *BMC Pregnancy and Childbirth*, *19*(1), 107. https://doi.org/10.1186/s12884-019-2258-y

152 Chasapis, C.T., Ntoupa, P.A., Spiliopoulou, C.A., & Stefanidou, M.E. (2020). Recent aspects of the effects of zinc on human health. *Archives of Toxicology*, *94*(5), 1443–1460. https://doi.org/10.1007/s00204-020-02702-9

153 Chausmer A.B. (1998). Zinc, Insulin and diabetes. *Journal of the American College of Nutrition*, *17*(2), 109–115. https://doi.org/10.1080/07315724.1998.10718735

154 Mistry, H.D., & Williams, P.J. (2011). The importance of antioxidant micronutrients in pregnancy. *Oxidative Medicine and Cellular Longevity*, *2011*, 841749. https://doi.org/10.1155/2011/841749

155 Schmidt, R.L., & Simonović, M. (2012). Synthesis and decoding of selenocysteine and human health. *Croatian Medical Journal*, *53*(6), 535–550. https://doi.org/10.3325/cmj.2012.53.535

156 Hogan, C., & Perkins, A.V. (2022). Selenoproteins in the human placenta: How essential is selenium to a healthy start to life?. *Nutrients*, *14*(3), 628. https://doi.org/10.3390/nu14030628

157 Habibi, N., Grieger, J.A., & Bianco-Miotto, T. (2020). A review of the potential interaction of selenium and iodine on placental and child health. *Nutrients*, *12*(9), 2678. https://doi.org/10.3390/nu12092678

158 Hubalewska-Dydejczyk, A., Duntas, L., & Gilis-Januszewska, A. (2020). Pregnancy, thyroid, and the potential use of selenium. *Hormones*, *19*(1), 47–53. https://doi.org/10.1007/s42000-019-00144-2

159 Polanska, K., Krol, A., Sobala, W., Gromadzinska, J., Brodzka, R., Calamandrei, G., Chiarotti, F., Wasowicz, W., & Hanke, W. (2016). Selenium status during pregnancy and child psychomotor development-Polish Mother and Child Cohort study. *Pediatric Research*, *79*(6), 863–869. https://doi.org/10.1038/pr.2016.32

160 Huang, Z., Rose, A.H., & Hoffmann, P.R. (2012). The role of selenium in inflammation and immunity: From molecular mechanisms to therapeutic opportunities. *Antioxidants & Redox Signaling*, *16*(7), 705–743. https://doi.org/10.1089/ars.2011.4145

161 Labunskyy, V.M., Hatfield, D.L., & Gladyshev, V.N. (2014). Selenoproteins: Molecular pathways and physiological roles. *Physiological Reviews*, *94*(3), 739–777. https://doi.org/10.1152/physrev.00039.2013

162 Rayman, M.P., Searle, E., Kelly, L., Johnsen, S., Bodman-Smith, K., Bath, S.C., Mao, J., & Redman, C.W. (2014). Effect of selenium on markers of risk of pre-eclampsia in UK pregnant women: A randomised, controlled pilot trial. *The British Journal of Nutrition*, *112*(1), 99–111. https://doi.org/10.1017/S0007114514000531

163 Lewandowska, M., Sajdak, S., & Lubiński, J. (2019). Serum selenium level in early healthy pregnancy as a risk marker of pregnancy induced hypertension. *Nutrients*, *11*(5), 1028. https://doi.org/10.3390/nu11051028

164 Qazi, I.H., Angel, C., Yang, H., Pan, B., Zoidis, E., Zeng, C.J., Han, H., & Zhou, G.B. (2018). Selenium, selenoproteins, and female reproduction: A review. *Molecules*, *23*(12), 3053. https://doi.org/10.3390/molecules23123053

165 Lewandowska, M., Sajdak, S., & Lubiński, J. (2019). The role of early pregnancy maternal selenium levels on the risk for small-for-gestational age newborns. *Nutrients*, *11*(10), 2298. https://doi.org/10.3390/nu11102298

166 Fanni, D., Gerosa, C., Nurchi, V.M., Manchia, M., Saba, L., Coghe, F., Crisponi, G., Gibo, Y., Van Eyken, P., Fanos, V., & Faa, G. (2021). The role of magnesium in

pregnancy and in fetal programming of adult diseases. *Biological Trace Element Research, 199*(10), 3647–3657. https://doi.org/10.1007/s12011-020-02513-0

167 Bullarbo, M., Ödman, N., Nestler, A., Nielsen, T., Kolisek, M., Vormann, J., & Rylander, R. (2013). Magnesium supplementation to prevent high blood pressure in pregnancy: A randomised placebo control trial. *Archives of Gynecology and Obstetrics, 288*(6), 1269–1274. https://doi.org/10.1007/s00404-013-2900-2

168 Dalton, L.M., Ní Fhloinn, D.M., Gaydadzhieva, G.T., Mazurkiewicz, O.M., Leeson, H., & Wright, C P. (2016). Magnesium in pregnancy. *Nutrition Reviews, 74*(9), 549–557. https://doi.org/10.1093/nutrit/nuw018

169 Morton, A. (2018). Hypomagnesaemia and pregnancy. *Obstetric Medicine, 11*(2), 67–72. https://doi.org/10.1177/1753495×17744478

170 Elliott, J.P., Morrison, J. C., & Bofill, J.A. (2016). Risks and benefits of magnesium sulfate tocolysis in preterm labor (PTL). *AIMS Public Health, 3*(2), 348–356. https://doi.org/10.3934/publichealth.2016.2.348

171 Zarean, E., & Tarjan, A. (2017). Effect of magnesium supplement on pregnancy outcomes: A randomized control trial. *Advanced Biomedical Research, 6*, 109. https://doi.org/10.41 03/2277–9175.213879

172 Jahnen-Dechent, W., & Ketteler, M. (2012). Magnesium basics. *Clinical Kidney Journal, 5*(Suppl 1), i3–i14. https://doi.org/10.1093/ndtplus/sfr163

173 Mesa, M.D., Loureiro, B., Iglesia, I., Fernandez Gonzalez, S., Llurba Olivé, E., García Algar, O., Solana, M.J., Cabero Perez, M.J., Sainz, T., Martinez, L., Escuder-Vieco, D., Parra-Llorca, A., Sánchez-Campillo, M., Rodriguez Martinez, G., Gómez Roig, D., Perez Gruz, M., Andreu-Fernández, V., Clotet, J., Sailer, S., Iglesias-Platas, I., & Cabañas, F. (2020). The evolving microbiome from pregnancy to early infancy: A comprehensive review. *Nutrients, 12*(1), 133. https://doi.org/10.3390/nu12010133

174 Reynolds, A., Mann, J., Cummings, J., Winter, N., Mete, E., & Te Morenga, L. (2019). Carbohydrate quality and human health: A series of systematic reviews and meta-analyses. *The Lancet, 393*(10170), 434–445. https://doi.org/10.1016/S0140–6736(18)31809-9

175 Pretorius, R.A., & Palmer, D.J. (2020). High-fiber diet during pregnancy characterized by more fruit and vegetable consumption. *Nutrients, 13*(1), 35. https://doi.org/10.3390/ nu13010035

176 Zerfu, T.A., & Mekuria, A. (2019). Pregnant women have inadequate fiber intake while consuming fiber-rich diets in low-income rural setting: Evidences from Analysis of common "ready-to-eat" stable foods. *Food Science & Nutrition, 7*(10), 3286–3292. https://doi.org/10.1002/fsn3.1188

177 Turjeman S., Collado M.C., & Koren O. (2021). The gut microbiome in pregnancy and pregnancy complications. *Current Opinion in Endocrine and Metabolic Research, 18*, 133–138. https://doi.org/10.1016/j.coemr.2021.03.004

178 Balci, S., Tohma, Y.A., Esin, S., Onalan, G., Tekindal, M.A., & Zeyneloglu, H.B. (2022). Gut dysbiosis may be associated with hyperemesis gravidarum. *The Journal of Maternal-Fetal & Neonatal Medicine, 35*, 11, 2041–2045. https://doi.org/10.1080/ 14767058.2020.1777268

179 Hasain, Z., Mokhtar, N.M., Kamaruddin, N.A., Mohamed Ismail, N.A., Razalli, N.H., Gnanou, J.V., & Raja Ali, R.A. (2020). Gut microbiota and gestational diabetes mellitus: A review of host-gut microbiota interactions and their therapeutic potential. *Frontiers in Cellular and Infection Microbiology, 10*, 188. https://doi.org/10.3389/ fcimb.2020.00188

180 Lv, L. J., Li, S. H., Li, S.C., Zhong, Z.C., Duan, H.L., Tian, C., Li, H., He, W., Chen, M.C., He, T.W., Wang, Y.N., Zhou, X., Yao, L., & Yin, A.H. (2019). Early-onset preeclampsia is associated with gut microbial alterations in antepartum and postpartum women. *Frontiers in Cellular and Infection Microbiology, 9*, 224. https://doi.org/ 10.3389/fcimb.2019.00224

181 Vuillermin, P.J., O'Hely, M., Collier, F., Allen, K.J., Tang, M., Harrison, L.C., Carlin, J.B., Saffery, R., Ranganathan, S., Sly, P.D., Gray, L., Molloy, J., Pezic, A., Conlon, M., Topping, D., Nelson, K., Mackay, C.R., Macia, L., Koplin, J., Dawson, S. L., BIS Investigator Group (2020). Maternal carriage of Prevotella during pregnancy associates with protection against food allergy in the offspring. *Nature Communications*, *11*(1), 1452. https://doi.org/10.1038/s41467-020-14552-1

182 Nyangahu, D.D., & Jaspan, H.B. (2019). Influence of maternal microbiota during pregnancy on infant immunity. *Clinical and Experimental Immunology*, *198*(1), 47–56. https://doi.org/10.1111/cei.13331

183 Pannaraj, P.S., Li, F., Cerini, C., Bender, J. M., Yang, S., Rollie, A., Adisetiyo, H., Zabih, S., Lincez, P.J., Bittinger, K., Bailey, A., Bushman, F. D., Sleasman, J.W., & Aldrovandi, G.M. (2017). Association between breast milk bacterial communities and establishment and development of the infant gut microbiome. *JAMA Pediatrics*, *171*(7), 647–654. https://doi.org/10.1001/jamapediatrics.2017.0378

184 Plaza-Díaz, J., Fontana, L., & Gil, A. (2018). Human milk oligosaccharides and immune system development. *Nutrients*, *10*(8), 1038. https://doi.org/10.3390/nu10081038

185 Van den Elsen L.W.J., Garssen J., Burcelin R., Verhasselt V. (2019). Shaping the gut microbiota by breastfeeding: The gateway to allergy prevention? *Frontiers in Pediatrics*, *47*(7), 2296–2360. https://doi.org/10.3389/fped.2019.00047

186 Kramer, M.S., & Kakuma, R. (2003). Energy and protein intake in pregnancy. *The Cochrane Database of Systematic Reviews*, (4), CD000032. https://doi.org/10.1002/14651858.CD000032

187 Thomas, D.M., Bredlau, C., Islam, S., Armah, K.A., Kunnipparampil, J., Patel, K., Redman, L.M., Misra, D., & Salafia, C. (2016). Relationships between misreported energy intake and pregnancy in the pregnancy, infection and nutrition study: New insights from a dynamic energy balance model. *Obesity Science & Practice*, *2*(2), 174–179. https://doi.org/10.1002/osp4.29

188 Most, J., Dervis, S., Haman, F., Adamo, K.B., & Redman, L.M. (2019). Energy intake requirements in pregnancy. *Nutrients*, *11*(8), 1812. https://doi.org/10.3390/nu11081812

189 Reynolds, R.M., Allan, K.M., Raja, E.A., Bhattacharya, S., McNeill, G., Hannaford, P.C., Sarwar, N., Lee, A. J., Bhattacharya, S., & Norman, J.E. (2013). Maternal obesity during pregnancy and premature mortality from cardiovascular event in adult offspring: Follow-up of 1 323 275 person years. *BMJ*, *347*, f4539. https://doi.org/10.1136/bmj.f4539

190 Elango, R., & Ball, R.O. (2016). Protein and amino acid requirements during pregnancy. *Advances in Nutrition*, *7*(4), 839S–44 S. https://doi.org/10.3945/an.115.011817

191 Herring, C.M., Bazer, F.W., Johnson, G.A., & Wu, G. (2018). Impacts of maternal dietary protein intake on fetal survival, growth, and development. *Experimental Biology and Medicine*, *243*(6), 525–533. https://doi.org/10.1177/1535370218758275

192 Rugină, C., Mărginean, C.O., Meliț, L.E., Giga, D.V., Modi, V., & Mărginean, C. (2020). Relationships between excessive gestational weight gain and energy and macronutrient intake in pregnant women. *The Journal of International Medical Research*, *48*(8), 300060520933808. https://doi.org/10.1177/0300060520933808

193 Levine, H., Jørgensen, N., Martino-Andrade, A., Mendiola, J., Weksler-Derri, D., Mindlis, I., Pinotti, R., & Swan, S.H. (2017). Temporal trends in sperm count: A systematic review and meta-regression analysis. *Human Reproduction Update*, *23*(6), 646–659. https://doi.org/10.1093/humupd/dmx022

194 Nordkap, L., Joensen, U.N., Blomberg Jensen, M., & Jørgensen, N. (2012). Regional differences and temporal trends in male reproductive health disorders: Semen quality may be a sensitive marker of environmental exposures. *Molecular and Cellular Endocrinology*, *355*(2), 221–230. https://doi.org/10.1016/j.mce.2011.05.048

195 Muciaccia, B., Boitani, C., Berloco, B.P., Nudo, F., Spadetta, G., Stefanini, M., de Rooij, D.G., & Vicini, E. (2013). Novel stage classification of human spermatogenesis based on acrosome development. *Biology of Reproduction, 89*(3), 60. https://doi.org/10.1095/biolreprod.113.111682

196 Cheah Y., & Yang W. (2011). Functions of essential nutrition for high quality spermatogenesis. *Advances in Bioscience and Biotechnology, 2*(4): 182–197 https://doi.org/10.4236/abb.2011.24029

197 Ding, G.L., Liu, Y., Liu, M.E., Pan, J.X., Guo, M.X., Sheng, J.Z., & Huang, H.F. (2015). The effects of diabetes on male fertility and epigenetic regulation during spermatogenesis. *Asian Journal of Andrology, 17*(6), 948–953. https://doi.org/10.4103/1008-682X.150844

198 Skoracka, K., Eder, P., Łykowska-Szuber, L., Dobrowolska, A., & Krela-Kaźmierczak, I. (2020). Diet and nutritional factors in male (in)fertility-underestimated factors. *Journal of Clinical Medicine, 9*(5), 1400. https://doi.org/10.3390/jcm9051400

199 Walczak-Jedrzejowska, R., Wolski, J.K., & Slowikowska-Hilczer, J. (2013). The role of oxidative stress and antioxidants in male fertility. *Central European Journal of Urology, 66*(1), 60–67. https://doi.org/10.5173/ceju.2013.01.art19

200 Salas-Huetos, A., Bulló, M., & Salas-Salvadó, J. (2017). Dietary patterns, foods and nutrients in male fertility parameters and fecundability: A systematic review of observational studies. *Human Reproduction Update, 23*(4), 371–389. https://doi.org/10.1093/humupd/dmx006

201 Ilacqua, A., Izzo, G., Emerenziani, G.P., Baldari, C., & Aversa, A. (2018). Lifestyle and fertility: The influence of stress and quality of life on male fertility. *Reproductive Biology and Endocrinology: RB&E, 16*(1), 115. https://doi.org/10.1186/s12958-018-0436-9

202 Irani, M., Amirian, M., Sadeghi, R., Lez, J.L., & Latifnejad Roudsari, R. (2017). The effect of folate and folate plus zinc supplementation on endocrine parameters and sperm characteristics in sub-fertile men: A systematic review and meta-analysis. *Urology Journal, 14*(5), 4069–4078. https://doi.org/10.22037/uj.v14i5.3772

203 Bottiglieri, T. (2013). Folate, vitamin B_{12}, and S-adenosylmethionine. *The Psychiatric Clinics of North America, 36*(1), 1–13. https://doi.org/10.1016/j.psc.2012.12.001

204 Martín-Calvo, N., Mínguez-Alarcón, L., Gaskins, A.J., Nassan, F.L., Williams, P.L., Souter, I., Hauser, R., Chavarro, J.E., & EARTH Study team (2019). Paternal preconception folate intake in relation to gestational age at delivery and birthweight of newborns conceived through assisted reproduction. *Reproductive Biomedicine Online, 39*(5), 835–843. https://doi.org/10.1016/j.rbmo.2019.07.005

205 Costanzo, P.R., & Knoblovits, P. (2016). Vitamin D and male reproductive system. *Hormone Molecular Biology and Clinical Investigation, 28*(3), 151–159. https://doi.org/10.1515/hmbci-2016-0049

206 Cito, G., Cocci, A., Micelli, E., Gabutti, A., Russo, G. I., Coccia, M.E., Franco, G., Serni, S., Carini, M., & Natali, A. (2020). Vitamin D and male fertility: An updated review. *The World Journal of Men's Health, 38*(2), 164–177. https://doi.org/10.5534/wjmh.190057

207 Jueraitetibaike, K., Ding, Z., Wang, D.D., Peng, L.P., Jing, J., Chen, L., Ge, X., Qiu, X.H., & Yao, B. (2019). The effect of vitamin D on sperm motility and the underlying mechanism. *Asian Journal of Andrology, 21*(4), 400–407. https://doi.org/10.4103/aja.aja_105_18

208 Surette, M.E. (2008). The science behind dietary omega-3 fatty acids. *Canadian Medical Association journal, 178*(2), 177–180. https://doi.org/10.1503/cmaj.071356

209 Safarinejad, M.R., & Safarinejad, S. (2012). The roles of omega-3 and omega-6 fatty acids in idiopathic male infertility. *Asian Journal of Andrology, 14*(4), 514–515. https://doi.org/10.1038/aja.2012.46

210 Safarinejad, M.R. (2011). Effect of omega-3 polyunsaturated fatty acid supplementation on semen profile and enzymatic anti-oxidant capacity of seminal plasma in infertile men with idiopathic oligoasthenoteratospermia: A double-blind, placebo-controlled, randomised study. *Andrologia*, *43*(1), 38–47. https://doi.org/10.1111/j.1439-0272.2009.01013.x

211 Esmaeili, V., Shahverdi, A.H., Moghadasian, M.H., & Alizadeh, A.R. (2015). Dietary fatty acids affect semen quality: A review. *Andrology*, *3*(3), 450–461. https://doi.org/10.1111/andr.12024

212 Jensen, T.K., Priskorn, L., Holmboe, S.A., Nassan, F.L., Andersson, A.M., Dalgård, C., Petersen, J.H., Chavarro, J.E., & Jørgensen, N. (2020). Associations of fish oil supplement use with testicular function in young men. *JAMA Network Open*, *3*(1), e1919462. https://doi.org/10.1001/jamanetworkopen.2019.19462

213 Fallah, A., Mohammad-Hasani, A., & Colagar, A.H. (2018). Zinc is an essential element for male fertility: A review of Zn roles in men's health, germination, sperm quality, and fertilization. *Journal of Reproduction & Infertility*, *19*(2), 69–81. https://www.ncbi.nlm.nih.gov/pmc/articles/PMC6010824/

214 Chu, D.S. (2018). Zinc: A small molecule with a big impact on sperm function. *PLoS Biology*, *16*(6), e2006204. https://doi.org/10.1371/journal.pbio.2006204

215 Albani, E., Castellano, S., Gurrieri, B., Arruzzolo, L., Negri, L., Borroni, E.M., & Levi-Setti, P.E. (2019). Male age: Negative impact on sperm DNA fragmentation. *Aging*, *11*(9), 2749–2761. https://doi.org/10.18632/aging.101946

216 Prasad, A S. (2014). Zinc is an antioxidant and anti-inflammatory agent: Its role in human health. *Frontiers in Nutrition*, *1*, 14. https://doi.org/10.3389/fnut.2014.00014

217 Allouche-Fitoussi, D., & Breitbart, H. (2020). The role of zinc in male fertility. *International Journal of Molecular Sciences*, *21*(20), 7796. https://doi.org/10.3390/ijms21207796

218 Salas-Huetos, A., Rosique-Esteban, N., Becerra-Tomás, N., Vizmanos, B., Bulló, M., & Salas-Salvadó, J. (2018). The effect of nutrients and dietary supplements on sperm quality parameters: A systematic review and meta-analysis of randomized clinical trials. *Advances in Nutrition (Bethesda, Md.)*, *9*(6), 833–848. https://doi.org/10.1093/advances/nmy057

219 Liu, Y., Peterson, K.E., Sánchez, B.N., Jones, A. D., Cantoral, A., Mercado-García, A., Solano-González, M., Ettinger, A.S., & Téllez-Rojo, M.M. (2019). Dietary intake of selenium in relation to pubertal development in Mexican children. *Nutrients*, *11*(7), 1595. https://doi.org/10.3390/nu11071595

220 Shetty, S., Marsicano, J.R., & Copeland, P.R. (2018). Uptake and utilization of selenium from selenoprotein P. *Biological Trace Element Research*, *181*(1), 54–61. https://doi.org/10.1007/s12011-017-1044-9

221 Foresta, C., Flohé, L., Garolla, A., Roveri, A., Ursini, F., & Maiorino, M. (2002). Male fertility is linked to the selenoprotein phospholipid hydroperoxide glutathione peroxidase. *Biology of Reproduction*, *67*(3), 967–971. https://doi.org/10.1095/biolreprod.102.003822

8 Tired All the Time

Most healthcare professionals are familiar with this. A patient slumps into a chair and says, "I am just so tired all the time". It's a pretty nebulous symptom, not least because tiredness and fatigue are so subjective.[1]

Of course, there are many possible clinical reasons for tiredness and fatigue. It could be an underactive thyroid, one of the various anaemias, diabetes, or a heart condition. It could be menopause. It may be related to a virus, for example, myalgic encephalomyelitis (ME) or post-viral fatigue. It could be about stress or depression which can create a poor sleeping pattern. Not getting enough sleep, or something else disrupting sleep, like sleep apnoea or scrolling a phone late at night will certainly cause fatigue. It may be that a patient is overloaded with sugar, and therefore insulin, which disrupts sleep.[2] It could be something as simple as mild dehydration because if we don't have enough water, none of our body processes work well[3] It could even be something more sinister like cancer. But if differential diagnosis fails to identify any of these (or other things) as causative factors, it is certainly worth considering nutrition.

This chapter dives into some nutritional biochemistry. Some readers may view this with all the enthusiasm of pushing a large rock uphill. However, it is necessary background for practitioners to understand how the provision of appropriate nutrition can benefit someone who is tired all the time. It is set out in as painless and streamlined a way as possible, without getting too bogged down in excessive intricate detail.

METABOLISM

Every second of every day, billions of enzymes transform billions of molecules of glucose, fat and protein into billions of other substances in the processes of energy creation.

Metabolism is either catabolic (breaking things down and generating heat) or anabolic (building things up and using heat). Energy metabolism, sometimes called cellular respiration, is primarily catabolic (which is why exercise makes us hot and sweaty) and catabolic metabolism is what this chapter explores. Energy is produced when the chemical bonds between atoms are broken, or when oxidation (the removal of an electron) or reduction (the addition of an electron) takes place.[4] Where oxidation and reduction reactions happen at the same time, this is called a redox reaction.

There are multiple energy metabolism processes, most of which take place inside the mitochondria, membrane-bound organelles within most cells. Cells with a high demand for energy, for example, liver or heart cells, contain thousands of mitochondria, in fact, mitochondria make up over 30% of the mass of cardiac cells.[5]

Mature red blood cells are the only cells in our bodies that do not have mitochondria.[6] Although they are present in stem cells that mature into red blood cells, it is not yet fully understood why these organelles are expelled during the maturation process.[7]

ENERGY SUBSTRATES

Most energy production is powered by glucose derived from the carbohydrates that we eat. However, if we are not getting enough calories from carbohydrates, the body will use alternative substances to create energy. These alternatives include dietary fats and body stores of fat; dietary proteins (the body will use protein from its own muscles only as a last resort) and even lactate and ketone bodies which are by-products of metabolic processes.[8,9] Different types of tissue have preferences for different fuel sources. Cardiac cells actually prefer using fat to generate energy.[10] The brain prefers glucose, but it can use ketone bodies to generate energy during periods of fasting, or after exercise when glucose is in short supply.[11] And in a lovely bit of circular economy, skeletal muscles produce lactate during periods of intense exercise, and then use that lactate to generate more energy for themselves.[12]

The various substrates of energy production may start their journey on different pathways, but they all feed into the Krebs cycle, which is sometimes called the citric acid cycle or tricarboxylic acid cycle, and then the electron transport chain, both of which are discussed in more detail below.

The aim of energy metabolism pathways is to create adenosine triphosphate (ATP). The bonds between the phosphate atoms in ATP store a particularly high level of energy which makes it the ideal energy currency for the body.[13] Energy is released when a single phosphate bond is broken, changing ATP to ADP (adenosine diphosphate).[14] ADP and ATP are recycled from one to the other, constantly adding and then removing phosphate molecules to generate energy.[13]

It is estimated that between ten million and one hundred million molecules of ATP are present in a typical cell at all times and, in a healthy cell where sufficient nutrition is present, this ATP is constantly being used and replaced every second.[15]

Energy production is entirely dependent on nutrition. Macronutrients (carbohydrates, fats, and, at a pinch, proteins) provide the fuel used in energy production. But the biochemical processes that create energy cannot happen without sufficient micronutrients. Vitamins, minerals, amino acids from protein breakdown, and other substances, enable energy production by providing the materials needed to synthesise the enzymes and co-enzymes which create the biochemical reactions that generate energy.[16] The micronutrients needed are noted for each biochemical process and are then discussed in more detail further down the chapter.

ENERGY PRODUCTION FROM GLUCOSE

The easiest way for our metabolism to produce energy is by using glucose, derived from the breakdown of the carbohydrates that we eat. If for some reason there is a lack of carbohydrates, our biochemistry will create glucose from fats, proteins, and metabolites such as lactate and ketone bodies through a process called gluconeogenesis (literally "making new glucose"), which takes place in the liver and kidneys.[17]

There are four different stages of energy production from glucose, all of which work continuously: glycolysis, the Link Reaction, the Krebs cycle and the electron transport chain. All of them are driven by a series of micronutrient-dependent enzymatic reactions. Glycolysis takes place in the cytoplasm of the cell, whilst the Link Reaction, the Krebs cycle, and the electron transport chain all take place inside the mitochondria.

The production of ATP within the mitochondria, in response to any increase or decrease in energy demand, is tightly regulated by calcium ions.[18] These flow through the mitochondrial membrane, ensuring that sufficient ATP is manufactured to meet the changing energy needs of cells. Low levels of calcium will result in lower energy production, which in turn will lead to increased feelings of fatigue.[19]

GLYCOLYSIS

Glycolysis is a ten-step process that is the starting point for energy metabolism. It is not particularly efficient at generating energy, but it is fast, and unlike most other energy-producing mechanisms, it can take place either aerobically or anaerobically.[20] This means that in high-intensity exercise situations, glycolysis can take place in an oxygen-free environment whilst available oxygen is directed to other energy-producing pathways.[21]

When glucose enters the cytoplasm of a cell a series of enzymatic reactions rearrange its molecules, splitting them into a number of other substances: two molecules of pyruvate, four molecules of ATP, and two molecules of NADH, (reduced nicotinamide adenine dinucleotide). Nicotinamide adenine dinucleotide (NAD^+) is a co-enzyme which is central to energy metabolism; the "H" shows that NAD^+ has had a hydrogen molecule added to it, creating the reduced form.[20]

The reactions in glycolysis need energy to fuel them, which uses up two of the ATP molecules. The pyruvate, and the remaining two molecules of ATP and NADH are transported into the mitochondria where the pyruvate enters the Link Reaction and the ATP and NADH enter the electron transport chain.[22] However, in anaerobic conditions (like intensive exercise) the pyruvate remains within the cell cytoplasm and is converted to lactate.[23] Most of this lactate is released into the bloodstream and circulates to the liver and kidneys where it is converted, through gluconeogenesis, back into glucose.[12]

The enzymes that split glucose molecules are dependent on magnesium, whilst the creation of NADH requires phosphate and niacin (B3).[24,25] Because red blood cells have no mitochondria, they can only generate energy through glycolysis.[26]

THE LINK REACTION

The Link Reaction links glycolysis with the Krebs cycle.

Within the mitochondrial matrix, yet more enzymatic reactions chop up the pyruvate produced in glycolysis. A carbon atom is removed and combines with two oxygen molecules, creating carbon dioxide (CO_2) which is exhaled when we breathe. And a hydrogen atom is removed and attached to NAD^+, creating NADH. The structure that emerges from these reactions is acetyl coenzyme A (acetyl-CoA). The chemical bonds in acetyl-CoA are so full of energy that they provide power for most of the chemical reactions in the next stage of energy production, the Krebs cycle.[27]

The enzymes that do the work in the Link Reaction are dependent on several B vitamins: thiamine (B1), riboflavin (B2), niacin, and pantothenic acid (B5). In fact, pantothenic acid's primary function in the body is as a component of coenzymes, particularly acetyl-CoA, which has a central role in the metabolism of carbohydrates, fats, and proteins.[28] Biotin, a substance that forms part of the B vitamin complex, is also needed for the formation of acetyl-CoA.[29]

The Krebs Cycle

When the acetyl-CoA produced in the Link Reaction enters the Krebs cycle it is combined with another compound, oxaloacetate, to form citric acid. In an eight-step process, a series of enzymatic reactions remove some bits, add others, stimulate both oxidation and reduction reactions, and generally rearrange all of the molecules. The final compound produced is oxaloacetate, which then cycles back into the first step to combine with acetyl-CoA. Over the course of the eight-step cycle, three molecules of NADH, one molecule of $FADH_2$, one molecule of guanosine triphosphate (GTP), and two molecules of CO_2 are produced. NADH and $FADH_2$ (the reduced form of flavin adenine dinucleotide (FAD), a coenzyme essential in energy metabolism, which carries two hydrogen atoms) are energy-carrying compounds which are passed on to the electron transport chain. GTP is a complex molecule that can act as an energy source but is also used as a building block for RNA and DNA. The CO_2 is exhaled when we breathe.[30,31]

The enzymatic reactions in the Krebs cycle are dependent on both vitamins and minerals. Six B vitamins, thiamine, riboflavin, niacin, pantothenic acid, cyanocobalamin (B12), and biotin are all co-factors to the enzymatic processes that drive the cycle. And the minerals iron, magnesium, and zinc are needed for the production and activation of many of the enzymes which trigger the redox reactions in the Krebs cycle.[32]

The Electron Transport Chain

The final stage in the straightforward process of energy creation from glucose is the electron transport chain. This takes the outputs of the Krebs cycle, glycolysis, and the Link Reaction and turns them into ATP via a process called oxidative phosphorylation.

The electron transport chain is made up of a series of protein complexes which collect electrons from donors and moves them along the chain like a complicated game of pass the parcel. The donor electrons are the hydrogen atoms attached to the reduced forms of NAD^+ (NADH) and FAD ($FADH_2$) which have come from the Krebs cycle.[33] As NADH and $FADH_2$ pass through the protein complexes, enzymes snip the hydrogen atoms off and attach them to oxygen, creating water (H_2O).

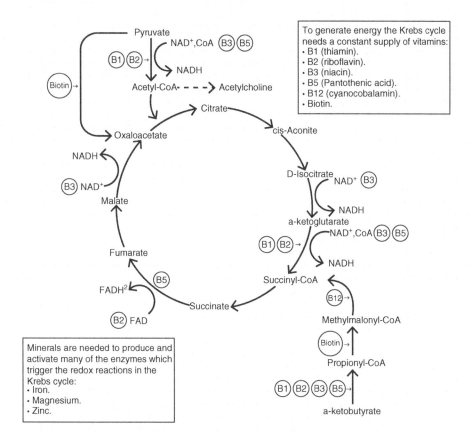

The Krebs cycle.

The oxidised NAD^+ and FAD are broken down by enzymes and their constituent parts are either recycled, repurposed, or eliminated via urine.[34,35]

The reactions that split the chemical bonds to release hydrogen also release energy. That energy is used to pump the hydrogen atoms backwards and forwards through mitochondrial membranes, where the enzyme ATP synthase triggers the formation ATP.[36] Some of the ATP created is cycled back to generate more energy but most is transported out of the mitochondria and into the cytoplasm of cells where it is used to power all of the functions of the body.[37]

Like all energy metabolism, the electron transport chain is driven by nutrition. When NADH (containing niacin) and $FADH_2$ (containing riboflavin) lose their electrons, another nutrient, Coenzyme Q10 (CoQ10), picks up those electrons and passes them down the chain of protein complexes. Two cytochromes (protein complexes containing iron), also transport hydrogen atoms across to the final acceptor molecule, oxygen.[38]

A zinc-dependent enzyme then combines hydrogen and oxygen to create water, which is expelled through breathing.[39] Vitamin C provides antioxidant protection for enzymatic reactions utilising iron and oxygen.[40]

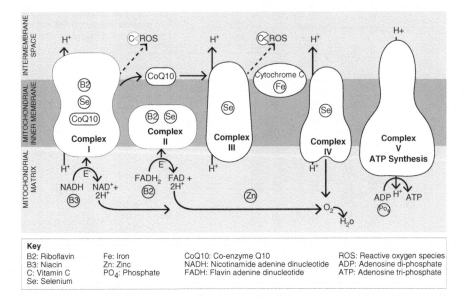

The electron transport chain.

IT GETS MORE COMPLICATED...

Using easily accessed glucose to generate energy through the pathways described above is the easiest way for our bodies to create the ATP that powers us. If we need a rapid boost of energy because we are doing some kind of intensive activity, a form of glucose which is stored in our muscles and liver, called glycogen, is released.[41] Glycogen can be rapidly broken down into glucose molecules which are then pushed through the four stages of ATP production.[42] The enzymes that snip glycogen up into separate glucose molecules require, among other things, the minerals phosphorus, calcium, magnesium, and manganese.[43]

If there is insufficient carbohydrate to break down into glucose, the body will turn to fat as a substrate for energy production. Fat contains more than double the calorific energy of carbohydrates but gaining energy from it is far more complex than the relatively straightforward four-stage process used to get energy from glucose.

There are two different sources of fat which the body can access to generate energy: dietary fat and body fat. Both types of fat are primarily found in the form of triglycerides. These have two main components; a glycerol "backbone" with three chains of carbons and hydrogens (fatty acid chains) attached to it. In order to gain energy from fats, the fatty acid chains need to be cut away from the glycerol "backbone", leaving four separate strands; the backbone and three free fatty acid chains.

This happens in different ways for dietary fats and body fats. Dietary fats are broken up during digestion when pancreatic enzymes in the duodenum split the bonds between the glycerol backbone and the fatty acid chains.[44] Body fat is more complex because fat cells need to be extracted from storage in adipocytes before lipolytic enzymes can snip the fatty acid chains away from the glycerol backbone of the triglycerides we store as fat cells.[45,46]

β-OXIDATION OF FATTY ACIDS

Once the glycerol and fatty acid chains have been split up, they go separate ways. The glycerol is converted to glucose through gluconeogenesis or is converted to lactate through a direct glycerol to lactate metabolism.[47] Both substances are then circulated back into energy metabolism.[8]

The fatty acid chains are used in a variety of ways, depending on their length and construction. Short-chain fatty acids (up to six carbons in length) may be used for energy generation by the microbiome within the gut, but may also be used as messenger molecules, particularly in gut-brain communications.[48] The essential fatty acids omega-3 and omega-6 are between 18 and 22 carbons in length.[49] These longer-chain fatty acids (up to 22 carbons in length, including some saturated fatty acids) are used structurally in cell membranes and are used to synthesise hormones, neuropeptides, and eicosanoids like prostaglandins, leukotrienes, and thromboxanes.[50,51] Everything else is either stored or used to generate energy from fat through the β-oxidation pathway.

As with all energy production, β-oxidation is a series of enzymatic reactions. Fatty acid chains are long strings of carbon atoms with hydrogen atoms attached laterally.[52] Once freed from the glycerol backbone, fatty acid chains destined for energy production are attached to the co-enzyme acyl-CoA, forming fatty acyl-CoA.[53] This is transported through the mitochondrial membrane by enzymes which are dependent on vitamin C, carnitine, and choline.[54,55]

Once inside the mitochondria, the fatty acyl-CoA undergoes a series of enzymatic cycles. Each cycle splits two carbon atoms off the chain at a time, and produces one unit of acetyl-CoA, one unit of $FADH_2$, one unit of NADH, one water molecule and around 12 molecules of ATP.[56] The acetyl-CoA enters the Krebs cycle whilst the NADH and $FADH_2$ go into the electron transport chain to be used in the generation of more energy.

β-oxidation of fatty acids also requires pantothenic acid, riboflavin, and niacin.[40]

PROTEIN METABOLISM

Amino acids, which are the building blocks of protein, are far more valuable to the body for use in repair and construction than they are in energy generation. But if the body is not getting enough calories from either carbohydrates or fats, for example, if someone is following one of the high protein, low carbohydrate diets which are currently popular for weight loss, it will use protein to generate energy.

Although protein contains the same amount of energy as carbohydrates, it is much more difficult for the body to use protein as an energy source because there are many different amino acids, all of which have their own breakdown pathway.

Therefore the body will only use protein to generate energy if there are insufficient calories from other sources.

To use protein to generate energy, it must first be broken up into its constituent amino acids. There are 20 different amino acids and all of them are made up of a carboxyl group consisting of one carbon atom, two oxygens and a hydrogen (CO_2H), and an amine group, which consists of one nitrogen and two hydrogen atoms (NH_2). Both carboxyl and amine groups are attached to a single carbon atom known as the α carbon. Also joined to the α carbon is a side chain; each side chain is a different size and shape, and it is this which determines which amino acid is which. Because of this variety in structure, each amino acid needs different enzymes to deconstruct it.[57]

When the body begins to break down amino acids to use for fuel, enzymes split the carboxyl and amine groups and the side chain away from the α carbon. Once split away, the carboxyl section is called the carbon skeleton. Enzymes shift bits around and add bits to turn it into pyruvate and acetyl-CoA, both of which feed into the Krebs cycle.[58] The amine component is converted into ammonia, which is then converted, in the liver and kidneys, to urea and excreted in urine.[59]

The use of protein as a primary energy source for any significant length of time can increase stress on the liver and kidneys.[60] This is partially because increasing the breakdown of protein also escalates the levels of highly toxic ammonia produced in the body, and partially because some amino acids contain sulphur and phosphate. Whilst both are essential to multiple body functions, excessive amounts put significant pressure on our detoxification and excretion pathways.[61]

Protein metabolism requires many of the B vitamins: thiamine, riboflavin, niacin, pantothenic acid, pyridoxine, vitamin B12, and biotin.[40]

Nutrients Needed for Energy Production

Nutrient	Energy Yielding Pathway
Vitamin B1 (thiamine)	Link reaction
	Krebs cycle
Vitamin B2 (riboflavin)	Link Reaction
	Krebs cycle
	Electron transport chain
	β-oxidation of fatty acids
	Protein metabolism
	Synthesis of CoQ10
Vitamin B3 (niacin)	Glycolysis
	Krebs cycle
	Electron transport chain
	Synthesis of CoQ10
Vitamin B5 (pantothenic acid)	Link reaction
	β-oxidation of fatty acids
	Krebs cycle
	Synthesis of CoQ10

Nutrients Needed for Energy Production

Nutrient	Energy Yielding Pathway
Vitamin B6 (pyridoxine)	Protein metabolism
	Synthesis of CoQ10
Vitamin B12 (cyanocobalamin)	Krebs cycle
	Synthesis of CoQ10
Folic acid	Electron transport chain
	Synthesis of CoQ10
Biotin	Krebs cycle
Choline	β-oxidation of fatty acids
Vitamin C	Electron transport chain
	β-oxidation of fatty acids
Calcium	Krebs cycle
	Electron transport chain
Iron	Krebs cycle
	Electron transport chain
Magnesium	Glycogen release
	Glycolysis
	Krebs cycle
	ATP functionality
Manganese	Gluconeogenesis
	Glycolysis
Phosphorus	Creation of ATP
	Synthesis of NAD^+
CoQ10	Electron transport chain
Vitamin D	Protects mitochondrial function and integrity

NUTRIENTS NEEDED FOR ENERGY PRODUCTION: VITAMINS

THIAMINE (VITAMIN B1)

Thiamine forms part of the coenzymes which are used in the enzymatic reactions that remove carboxyl groups and release carbon dioxide in the Link Reaction and the Krebs cycle, as well as in the metabolism of protein for energy.[40,62] Dietary sources of vitamin B1 can be found in the nutrient cheat sheets at the end of this book.

The UK RNI for thiamine is below that of both the United States and the European Union (0.8 mg/d as opposed to 1.1 mg/d), was set in 1991, and has not been reviewed since.[63] A significant proportion of pregnant women are found to suffer from thiamine deficiency.[64] Obese individuals and those with type II diabetes are also often deficient in vitamin B1.[65,66] Thiamine deficiency has also been noted in the elderly and in individuals with psychiatric disorders.[67] Persistently low levels of thiamine have been linked with the development of Alzheimer's disease and other dementias, as well as Parkinson's disease.[68,69,70] It is possible that the mechanisms behind this relate to energy production.

Riboflavin (Vitamin B2)

Riboflavin forms part of the coenzyme flavin adenine dinucleotide (FAD) which is used in the Link Reaction, Krebs cycle, and electron transport chain, during the β-oxidation of fatty acids and in protein metabolism.[40] It is also a key nutrient required in the synthesis of CoQ10, which is discussed in detail below. Dietary sources of vitamin B2 can be found in the nutrient cheat sheets at the end of this book.

Intakes of riboflavin in the UK have fallen significantly over the last two decades.[71] Women appear to have particularly low intakes of riboflavin, with 10% of women aged 20–59 having such low intakes that they are at risk of deficiency.[72] This is particularly concerning as riboflavin has a role in the absorption of iron.[73] And iron itself is a key nutrient in energy metabolism, as well as being essential in the prevention of iron deficiency anaemia, a significant issue among women of childbearing age in the UK.[74]

Niacin (Vitamin B3)

Niacin forms part of the coenzyme NAD^+ which plays a key role in glycolysis, the Krebs cycle, and the electron transport chain.[40] It is also required in the synthesis of CoQ10. Dietary sources of vitamin B3 can be found in the nutrient cheat sheets at the end of this book.

Where niacin occurs in plant foods it is often bound to sugars that reduce its bioavailability, preventing it from being absorbed.[75] However, the levels of niacin in some foods reported in national food composition databases are for the entirety of niacin within a food, rather than the amount that is bioavailable.[76] So we may all be consuming less niacin than has been thought.

Whilst intakes in the UK do not appear to be of concern, the lower bioavailability of niacin from plant foods may put vegetarians and vegans at risk of deficiency.[77] Intakes of niacin in these groups, even at the levels currently noted in national food composition databases, are less than adequate and about of third of vegetarians and vegans are deficient in niacin.[78]

Pantothenic Acid (Vitamin B5)

Pantothenic acid is essential to the coenzyme acetyl-CoA which is formed in both the Link Reaction and in the β-oxidation of fatty acids and which then feeds into the Krebs cycle. It is also needed for the synthesis of CoQ10.[40] Dietary sources of vitamin B5 can be found in the nutrient cheat sheets at the end of this book.

Unlike several other B vitamins, there is no specific deficiency disease associated with pantothenic acid. The UK has never set an RNI for pantothenic acid and does not track intakes of it within the Nation Diet and Nutrition Survey (NDNS), therefore it is not possible to determine whether intakes are adequate or not.

Pyridoxine (Vitamin B6)

Pyridoxin is an essential cofactor in protein metabolism, as well as in the synthesis of CoQ10.[40] Dietary sources of vitamin B6 can be found in the nutrient cheat sheets at the end of this book.

Deficiency of pyridoxine is rare, and the UK does not track or report intakes of this nutrient. Therefore it is not possible to determine whether UK intakes are adequate.

Cyanocobalamin (Vitamin B12)

Vitamin B12 forms part of a coenzyme that produces one of the Krebs cycle substrates; it is also needed for the synthesis of CoQ10.[79,80] Dietary sources of vitamin B12 can be found in the nutrient cheat sheets at the end of this book.

Although vitamin B12 intakes in most of the UK population are good, around 5% have intakes of vitamin B12 that fall below the lower reference nutrient intake (LRNI), which puts them at risk of deficiency.[72] There are also concerns about intakes among vegetarians, particularly vegans, as the primary sources of this nutrient are animal based.[81]

Folic Acid

Folic acid is primarily known for its functions relating to the closure of the neural tube in foetal development, however, it is also needed for the synthesis of CoQ10, one of the acceptor molecules in the electron transport chain.[80] Dietary sources of folic acid can be found in the nutrient cheat sheets at the end of this book.

Intakes of folic acid have fallen consistently over the last few decades. Data from the most recent NDNS shows that 90% of women of childbearing age have intakes of folic acid below that which would be needed to prevent neural tube defects.[71] The announcement in 2021 of the intention of the government to fortify white flour with folic acid may help raise blood folate levels.[82] However, as the government has not announced when this will be implemented, what level fortification will be at, nor how much this will increase daily intake, it is difficult to tell how valid or effective this policy will be.

Biotin

Biotin is classified as part of the B complex of vitamins, and it is sometimes known as vitamin B7. It is used in the formation of acetyl-CoA and in the formation of the enzyme pyruvate carboxylase which is needed for the synthesis of oxaloacetate in the Krebs cycle.[40] Dietary sources of biotin can be found in the nutrient cheat sheets at the end of this book.

Biotin cannot be synthesised in the body in sufficient quantities to fulfil all of its functions and therefore both the European Union and the United States recognise biotin as essential. However the UK does not and so it is not included it in the national food composition database (McCance and Widdowson), nor are there any official recommended intakes. Intakes of biotin are not monitored in the UK, and it is not possible to determine whether UK intakes are adequate or not.

Choline

Choline is an essential component of the mitochondrial membrane and is used in the transportation of fatty acyl-CoA during the β-oxidation of fatty acids.[83] Dietary sources of choline can be found in the nutrient cheat sheets at the end of this book.

As with biotin, both the European Union and the United States accept that choline is an essential nutrient because our bodies cannot make it in the amounts needed for health. But once again, the UK government does not accept that this nutrient is essential. Therefore, it is not included in food composition databases, intakes are not monitored in the NDNS, and there are no official UK intake recommendations.[84]

The European Food Safety Authority (EFSA) has set a level of 400 mg per day for all adults, whilst the American Institute of Medicine (IOM) has set an adequate intake of 550 mg/d for males and 425 mg/d for non-pregnant females.[85,86] However average daily intakes in the UK for men are just over 300 mg, and around 250 mg for women, meaning there is an unacknowledged shortfall of choline in the UK.[84]

Vitamin C

Vitamin C is used to protect against oxidation within the electron transport chain and in the formation of enzymes that transport fatty acyl-CoA in the β-oxidation of fats.[40]

As with all nutrients, dietary sources of vitamin C can be found in the nutrient cheat sheets at the back of this book. As vitamin C is found only in fruit and vegetables, it is worth noting that intake of these has fallen consistently over the last two decades in the UK.[71] Despite nearly 20 years of the Five-A-Day message from the UK government, 86% of the UK population eat less than 3.5 portions of fruit and vegetables a day and, even more concerning, 21% are eating less than one portion per day.[87]

The UK RNI for vitamin C was set at 40 mg a day in 1991 and has not been reviewed since.[88] In 2012, a peer review of available evidence proposed an optimum intake of vitamin C in healthy people of 200 mg a day.[89] If this were the recommended intake in the UK, virtually everyone in the population would be classified as severely deficient. Although data from the NDNS shows only a very small percentage of individuals with intakes that fall below the LRNI (10 mg), the 2019 survey found a significant proportion of women have plasma vitamin C levels so low that they are at risk of deficiency.[90]

Authorities in the UK have been aware of many years that poor vitamin C status is common among individuals living on a low income.[91] The only reason not more of the population were found to be at risk is because of the extremely low bar set by the British government. Frankly, it is remarkable that more cases of scurvy are not being reported (171 cases in 2020–2021).[92]

NUTRIENTS NEEDED FOR ENERGY PRODUCTION: MINERALS

CALCIUM

Calcium is used as a messenger molecule in the regulation of ATP production.[93] It is also central to the conversion of glycogen, released from the muscles and liver, into glucose which can then enter glycolysis.[94] Dietary sources of calcium can be found in the nutrient cheat sheets at the end of this book.

As with most micronutrients, the UK RNI for calcium was set in 1991 and has not been reviewed since. It is set at 700 mg, significantly lower than the recommended intakes from both IOM and EFSA (1000 mg and 800 mg, respectively). It is concerning therefore that calcium intakes in the UK have fallen steadily over the last two decades, leaving 11% of the adult population at risk of deficiency, based on the already low expectations of the UK RNI.[71,72]

IRON

Iron is needed for the synthesis of the enzyme succinate dehydrogenase which is used in the Krebs cycle and the electron transport chain.[95] It is also needed for the formation and function of the cytochromes within the electron transport chain.[96] Dietary sources of iron can be found in the nutrient cheat sheets at the end of this book whilst the complexities of iron absorption are discussed in Chapter 3.

UK intakes have fallen significantly over the last 20 years, particularly among women.[71] Indeed, around 27% of women aged between 20 and 50 have iron intakes that are so low they are at risk of deficiency.[97] At the same time, consumption of red meat has also fallen, particularly among women, which may correlate with reduced iron intakes.[98]

MAGNESIUM

Magnesium shows up all over the place in energy production. When glycogen is released from the muscles or the liver, magnesium regulates the enzymes that split it into glucose molecules.[99] Magnesium is needed by more than half of the enzymes that push those glucose molecules through glycolysis.[24] And magnesium is also needed for the production and activation of enzymes that drive redox reactions in the Krebs cycle.[32] The relevance of magnesium to energy production goes even further; every molecule of ATP is bound to a magnesium ion in order to create its functional form; without magnesium ATP simply doesn't work.[100]

As with all other micronutrients discussed here, dietary sources of magnesium can be found in the nutrient cheat sheets at the end of this book. Magnesium is pretty ubiquitous, being widely available in different foods of both plant and animal origin. Yet despite that, magnesium consumption has been falling for the last two decades and nearly 26% of UK adults aged 20–59 have intakes that are so low that they are at potential risk of deficiency.[71,72]

MANGANESE

The trace element manganese is used in enzymes needed for gluconeogenesis.[101] It is also a cofactor in the function of enzymes that split glycogen into glucose molecules.[102] Dietary sources of manganese can be found in the nutrient cheat sheets at the end of this book.

Although manganese content of food is listed in the UK's national food composition database, the National Diet and Nutrition Survey does not measure intakes for this nutrient. Therefore, there is no data on whether UK intakes are adequate or not. However, deficiency is extremely rare, other than in experimental settings.[103]

PHOSPHORUS

Energy is generated when the bonds holding phosphorus within the structure of ATP are broken, meaning that what was ATP becomes ADP – adenosine diphosphate. In order to produce energy, a new molecule of phosphorus must be attached, which occurs in the electron transport chain.[14] The synthesis of NAD^+ also requires phosphorus as the structure of the cofactor is held together with phosphate groups.[104] Dietary sources of phosphorus can be found in the nutrient cheat sheets at the end of this book.

Phosphorus from animal products is easier to absorb than phosphorus from plant foods because phosphorus in plants is bound to phytates, which our digestive system cannot break down.[105] There are no concerns about phosphorus intakes in the UK.[106]

OTHER NUTRIENTS NEEDED FOR ENERGY PRODUCTION

COENZYME Q10

CoQ10 is a key nutrient in the electron transport chain.[107] It is synthesised within the body and therefore it is not classified as "essential". The greatest synthesis occurs in those tissues which have the highest metabolic energy usage; the heart, liver, kidneys, and skeletal muscle.[108] Dietary sources of CoQ10 can be found in the nutrient cheat sheets at the end of this book.

Because CoQ10 has not been classified as essential recommended levels have not been set, it is not included in the UK national food composition databases, and its intake is not tracked. It is therefore impossible to determine if intakes in the UK are adequate.

The synthesis of CoQ10 is dependent on a sufficient supply of the amino acid tyrosine, vitamins B2, B3, B5, B6, B12, folic acid and vitamin C and cholesterol.[109] Intake of many of these nutrients is far from optimum in the UK. Synthesis peaks at around age 25 and then, regardless of nutrient status, declines with age, with production at age 65 being only around 50% of that at age 25.[110]

Several things can disrupt CoQ10 synthesis: cardiovascular and kidney disease, metabolic syndrome and type II diabetes, as well as some pharmaceuticals, particularly statins and amitriptyline anti-depressants.[111] CoQ10 in serum is bound to low-density lipoprotein (LDL), where it protects it from peroxidation. When statins reduce cholesterol, they also reduce CoQ10.[112] In addition, statins actively inhibit the CoQ10 synthesis pathway because enzymes that synthesise cholesterol also synthesise CoQ10.[113]

Many of the side effects of statins come into focus when viewed in relation to the actions of CoQ10, particularly things like fatigue and muscle weakness. Advising patients who are taking statins to supplement with a minimum of 100 mg a day of CoQ10 could well mitigate some of the side effects of the medication; it is an extremely safe substance with no recorded adverse effects, and it could provide significant benefits to patients.[114]

VITAMIN D

Recent investigations into the genome suggest that vitamin D's original function was in the regulation of genes involved in energy metabolism.[115] Like all body tissues, the mitochondria are well supplied with vitamin D receptors and, although vitamin D is not directly involved in the energy production pathways, there is growing evidence that it is essential to the function of the mitochondria, where all synthesis of ATP takes place.[116]

Vitamin D deficiency decreases the numbers of mitochondria in muscle tissues whilst supplementation increases both density and function.[117] Although the exact mechanisms behind this are not yet fully understood, vitamin D is known to modulate inflammatory responses and protect against oxidative stress and cell damage.[118] It seems that these functions may be behind vitamin D's action within the mitochondria, and this may be why fatigue is often associated with vitamin D deficiency.[119]

The dire state of vitamin D status in the UK, and the wider functions of the nutrient have been discussed at length in Chapter 6.

WATER

Mild dehydration makes us tired.[120] Which is not really surprising as our cells are mostly made up of water and so it makes sense that our biochemical processes have evolved to work in a liquid environment. A loss of even 1% of our body water can have a significant negative impact on our ability to function, and this includes energy metabolism.[121]

Water intake requirements vary, depending on a range of factors including age, gender, activity and physical environment. However it seems that consuming less than 1.8 litres of fluid from all sources (including tea, coffee, soft drinks, and food) is likely to be detrimental.[122] A survey by the drinks brand Aqua Pura found that average UK intake is only around 850 ml of fluid a day.[123]

UK guidelines are somewhat imprecise on how much we should drink. The recommendation is to drink 6–8 glasses of water, but the size of the glass is not specified.[124]

NUTRITIONAL MANAGEMENT OF FATIGUE

As noted at the beginning of this chapter, there are multiple causes of fatigue. It may be a single factor, or it may be a combination of things. Some of these may be easy to address, others may be far more complex.

From a nutrition perspective, at the more complex end of the scale are dietary interventions. As discussed in Chapter 4 on obesity, our individual relationship with food is so deep rooted that changing the way we eat is one of the most difficult things we can do. However, given the nutritional implications of fatigue, a discussion around diet and eating patterns could be a useful place to start if other things have been eliminated.

We know that the UK diet contains far too much ultra-processed food. The nutrient poor but calorie dense status of ultra-processed foods means that it does not provide the nutrition needed to process the calories it contains. Diets high in sugar can disrupt sleep; so do diets high in fat.[125,126] Both sugar and fat are found in copious quantities in ultra-processed foods and disrupted sleep can lead to ongoing fatigue.

It would be helpful to find out if the patient is eating regularly. If eating patterns are irregular, then it is possible that the patient is simply not consuming enough calories at the right time. This is particularly relevant if meals are being missed on a regular basis.[127] Equally, if fruit and vegetable intake is low, and/or if ultra-processed food makes up a significant proportion of their diet, they may be suffering micronutrient insufficiency because energy production is about far more than just calories.[32] But rather than simply telling a patient to cut out all of the ultra-processed food, suggest adding in some fruit and vegetables and some whole grains. Increasing the scope of a diet makes people feel better than if they feel they have to restrict what they eat and they may well end up substituting some of the ultra-processed stuff for real food.

ALWAYS READ THE LABEL

It is also important to remember that no single nutrient will resolve fatigue (or any other issue unless the patient is suffering from a specific deficiency disease). If a patient's diet is poor, it would be worth considering recommending the use of food supplements, to increase their micronutrient intake across a broad spectrum of vitamins and minerals. Whilst the use of food supplements is not necessarily a long-term solution, it can certainly be part of a transition to a more broadly balanced diet.

There are hundreds of multivitamin and mineral products on the market in the UK. The market is huge and confusing. There are age specific multivitamin products, products for pregnancy and conception, gender-specific products and products designed for hair, skin, and nails. There are even products specifically targeted at tiredness and fatigue. They range from expensive branded varieties to relatively inexpensive own brands. They are sold in supermarkets, pharmacies, and health food stores.

One of the most important things to do when looking at multivitamin and mineral products is to read the label. A detailed infographic of how to read a food supplement label can be found in the introduction to this book.

It is important to make sure that the amount of any vitamin or mineral contained within the product is at least 100% of the daily requirement. Current labelling legislation requires this to be listed as Nutrient Reference Value (NRV) or Reference Intake (RI); both mean the same thing; they are just different nomenclatures. 100% of NRV will not pose any risk of overdose to consumers but it may well make a significant difference to their overall energy levels. If some vitamins or minerals in a product exceed the NRV it should not raise any safety concerns as the UK food supplement industry formulate products with safety in mind. However, if a patient is taking multiple different products, it would be advisable to have a discussion about safe upper levels for vitamins and minerals. Where safe intake levels have been set, these are listed in the nutrient cheat sheets at the back of this book.

Of course nutrition is not the answer to everything. But a good diet is an excellent place to start.

REFERENCES

1 NICE (2020). Tiredness/fatigue in adults. https://cks.nice.org.uk/topics/tiredness-fatigue-in-adults/

2 Breymeyer, K.L., Lampe, J.W., McGregor, B.A., & Neuhouser, M.L. (2016). Subjective mood and energy levels of healthy weight and overweight/obese healthy adults on high- and low-glycemic load experimental diets. *Appetite, 107,* 253–259. https://doi.org/10.1016/j.appet.2016.08.008

3 Benton, D., & Young, H.A. (2015). Do small differences in hydration status affect mood and mental performance? *Nutrition Reviews, 73 Suppl 2,* 83–96. https://doi.org/10.1093/nutrit/nuv045

4 Judge, A., & Dodd, M.S. (2020). Metabolism. *Essays in Biochemistry, 64*(4), 607–647. https://doi.org/10.1042/EBC20190041

5 Tahrir, F.G., Langford, D., Amini, S., Mohseni Ahooyi, T., & Khalili, K. (2019). Mitochondrial quality control in cardiac cells: Mechanisms and role in cardiac cell injury and disease. *Journal of Cellular Physiology, 234*(6), 8122–8133. https://doi.org/10.1002/jcp.27597

6 Zhang, Z.W., Cheng, J., Xu, F., Chen, Y.E., Du, J.B., Yuan, M., Zhu, F., Xu, X.C., & Yuan, S. (2011). Red blood cell extrudes nucleus and mitochondria against oxidative stress. *IUBMB Life, 63*(7), 560–565. https://doi.org/10.1002/iub.490

7 Moras, M., Lefevre, S.D., & Ostuni, M.A. (2017). From erythroblasts to mature red blood cells: Organelle clearance in mammals. *Frontiers in Physiology, 8,* 1076. https://doi.org/10.3389/fphys.2017.01076

8 Brooks G. A. (2020). Lactate as a fulcrum of metabolism. *Redox Biology, 35,* 101454. https://doi.org/10.1016/j.redox.2020.101454

9 Jensen, N.J., Wodschow, H.Z., Nilsson, M., & Rungby, J. (2020). Effects of ketone bodies on brain metabolism and function in neurodegenerative diseases. *International Journal of Molecular Sciences, 21*(22), 8767. https://doi.org/10.3390/ijms21228767

10 Pascual, F., & Coleman, R.A. (2016). Fuel availability and fate in cardiac metabolism: A tale of two substrates. *Biochimica et Biophysica Acta – Molecular and Cell Biology of Lipids, 1861*(10), 1425–1433. https://doi.org/10.1016/j.bbalip.2016.03.014

11 Puchalska, P., & Crawford, P.A. (2017). Multi-dimensional roles of ketone bodies in fuel metabolism, signaling, and therapeutics. *Cell Metabolism, 25*(2), 262–284. https://doi.org/10.1016/j.cmet.2016.12.022

12 Rabinowitz, J.D., & Enerbäck, S. (2020). Lactate: The ugly duckling of energy metabolism. *Nature Metabolism, 2*(7), 566–571. https://doi.org/10.1038/s42255-020-0243-4

13 Dunn, J., & Grider, M.H. (2021). *Physiology, Adenosine Triphosphate.* In: *StatPearls* [Internet]. Treasure Island (FL): StatPearls Publishing; Available from: https://www.ncbi.nlm.nih.gov/books/NBK553175/

14 Bonora, M., Patergnani, S., Rimessi, A., De Marchi, E., Suski, J.M., Bononi, A., Giorgi, C., Marchi, S., Missiroli, S., Poletti, F., Wieckowski, M.R., & Pinton, P. (2012). ATP synthesis and storage. *Purinergic Signalling, 8*(3), 343–357. https://doi.org/10.1007/s11302-012-9305-8

15 Flamholz, A., Phillips, R., & Milo, R. (2014). The quantified cell. *Molecular Biology of the Cell, 25*(22), 3497–3500. https://doi.org/10.1091/mbc.E14-09-1347.

16 Lewis, T., & Stone, W.L. *Biochemistry, Proteins Enzymes.* (2021). In: *StatPearls* [Internet]. Treasure Island (FL): StatPearls Publishing. Available from: https://www.ncbi.nlm.nih.gov/books/NBK554481/

17 Chourpiliadis, C., & Mohiuddin, S.S. (2022). *Biochemistry, Gluconeogenesis.* In: *StatPearls* [Internet]. Treasure Island (FL): StatPearls Publishing; Available from: https://www.ncbi.nlm.nih.gov/books/NBK544346/

18 Griffiths, E.J., & Rutter, G.A. (2009). Mitochondrial calcium as a key regulator of mitochondrial ATP production in mammalian cells. *Biochimica et Biophysica Acta-Bioenergetics, 1787*(11), 1324–1333. https://doi.org/10.1016/j.bbabio.2009.01.019

19 Fink, B.D., Bai, F., Yu, L., & Sivitz, W.I. (2017). Regulation of ATP production: Dependence on calcium concentration and respiratory state. *American Journal of Physiology. Cell physiology, 313*(2), C146–C153. https://doi.org/10.1152/ajpcell.00086.2017

20 Chaudhry, R., & Varacallo, M. *Biochemistry, Glycolysis.* (2021). In: *StatPearls* [Internet]. Treasure Island (FL): StatPearls Publishing. Available from: https://www.ncbi.nlm.nih.gov/books/NBK482303/

21 Park, S.B., Park, D.S., Kim, M., Lee, E., Lee, D., Jung, J., Son, S.J., Hong, J., & Yang, W. H. (2021). High-intensity warm-up increases anaerobic energy contribution during 100-m sprint. *Biology, 10*(3), 198. https://doi.org/10.3390/biology10030198

22 Berg, J.M., Tymoczko, J.L., & Stryer, L. (2002). *Biochemistry.* 5th edition. New York: W H Freeman. Section 16.1, Glycolysis Is an Energy-Conversion Pathway in Many Organisms. Available from: https://www.ncbi.nlm.nih.gov/books/NBK22593/

23 Xiong, Y., Lei, Q.Y., Zhao, S., & Guan, K.L. (2011). Regulation of glycolysis and gluconeogenesis by acetylation of PKM and PEPCK. *Cold Spring Harbor Symposia on Quantitative Biology, 76,* 285–289. https://doi.org/10.1101/sqb.2011.76.010942

24 Pilchova, I., Klacanova, K., Tatarkova, Z., Kaplan, P., & Racay, P. (2017). The involvement of Mg^{2+} in regulation of cellular and mitochondrial functions. *Oxidative Medicine and Cellular Longevity, 2017,* 6797460. https://doi.org/10.1155/2017/6797460

25 Makarov, M.V., Trammell, S., & Migaud, M.E. (2019). The chemistry of the vitamin B3 metabolome. *Biochemical Society Transactions, 47*(1), 131–147. https://doi.org/10.1042/BST20180420

26 McMahon, T.J., Darrow, C.C., Hoehn, B.A., & Zhu, H. (2021). Generation and export of red blood cell ATP in health and disease. *Frontiers in Physiology, 12,* 754638. https://doi.org/10.3389/fphys.2021.754638

27 Berg, J.M., Tymoczko, J.L., & Stryer, L. (2002). *Biochemistry.* 5th edition. New York: W H Freeman. Section 17.1, The Citric Acid Cycle Oxidizes Two-Carbon Units. Available from: https://www.ncbi.nlm.nih.gov/books/NBK22427/

28 Leonardi, R., & Jackowski, S. (2007). Biosynthesis of pantothenic acid and coenzyme A. *EcoSal Plus*, *2*(2). 10.1128/ecosalplus.3.6.3.4. https://doi.org/10.1128/ecosalplus. 3.6.3.4

29 Zempleni, J., Wijeratne, S.S., & Hassan, Y.I. (2009). Biotin. *BioFactors (Oxford, England)*, *35*(1), 36–46. https://doi.org/10.1002/biof.8

30 Berg, J.M., Tymoczko, J.L., & Stryer, L. (2002). *Biochemistry*. 5th edition. New York: W H Freeman. Chapter 17, The Citric Acid Cycle. Available from: https://www.ncbi. nlm.nih.gov/books/NBK21163/

31 Sasaki, A.T. (2016). Dynamic role of the GTP energy metabolism in cancers. *The Keio Journal of Medicine*, *65*(1), 21. https://doi.org/10.2302/kjm.65–001-ABST

32 Tardy, A.L., Pouteau, E., Marquez, D., Yilmaz, C., & Scholey, A. (2020). Vitamins and minerals for energy, fatigue and cognition: A narrative review of the biochemical and clinical evidence. *Nutrients*, *12*(1), 228. https://doi.org/10.3390/ nu12010228

33 Guo, R., Gu, J., Zong, S., Wu, M., & Yang, M. (2018). Structure and mechanism of mitochondrial electron transport chain. *Biomedical Journal*, *41*(1), 9–20. https://doi.org/ 10.1016/j.bj.2017.12.001

34 Gasparrini, M., Sorci, L. & Raffaelli, N. (2021). Enzymology of extracellular NAD metabolism. *Cellular and Molecular Life Sciences*. *78*, 3317–3331. https://doi.org/ 10.1007/s00018–020-03742-1

35 Giancaspero, T.A., Busco, G., Panebianco, C., Carmone, C., Miccolis, A., Liuzzi, G.M., Colella, M., & Barile, M. (2013). FAD synthesis and degradation in the nucleus create a local flavin cofactor pool. *The Journal of Biological Chemistry*, *288*(40), 29069–29080. https://doi.org/10.1074/jbc.M113.500066

36 Zhao, R.Z., Jiang, S., Zhang, L., & Yu, Z.B. (2019). Mitochondrial electron transport chain, ROS generation and uncoupling (Review). *International Journal of Molecular Medicine*, *44*(1), 3–15. https://doi.org/10.3892/ijmm.2019.4188

37 Ruprecht, J.J., King, M.S., Zögg, T., Aleksandrova, A.A., Pardon, E., Crichton, P.G., Steyaert, J., & Kunji, E. (2019). The molecular mechanism of transport by the mitochondrial ADP/ATP carrier. *Cell*, *176*(3), 435–447.e15. https://doi.org/10.1016/ j.cell.2018.11.025

38 Deshpande, O.A., & Mohiuddin, S.S. (2022). *Biochemistry, Oxidative Phosphorylation*. In: StatPearls [Internet]. Treasure Island (FL): StatPearls Publishing; Available from: https://www.ncbi.nlm.nih.gov/books/NBK553192/

39 Rustin, P., Munnich, A., & Rötig, A. (2002). Succinate dehydrogenase and human diseases: New insights into a well-known enzyme. *European Journal of Human Genetics: EJHG*, *10*(5), 289–291. https://doi.org/10.1038/sj.ejhg.5200793

40 Eastwood, M. (2003). *Principles of Human Nutrition* (2nd ed.). Hoboken, New Jersey: Wiley-Blackwell.

41 Murray, B., & Rosenbloom, C. (2018). Fundamentals of glycogen metabolism for coaches and athletes. *Nutrition Reviews*, *76*(4), 243–259. https://doi.org/10.1093/nutrit/ nuy001

42 Berg, J.M., Tymoczko, J.L., & Stryer, L. (2002). *Biochemistry*. 5th edition. New York: W H Freeman. Chapter 21, Glycogen Metabolism. Available from: https://www.ncbi. nlm.nih.gov/books/NBK21190/

43 Adeva-Andany, M.M., González-Lucán, M., Donapetry-García, C., Fernández-Fernández, C., & Ameneiros-Rodríguez, E. (2016). Glycogen metabolism in humans. *BBA Clinical*, *5*, 85–100. https://doi.org/10.1016/j.bbacli.2016.02.001

44 Talley, J.T., & Mohiuddin, S.S. (2022). *Biochemistry, Fatty Acid Oxidation*. In: *StatPearls* [Internet]. Treasure Island (FL): StatPearls. Available from: https://www. ncbi.nlm.nih.gov/books/NBK556002/

45 Choe, S.S., Huh, J.Y., Hwang, I.J., Kim, J.I., & Kim, J.B. (2016). Adipose tissue remodeling: Its role in energy metabolism and metabolic disorders. *Frontiers in Endocrinology, 7*, 30. https://doi.org/10.3389/fendo.2016.00030

46 Lass, A., Zimmermann, R., Oberer, M., & Zechner, R. (2011). Lipolysis – A highly regulated multi-enzyme complex mediates the catabolism of cellular fat stores. *Progress in Lipid Research, 50*(1), 14–27. https://doi.org/10.1016/j.plipres.2010.10.004

47 Shah, A., Wang, Y., Su, X., & Wondisford, F.E. (2022). Glycerol's contribution to lactate production outside of a glucose intermediate in fasting humans. *Metabolism: Clinical and Experimental, 132*, 155214. https://doi.org/10.1016/j.metabol.2022.155214

48 Silva, Y.P., Bernardi, A., & Frozza, R.L. (2020). The role of short-chain fatty acids from gut microbiota in gut-brain communication. *Frontiers in Endocrinology, 11*, 25. https://doi.org/10.3389/fendo.2020.00025

49 Erasmus, U., (1993). *Fats that Heal Fats that Kill*; Section 3:16. Burnaby BC Canada: Alive Books.

50 de Carvalho, C., & Caramujo, M.J. (2018). The various roles of fatty acids. *Molecules, 23*(10), 2583. https://doi.org/10.3390/molecules23102583

51 Bhathena, S.J. (2006). Relationship between fatty acids and the endocrine and neuroendocrine system. *Nutritional Neuroscience, 9*(1–2), 1–10. https://doi.org/10.1080/10284150600627128

52 Erasmus, U. (1993). *Fats that Heal Fats that Kill*; Section 2:3. Burnaby BC Canada: Alive Books.

53 Grevengoed, T.J., Klett, E.L., & Coleman, R.A. (2014). Acyl-CoA metabolism and partitioning. *Annual Review of Nutrition, 34*, 1–30. https://doi.org/10.1146/annurev-nutr-071813-105541

54 Lee, H., Ahn, J., Shin, S.S., & Yoon, M. (2019). Ascorbic acid inhibits visceral obesity and nonalcoholic fatty liver disease by activating peroxisome proliferator-activated receptor α in high-fat-diet-fed C57BL/6 J mice. *International Journal of Obesity, 43*, 1620–1630. https://doi.org/10.1038/s41366-018-0212-0

55 Zhu, J., Wu, Y., Tang, Q., Leng, Y., & Cai, W. (2014). The effects of choline on hepatic lipid metabolism, mitochondrial function and antioxidative status in human hepatic C3A cells exposed to excessive energy substrates. *Nutrients, 6*(7), 2552–2571. https://doi.org/10.3390/nu6072552

56 Spinelli, J.B., & Haigis, M.C. (2018). The multifaceted contributions of mitochondria to cellular metabolism. *Nature Cell Biology, 20*(7), 745–754. https://doi.org/10.1038/s41556-018-0124-1

57 Alberts, B., Johnson, A., Lewis, J., et al. (2002). *Molecular Biology of the Cell.* 4th edition. New York: Garland Science. The Shape and Structure of Proteins. Available from: https://www.ncbi.nlm.nih.gov/books/NBK26830/

58 Watford, M., & Wu, G. (2018). Protein. *Advances in Nutrition, 9*(5), 651–653. https://doi.org/10.1093/advances/nmy027

59 Gurina, T.S., & Mohiuddin, S.S. *Biochemistry, Protein Catabolism.* (2021). In: *StatPearls* [Internet]. Treasure Island (FL): StatPearls Publishing. Available from: https://www.ncbi.nlm.nih.gov/books/NBK556047/

60 Wyka, J., Malczyk, E., Misiarz, M., Zołoteńka-Synowiec, M., Całyniuk, B., & Baczyńska, S. (2015). Assessment of food intakes for women adopting the high protein Dukan diet. *Roczniki Panstwowego Zakladu Higieny, 66*(2), 137–142. PMID: 26024402. http://wydawnictwa.pzh.gov.pl/roczniki_pzh/download-article?id=1073

61 Pesta, D.H., & Samuel, V.T. (2014). A high-protein diet for reducing body fat: Mechanisms and possible caveats. *Nutrition & Metabolism, 11*(1), 53. https://doi.org/10.1186/1743-7075-11-53

62 Kerns, J.C., & Gutierrez, J.L. (2017). Thiamin. *Advances in Nutrition, 8*(2), 395–397. https://doi.org/10.3945/an.116.013979

63 Mason, P. (2007). *Dietary Supplements* (Third Edition). London: Pharmaceutical Press.

64 Baker, H., DeAngelis, B., Holland, B., Gittens-Williams, L., & Barrett, T., Jr (2002). Vitamin profile of 563 gravidas during trimesters of pregnancy. *Journal of the American College of Nutrition, 21*(1), 33–37. https://doi.org/10.1080/07315724.2002.10719191

65 Kerns, J.C., Arundel, C., & Chawla, L.S. (2015). Thiamin deficiency in people with obesity. *Advances in Nutrition, 6*(2), 147–153. https://doi.org/10.3945/an.114.007526

66 Nix, W.A., Zirwes, R., Bangert, V., Kaiser, R.P., Schilling, M., Hostalek, U., & Obeid, R. (2015). Vitamin B status in patients with type 2 diabetes mellitus with and without incipient nephropathy. *Diabetes Research and Clinical Practice, 107*(1), 157–165. https://doi.org/10.1016/j.diabres.2014.09.058

67 Marrs, C., & Lonsdale, D., (2021) Hiding in plain sight: Modern thiamine deficiency. *Cells, 10*(10), 2595. https://doi.org/10.3390/cells10102595

68 Sang, S., Pan, X., Chen, Z., Zeng, F., Pan, S., Liu, H., Jin, L., Fei, G., Wang, C., Ren, S., Jiao, F., Bao, W., Zhou, W., Guan, Y., Zhang, Y., Shi, H., Wang, Y., Yu, X., Wang, Y., & Zhong, C. (2018). Thiamine diphosphate reduction strongly correlates with brain glucose hypometabolism in Alzheimer's disease, whereas amyloid deposition does not. *Alzheimer's Research & Therapy, 10*(1), 26. https://doi.org/10.1186/s13195-018-0354-2

69 Gibson, G.E., Hirsch, J.A., Fonzetti, P., Jordan, B.D., Cirio, R.T., & Elder, J. (2016). Vitamin B1 (thiamine) and dementia. *Annals of the New York Academy of Sciences, 1367*(1), 21–30. https://doi.org/10.1111/nyas.13031

70 Håglin, L., Domellöf, M., Bäckman, L., & Forsgren, L. (2020). Low plasma thiamine and phosphate in male patients with Parkinson's disease is associated with mild cognitive impairment. *Clinical Nutrition ESPEN, 37*, 93–99. https://doi.org/10.1016/j.clnesp.2020.03.012

71 Derbyshire, E. (2019). UK dietary changes over the last two decades: A focus on vitamin and mineral intakes. *Journal of Vitamins and Minerals, 2*(2), 104. https://www.gavinpublishers.com/articles/research-article/Journal-of-Vitamins-Minerals/uk-dietary-changes-over-the-last-two-decades-a-focus-on-vitamin-mineral-intakes

72 Derbyshire, E. (2018). Micronutrient intakes of British adults across mid-life: A secondary analysis of the UK National Diet and Nutrition Survey. *Frontiers in Nutrition, 5*, 55. https://doi.org/10.3389/fnut.2018.00055

73 Sepúlveda Cisternas, I., Salazar, J.C., & García-Angulo, V.A. (2018). Overview on the bacterial iron-riboflavin metabolic axis. *Frontiers in Microbiology, 9*, 1478. https://doi.org/10.3389/fmicb.2018.01478

74 NICE (2021). Anaemia – Iron deficiency: How common is it? https://cks.nice.org.uk/topics/anaemia-iron-deficiency/background-information/prevalence/

75 Wall, J.S., Carpenter, K.J. (1988). Variation in availability of niacin in grain products; Changes in chemical composition during grain development and processing affect the nutritional availability of niacin. *Food Technology,* October, 198–204. https://pubag.nal.usda.gov/download/23799/pdf

76 Chamlagain, B., Rautio, S., Edelmann, M., Ollilainen, V., & Piironen, V. (2020). Niacin contents of cereal-milling products in food-composition databases need to be updated. *Journal of Food Composition and Analysis, 91*, 103518. https://doi.org/10.1016/j.jfca.2020.103518

77 Bakaloudi, D.R., Halloran, A., Rippin, H.L., Oikonomidou, A.C., Dardavesis, T.I., Williams, J., Wickramasinghe, K., Breda, J., & Chourdakis, M. (2021). Intake and adequacy of the vegan diet. A systematic review of the evidence. *Clinical Nutrition, 40*(5), 3503–3521. https://doi.org/10.1016/j.clnu.2020.11.035

78 Schüpbach, R., Wegmüller, R., Berguerand, C., Bui, M., & Herter-Aeberli, I. (2017). Micronutrient status and intake in omnivores, vegetarians and vegans in Switzerland. *European Journal of Nutrition, 56*(1), 283–293. https://doi.org/10.1007/s00394-015-1079-7

79 Janssen, J., Grefte, S., Keijer, J., & de Boer, V. (2019). Mito-nuclear communication by mitochondrial metabolites and its regulation by B-vitamins. *Frontiers in Physiology, 10*, 78. https://doi.org/10.3389/fphys.2019.00078

80 Folkers, K. (1996). Relevance of the biosynthesis of coenzyme Q10 and of the four bases of DNA as a rationale for the molecular causes of cancer and a therapy. *Biochemical and Biophysical Research Communications, 224*(2), 358–361. https://doi.org/10.1006/bbrc.1996.1033

81 Rizzo, G., Laganà, A.S., Rapisarda, A.M., La Ferrera, G.M., Buscema, M., Rossetti, P., Nigro, A., Muscia, V., Valenti, G., Sapia, F., Sarpietro, G., Zigarelli, M., & Vitale, S.G. (2016). Vitamin B12 among vegetarians: Status, assessment and supplementation. *Nutrients, 8*(12), 767. https://doi.org/10.3390/nu8120767

82 Department of Health and Social Care (2021). Folic acid to be added to flour to prevent spinal conditions in babies. https://www.gov.uk/government/news/folic-acid-added-to-flour-to-prevent-spinal-conditions-in-babies

83 Corbin, K.D., & Zeisel, S.H. (2012). Choline metabolism provides novel insights into nonalcoholic fatty liver disease and its progression. *Current Opinion in Gastroenterology, 28*(2), 159–165. https://doi.org/10.1097/MOG.0b013e32834e7b4b

84 Derbyshire, E. (2019). Could we be overlooking a potential choline crisis in the United Kingdom?. *BMJ Nutrition, Prevention & Health, 2*(2), 86–89. https://doi.org/10.1136/bmjnph-2019-000037

85 Vennemann, F.B., Ioannidou, S., Valsta, L.M., Dumas, C., Ocké, M.C., Mensink, G.B., Lindtner, O., Virtanen, S.M., Tlustos, C., D'Addezio, L., Mattison, I., Dubuisson, C., Siksna, I., & Héraud, F. (2015). Dietary intake and food sources of choline in European populations. *The British Journal of Nutrition, 114*(12), 2046–2055. https://doi.org/10.1017/S0007114515003700

86 Institute of Medicine (US) Standing Committee on the Scientific Evaluation of Dietary Reference Intakes and its Panel on Folate, Other B Vitamins, and Choline. (1998). *Dietary Reference Intakes for Thiamin, Riboflavin, Niacin, Vitamin B6, Folate, Vitamin B12, Pantothenic Acid, Biotin, and Choline*. National Academies Press (US). Washington DC. https://nap.nationalacademies.org/catalog/6015/dietary-reference-intakes-for-thiamin-riboflavin-niacin-vitamin-b6-folate-vitamin-b12-pantothenic-acid-biotin-and-choline

87 Veg Facts 2021 (2021). The Food Foundation. https://foodfoundation.org.uk/publication/veg-facts-2021/

88 Department of Health (1991). *Dietary Reference Values: A Guide.* https://assets.publishing.service.gov.uk/government/uploads/system/uploads/attachment_data/file/743790/Dietary_Reference_Values_-_A_Guide__1991_.pdf

89 Frei, B., Birlouez-Aragon, I., & Lykkesfeldt, J. (2012). Authors' perspective: What is the optimum intake of vitamin C in humans?. *Critical Reviews in Food Science and Nutrition, 52*(9), 815–829. https://doi.org/10.1080/10408398.2011.649149

90 Public Health England (2019). NDNS: Time trend and income analyses for Years 1 to 9: Report. https://assets.publishing.service.gov.uk/government/uploads/system/uploads/attachment_data/file/772434/NDNS_UK_Y1–9_report.pdf

91 Mosdøl, A., Erens, B., & Brunner, E.J. (2008). Estimated prevalence and predictors of vitamin C deficiency within UK's low-income population. *Journal of Public Health, 30*(4), 456–460. https://doi.org/10.1093/pubmed/fdn076

92 NHS Digital (2021). Admissions for scurvy, rickets and malnutrition, 2007–08 to 2020–21. https://digital.nhs.uk/binaries/content/assets/website-assets/supplementary-information/supplementary-info-2021/10977_scurvy_rickets_malnutrition_update_oct2021.xlsx

93 Clapham, D.E. (2007). Calcium signalling. *Cell 13*(6), 1047–1058. https://doi.org/10.1016/j.cell.2007.11.028

94 Tammineni, E.R., Kraeva, N., Figueroa, L., Manno, C., Ibarra, C. A., Klip, A., Riazi, S., & Rios, E. (2020). Intracellular calcium leak lowers glucose storage in human muscle, promoting hyperglycemia and diabetes. *eLife, 9*, e53999. https://doi.org/10.7554/eLife.53999

95 Oexle, H., Gnaiger, E., & Weiss, G. (1999). Iron-dependent changes in cellular energy metabolism: Influence on citric acid cycle and oxidative phosphorylation. *Biochimica et Biophysica Acta, 1413*(3), 99–107. https://doi.org/10.1016/s0005-2728(99)00088-2

96 Paul, B.T., Manz, D.H., Torti, F.M., & Torti, S.V. (2017). Mitochondria and Iron: Current questions. *Expert Review of Hematology, 10*(1), 65–79. https://doi.org/10.1080/17474086.2016.1268047

97 Milman, N.T. (2019). Dietary iron intake in women of reproductive age in Europe: A review of 49 studies from 29 countries in the period 1993–2015. *Journal of Nutrition and Metabolism, 2019*, 7631306. https://doi.org/10.1155/2019/7631306

98 Derbyshire, E. (2017). Associations between red meat intakes and the micronutrient intake and status of UK females: A secondary analysis of the UK National Diet and Nutrition Survey. *Nutrients, 9*(7), 768. https://doi.org/10.3390/nu9070768

99 Fiorentini, D., Cappadone, C., Farruggia, G., & Prata, C. (2021). Magnesium: Biochemistry, nutrition, detection, and social impact of diseases linked to its deficiency. *Nutrients, 13*(4), 1136. https://doi.org/10.3390/nu13041136

100 Yamanaka, R., Tabata, S., Shindo, Y., Hotta, K., Suzuki, K., Soga, T., & Oka, K. (2016). Mitochondrial Mg(2+) homeostasis decides cellular energy metabolism and vulnerability to stress. *Scientific Reports, 6*, 30027. https://doi.org/10.1038/srep30027

101 Li, L., & Yang, X. (2018). The essential element manganese, oxidative stress, and metabolic diseases: Links and interactions. *Oxidative Medicine and Cellular Longevity, 2018*, 7580707. https://doi.org/10.1155/2018/7580707

102 Chen, P., Bornhorst, J., & Aschner, M. (2018). Manganese metabolism in humans. *Frontiers in Bioscience (Landmark edition), 23*, 1655–1679. https://doi.org/10.2741/4665

103 Aschner, M., & Erikson, K. (2017). Manganese. *Advances in Nutrition, 8*(3), 520–521. https://doi.org/10.3945/an.117.015305

104 Xie, N., Zhang, L., Gao, W., Huang, C., Huber, P.E., Zhou, X., Li, C., Shen, G., & Zou, B. (2020). NAD$^+$ metabolism: Pathophysiologic mechanisms and therapeutic potential. *Signal Transduction and Targeted Therapy, 5*(1), 227. https://doi.org/10.1038/s41392-020-00311-7

105 Yee, J., Rosenbaum, D., Jacobs, J.W., & Sprague, S.M. (2021). Small intestinal phosphate absorption: Novel therapeutic implications. *American Journal of Nephrology, 52*(7), 522–530. https://doi.org/10.1159/000518110

106 St-Jules, D.E., Jagannathan, R., Gutekunst, L., Kalantar-Zadeh, K., & Sevick, M.A. (2017). Examining the proportion of dietary phosphorus from plants, animals, and food additives excreted in urine. *Journal of Renal Nutrition, 27*(2), 78–83. https://doi.org/10.1053/j.jrn.2016.09.003

107 Saini, R. (2011). Coenzyme Q10: The essential nutrient. *Journal of Pharmacy & Bio-Allied Sciences, 3*(3), 466–467. https://doi.org/10.4103/0975-7406.84471

108 Pravst, I., Zmitek, K., & Zmitek, J. (2010). Coenzyme Q10 contents in foods and fortification strategies. *Critical Reviews in Food Science and Nutrition, 50*(4), 269–280. https://doi.org/10.1080/10408390902773037

109 Alcázar-Fabra, M., Navas, P., & Brea-Calvo, G. (2016). Coenzyme Q biosynthesis and its role in the respiratory chain structure. *Biochimica et Biophysica Acta, 1857*(8), 1073–1078. https://doi.org/10.1016/j.bbabio.2016.03.010

110 Barcelos, I.P., & Haas, R.H. (2019). CoQ10 and aging. *Biology, 8*(2), 28. https://doi.org/10.3390/biology8020028

111 Hargreaves, I., Heaton, R.A., & Mantle, D. (2020). Disorders of human coenzyme Q10 metabolism: An overview. *International Journal of Molecular Sciences, 21*(18), 6695. https://doi.org/10.3390/ijms21186695

112 Deichmann, R., Lavie, C., & Andrews, S. (2010). Coenzyme q10 and statin-induced mitochondrial dysfunction. *The Ochsner Journal, 10*(1), 16–21.

113 Derosa, G., D'Angelo, A., & Maffioli, P. (2019). Coenzyme q10 liquid supplementation in dyslipidemic subjects with statin-related clinical symptoms: A double-blind, randomized, placebo-controlled study. *Drug Design, Development and Therapy, 13*, 3647–3655. https://doi.org/10.2147/DDDT.S223153

114 Arenas-Jal, M., Suñé-Negre, J.M., & García-Montoya, E. (2020). Coenzyme Q10 supplementation: Efficacy, safety, and formulation challenges. *Comprehensive Reviews in Food Science and Food Safety, 19*(2), 574–594. https://doi.org/10.1111/1541-4337.12539

115 Hanel, A., & Carlberg, C. (2020). Vitamin D and evolution: Pharmacologic implications. *Biochemical Pharmacology, 173*, 113595. https://doi.org/10.1016/j.bcp.2019.07.024

116 Ricca, C., Aillon, A., Bergandi, L., Alotto, D., Castagnoli, C., & Silvagno, F. (2018). Vitamin D receptor is necessary for mitochondrial function and cell health. *International Journal of Molecular Sciences, 19*(6), 1672. https://doi.org/10.3390/ijms19061672

117 Latham, C.M., Brightwell, C.R., Keeble, A.R., Munson, B.D., Thomas, N.T., Zagzoog, A.M., Fry, C.S., & Fry, J.L. (2021). Vitamin D promotes skeletal muscle regeneration and mitochondrial health. *Frontiers in Physiology, 12*, 660498. https://doi.org/10.3389/fphys.2021.660498

118 Wimalawansa, S.J. (2019). Vitamin D deficiency: Effects on oxidative stress, epigenetics, gene regulation, and aging. *Biology, 8*(2), 30. https://doi.org/10.3390/biology8020030

119 Roy, S., Sherman, A., Monari-Sparks, M.J., Schweiker, O., & Hunter, K. (2014). Correction of low vitamin D improves fatigue: Effect of correction of low vitamin D in Fatigue Study (EViDiF Study). *North American Journal of Medical Sciences, 6*(8), 396–402. https://doi.org/10.4103/1947-2714.139291

120 Shaheen, N.A., Alqahtani, A.A., Assiri, H., Alkhodair, R., & Hussein, M.A. (2018). Public knowledge of dehydration and fluid intake practices: Variation by participants' characteristics. *BMC Public Health, 18*(1), 1346. https://doi.org/10.1186/s12889-018-6252-5

121 Jéquier, E., & Constant, F. (2010). Water as an essential nutrient: The physiological basis of hydration. *European Journal of Clinical Nutrition, 64*(2), 115–123. https://doi.org/10.1038/ejcn.2009.111

122 Armstrong, L.E., & Johnson, E.C. (2018). Water intake, water balance, and the elusive daily water requirement. *Nutrients, 10*(12), 1928. https://doi.org/10.3390/nu10121928

123 Briggs, F. (2021). New study by Aqua Pura reveals majority of UK is dehydrated. *Retail Times.* https://www.retailtimes.co.uk/new-study-by-aqua-pura-reveals-majority-of-uk-is-dehydrated/

124 NHS Live Well (2021). Water, drinks and your health. https://www.nhs.uk/live-well/eat-well/food-guidelines-and-food-labels/water-drinks-nutrition/

125 Alahmary, S.A., Alduhaylib, S.A., Alkawii, H.A., Olwani, M.M., Shablan, R.A., Ayoub, H.M., Purayidathil, T.S., Abuzaid, O.I., & Khattab, R.Y. (2019). Relationship between added sugar intake and sleep quality among university students: A cross-sectional study. *American Journal of Lifestyle Medicine, 16*(1), 122–129. https://doi.org/10.1177/1559827619870476

126 St-Onge, M.P., Mikic, A., & Pietrolungo, C.E. (2016). Effects of diet on sleep quality. *Advances in Nutrition, 7*(5), 938–949. https://doi.org/10.3945/an.116.012336

127 Tanaka, M., Mizuno, K., Fukuda, S., Shigihara, Y., & Watanabe, Y. (2008). Relationships between dietary habits and the prevalence of fatigue in medical students. *Nutrition, 24*(10), 985–989. https://doi.org/10.1016/j.nut.2008.05.003

9 Different Ways of Eating

There are more than seven and a half billion people on the planet. Most of them eat a mixed diet of meat, fish, poultry, other animal products, fruit, vegetables, and starchy foods, generally grains and or tubers. Although that is starting to change. Globally sales of ultra-processed food are booming, across all age groups, in wealthy and middle-income countries, and even in some lower-income countries in Asia, Africa and Latin America.[1] And, as discussed in Chapter 4, these sales are driving an obesity crisis. But only in the privileged, affluent West do we see entire industries seeking to sell us an idea of the "right" way to eat.

Even though changing our eating patterns is not easy, different ways of eating are on the rise. Over the last decade, increasing numbers of people in the UK have started to revise the way they eat, changing the foods they chose to eat, as well as the timing and patterns of consumption. Sometimes changes are short-term, seeking weight loss. Sometimes people make a real commitment to transform their diet long term. And sometimes, what started as a short-term effort can evolve into long-term change.

The trouble is, when people move away from traditional eating patterns, dietary changes can be made without really thinking them through. All too often there is no clear understanding that whilst benefits may emerge from the changes being made, there can also be risks. This chapter looks at some of the more popular "new" ways of eating that are currently gaining ground in the UK.

MEDITERRANEAN DIET

In the early 1950s, the American biologist Ancel Keys noticed that comparatively poor people living in Italy were far healthier than their relations who happened to be living in the far wealthier United States. His investigations led, in 1975, to the publication of a book, *How to Eat Well and Stay Well, the Mediterranean Way.*[2] But it wasn't until the 1990s, when vested interests, including the International Olive Oil Council, started to promote it, that the diet began to gain ground and become widely popular.[3]

The Mediterranean diet as we now know it is an amalgamation of the traditional diets of many different cultures from the countries around the Mediterranean. It is not as prescriptive as many other "diets". It advocates high consumption of fruit, vegetables, whole grains, legumes, fish, eggs, some dairy products, moderate intake of meat, olive oil, and wine, and the avoidance of processed foods.[4] It is promoted as one of the healthiest ways to eat and it does appear to be protective against cardiovascular disease, type II diabetes and metabolic syndrome, and obesity.[5] It may also reduce the incidence of some cancers

DOI: 10.1201/b22900-10

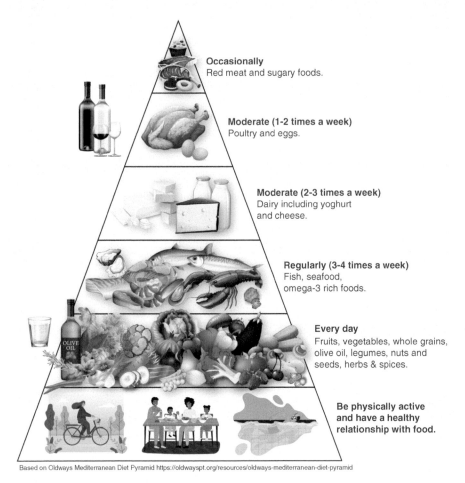

Occasionally
Red meat and sugary foods.

Moderate (1-2 times a week)
Poultry and eggs.

Moderate (2-3 times a week)
Dairy including yoghurt
and cheese.

Regularly (3-4 times a week)
Fish, seafood,
omega-3 rich foods.

Every day
Fruits, vegetables, whole grains,
olive oil, legumes, nuts and
seeds, herbs & spices.

**Be physically active
and have a healthy
relationship with food.**

Based on Oldways Mediterranean Diet Pyramid https://oldwayspt.org/resources/oldways-mediterranean-diet-pyramid

The Mediterranean diet food pyramid.

and protect cognitive function.[6] It is ironic that, as the Mediterranean diet is gaining ground in many western countries, it is currently under threat in the countries it originated in because ultra-processed food is seen by too many as easier and more convenient.[7]

Because it has few definitive "rules" and focuses less on the quantity of food consumed and more on the quality many people find it relatively easy to maintain over the long term. However, some elements of the diet, such as the inclusion of legumes and fish, are seen as problematic in the UK because these foods are not widely consumed here.[8] It can also be viewed as expensive because of the emphasis on fresh ingredients.[9]

The Mediterranean diet is beneficial to overall health and wellbeing without being overly restrictive. Its broad spectrum of foods means that it is one of the very few "diets" that can be considered both varied and balanced and is easy to maintain over the long term.

THE FLEXITARIAN DIET

Flexitarian eating is a relatively recent idea, devised by a dietician in 2008. The idea of flexible eating is very appealing, and it has been growing steadily ever since. The desire to reduce meat intakes because of perceived health benefits, and or environmental concerns seem to be key drivers to its growth.[10]

The flexitarian diet is sometimes called a semi-vegetarian diet because it allows some limited meat, poultry, and fish consumption. It is all about flexibility; there are no hard and fast rules, no calorie counting and no prohibited foods, although sweets and foods with added sugar are not encouraged. Instead, flexitarianism advocates eating the least processed food possible, with lots of fruit, vegetables, legumes, whole grains, eggs, dairy, and occasional meat, poultry, and fish.

Intake of meat in the UK has reduced by 17% over the last decade and this downward trend looks set to continue.[11] It is partially driven by British consumers seeking to make their diet more sustainable by reducing their intake of animal products, as well as concerns about animal welfare and a belief that reducing meat intake will be beneficial to health.[12,13] Indeed 13% of UK consumers consider themselves to be flexitarian, whilst 68% are actively trying to reduce their meat intake.[14]

There are some clear health benefits to following a flexitarian diet. Increasing intakes of plant foods and reducing intakes of red meat reduces the risk of all-cause mortality.[15] A flexitarian diet is effective in stimulating and sustaining weight loss, in supporting metabolic health, and in maintaining blood pressure at healthy levels.[16] Flexitarian diets may also reduce the risk of type II diabetes and cardiovascular disease.[17,18] And eating a flexitarian diet may be more protective against colorectal cancers than any other dietary pattern, including following a vegan or vegetarian diet.[19] This may be because the consumption of dairy products is generally protective against all forms of colorectal cancers.[20]

As with most significant dietary changes, there are some potential risks. Reducing intakes of animal products can also mean reducing intakes of some key micronutrients.[21] But because a flexitarian diet includes animal products, the risk is small.

The flexitarian diet also has a positive impact on the microbiome.[22] Flexitarian intake of plant foods is far higher than an average omnivorous diet and increases the overall intake of fibre, which is key to the health and wellbeing of the microbiome.[23]

There is not, as yet, a huge amount of research on the flexitarian diet, but what there is appears to be extremely positive. Because animal products are not prohibited there is less consumption of ultra-processed plant-based meat alternatives. And, unlike many diets, it seems to be sustainable in the long term.

VEGETARIANISM AND VEGANISM

Vegetarianism and veganism have a long tradition on the Indian subcontinent, particularly among Hindus, Jains, Sikhs, and Buddhists. East Asia and Europe also have traditions of abstaining from eating meat, but these were more limited, generally restricted to specific days or periods within a religious calendar. In the modern world, the motivating factors for vegetarianism and veganism include mitigating climate change, concerns about animal welfare, and the claimed health benefits of a plant-based diet.

Our ancestors spent several million years eating animals; long before *Homo sapiens* were hunting, they were scavenging kills made by larger animals. We know this because there are thousands of stone tools associated with the bones of those scavenged kills.[24] Initially hunting was probably opportunistic, but it became increasingly deliberate and efficient.[25] And around 11,000 years ago we started domesticating animals, which changed most of human society forever.[26]

The design, volume, and function of our digestive tract is adapted to enable us to consume almost anything that is not toxic. Our teeth evolved to accommodate a diet consisting of both animal- and plant-based foods.[27] Acidity in the human stomach is higher than most omnivores, and new research suggests that humanity's diet during our early evolution was meat heavy.[28] Eating lots of difficult to digest bulky plant foods needs sizable stomachs (sometimes two) and intestines to ferment cellulose-based foods, making nutrients more available. Eating easier to digest, nutrient dense animal foods requires a much smaller, less energy demanding, gut.[29] The overall size of *Homo sapiens'* GI tract is the smallest of the great apes, suggesting that plant food was a secondary source of nutrition through much of humanity's evolution.[30]

In the last century civilisation and society have changed and developed in extraordinary ways. But our biochemical and nutritional requirements remain the same as they have always been.

JUNK FOOD VEGETARIANS

Being a vegetarian is supposed to mean that you eat actual vegetables. Plus nuts and seeds and legumes and tubers and whole grains and fruit and seaweeds, and even more vegetables. But the modern version of plant-based eating does not necessarily lead to an increase of fruit and vegetable intake.

Contemporary vegetarians and vegans often eat pre-prepared, highly processed meat substitutes and ready meals. Many plant-based meat alternatives (PBMAs) are ultra-processed, containing up to 30 different factory produced ingredients instead of a single natural ingredient (meat). Vegans and vegetarians often eat a far higher proportion of ultra-processed foods than omnivores or pescatarians (who eat plant foods and fish, but no meat).[31]

The growth in PBMAs is concerning because, from a nutrition perspective, these alternatives are not equivalent to actual meat. Some substances found in meat do not occur in PBMAs, whilst some substances in PBMAs are not found in meat.[32] A recent evaluation of PBMAs found that most contained too little calcium, potassium, magnesium, zinc, and B12, but contained high levels of highly processed fat, salt, and sugar.[33] And not only is protein from PBMAs not as well absorbed as protein from animals, PBMAs also contain fewer essential and non-essential amino acids than animal products.[34]

POTENTIAL NUTRIENT SHORTFALLS IN VEGETARIAN DIETS

There are concerns about nutrient shortfalls in vegetarian and vegan diets, particularly vitamins A, B2, B3, B6, B12, and D and the minerals iron, calcium, iodine, selenium, and zinc.[35] In addition, intakes of the phospholipid choline and the omega-3 fatty acids can be low in vegan and vegetarian diets.

VITAMIN A

Within a vegan or vegetarian diet, only the β-carotene form of vitamin A, from brightly coloured plant foods, can form part of the diet. The body converts β-carotene to retinol, but high fibre intake with any food containing β-carotene, and low levels of zinc and iron can reduce, or even prevent the conversion of β-carotene to retinol.[36] In addition, the conversion of β-carotene to retinol decreases as levels of β-carotene increase – so the more β-carotene that is consumed, the less will be converted into retinol.[37] Vegans in particular often have low plasma levels of vitamin A.[38,39]

B VITAMINS

Vitamin B12 only occurs in foods of animal origin and artificially fortified foods like breakfast cereals or nutritional yeast. Up to 80% of vegans, and 40% of vegetarians who do not eat fortified foods or take food supplements, are deficient in B12.[40] Although many vegetarians and vegans are aware of concerns around B12, most are not aware of other B vitamins. Riboflavin, niacin, and pyridoxine derive primarily from animal foods and vegetarians and vegans are particularly vulnerable to deficiency in these nutrients.[41,42] The phospholipid choline can also be difficult to obtain from plant-based diets and both vegetarians and vegans are at risk of inadequate intakes of this nutrient.[43,44]

VITAMIN D

There are two forms of dietary vitamin D: vitamin D3 from animals and vitamin D2 from plants. D3 is more effective at raising blood levels of the active form of vitamin D.[45] Intakes of vitamin D is low in all UK populations.[46] However, the limited availability of vitamin D from plant foods means many vegetarians and vegans have particularly low intakes, and vitamin D deficiency is often reported in vegan populations.[47]

OMEGA-3

Of the three key omega-3 fatty acids, alpha-linolenic acid (ALA) is the only one widely found in plant foods. Eicosapentaenoic acid (EPA) and docosahexaenoic acid (DHA) are primarily found in oily fish, although some varieties of seaweed and marine algae do contain a limited amount.[48] ALA provides the substrate for EPA and DHA synthesis, but conversion is very inefficient in humans and when conversion is successful, levels of EPA increase slightly, but levels of DHA decline.[49,50] UK intakes of EPA and DHA are inadequate even in non-vegetarian populations, but plasma levels of EPA and DHA in vegetarians and vegans are significantly lower than those seen in omnivores.[51,52]

IRON

Although iron is widely found in plant foods, meat is a far richer source. 200 g of spinach contains around the same amount of iron as 50 g of red meat, and iron from plants is not as well absorbed as iron from meat.[53] The two forms of iron, haem in meat, and non-haem in plants, have very different absorption pathways with the non-haem pathway being more complex and less efficient than the haem pathway. Non-haem iron does not have specific transporters to facilitate absorption, and chemicals called phytates bond with it, forming chelates which prevent absorption.[54,55] Low iron levels are common among vegetarians, even more prevalent among vegans, and particularly concerning among vegetarian and vegan women.[56]

CALCIUM

Plant foods contain plenty of calcium, but plants also contain oxalates and phytates which form chelates with minerals, preventing absorption.[57] Vegetarians and vegans have a lower bone mineral density (BMD) and higher rates of femoral head fracture than omnivores, whilst vegans have lower BMD of the lumbar spine than omnivores or vegetarians.[58,59]

IODINE

The only reliable source of plant-based iodine is seaweed, but levels are widely variable, and eating seaweed can lead to excessive iodine intake.[60] Iodised salt can be a good source, but as there is no UK government policy to ensure deficiency is prevented, it is not readily available here.[61] Intakes of iodine in the UK across all populations tend to be low, but they are particularly low in vegetarians and vegans.[62,63] Iodine intakes among vegan and vegetarian women in the UK are so low that the development and cognitive ability of any children they may have, is at risk.[64]

SELENIUM

The mineral content of plants is dependent on how much of that mineral is in the soil that plants grow in. The soil across Europe, including the UK, is generally selenium poor.[65] Selenium uptake by plants is also dependent on what form the selenium is in, whether it is bound to organic matter which can facilitate uptake, and the microbial communities in the soil which can either block or assist absorption by the plant.[66] Selenium intakes in the UK are generally poor, however, vegetarians and vegans are at particular risk of deficiency because they do not eat animal products and seafood which are some of the richest sources of selenium.[64,67]

ZINC

Although zinc is widely available in plant foods, it needs good quality protein to be absorbed, transported, and utilised.[68] Unfortunately, plant-based protein is often high in phytates, which inhibit zinc absorption.[69] Zinc insufficiency is common in both vegans and vegetarians, although vegans seem particularly at risk of outright zinc deficiency.[59,69] Zinc is needed for iron absorption, so zinc insufficiency will also impact iron status.[70]

Being a healthy vegetarian takes work, cooking real food, and a lot of chewing. Anyone deciding to move to a vegetarian or vegan diet should be advised to include a good quality multivitamin and multimineral, and an algal omega-3 supplement in their daily diet to ensure sufficient micronutrient intakes, at least until they are more confident of the adequacy of their diet.

THE KETO DIET

The keto (ketogenic) diet is a very low carbohydrate diet that restricts carbohydrate intake to less than 50 g/day. It was originally developed in the 1920s to manage epilepsy, and it continues to be used today in patients that do not respond well to pharmaceutical management of the condition.[71]

The idea of low carbohydrate diets for weight loss was popularised in the early 1970s when the book *Dr Atkins' Diet Revolution* became a best seller.[72] Dr Atkins advocated very low carbohydrate, modest protein, and high-fat intakes. Since then interest in ketogenic diets has fluctuated, but in recent years it has become increasingly popular.

Energy from fat is generated through β-oxidation. This produces Acetyl-CoA which enters the Krebs cycle; the molecules NADH and $FADH_2$, which enter the electron transport chain to generate ATP; and the ketone bodies acetoacetate and β-hydroxybutyrate.[73] Through a series of enzymatic reactions, the ketone bodies are converted to acetyl-CoA, which enters the Krebs cycle, and acetone, which is excreted, either through exhalation or urine.[74] The hormones glucagon, cortisol, and thyroxin play a part in this, but the process is primarily regulated by insulin.[75] Low intakes of carbohydrates reduce the levels of circulating insulin. Low levels of circulating insulin promote lipolysis (the metabolic breakdown of fat) and this, in turn, stimulates the production of ketone bodies through β-oxidation.[76]

We produce ketone bodies all the time, they provide energy substrates for the heart, brain, and muscles when other fuel sources are limited, for example, during sleep or during intensive exercise.[77] But the keto diet significantly increases their production, which can create some risks. Although cases are rare, there are reports of starvation ketoacidosis occurring in some individuals (both diabetic and non-diabetic) who have pushed the diet too far.[78,79,80,81]

The body prefers to make use of carbohydrates to generate energy because it is the least metabolically expensive route. Second choice for energy metabolism is fat because, although β-oxidation is more complex than "standard" energy metabolism, fat contains more than double the number of calories of either

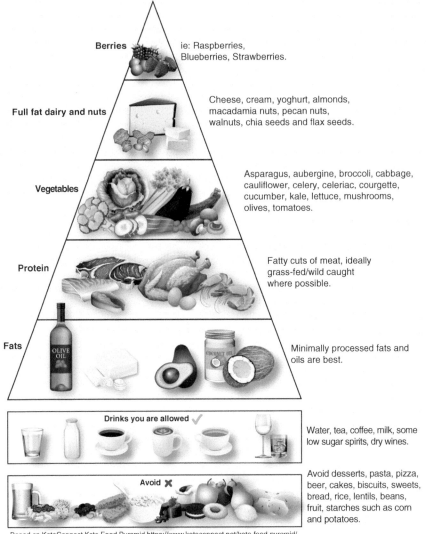

Berries — ie: Raspberries, Blueberries, Strawberries.

Full fat dairy and nuts — Cheese, cream, yoghurt, almonds, macadamia nuts, pecan nuts, walnuts, chia seeds and flax seeds.

Vegetables — Asparagus, aubergine, broccoli, cabbage, cauliflower, celery, celeriac, courgette, cucumber, kale, lettuce, mushrooms, olives, tomatoes.

Protein — Fatty cuts of meat, ideally grass-fed/wild caught where possible.

Fats — Minimally processed fats and oils are best.

Drinks you are allowed ✓ — Water, tea, coffee, milk, some low sugar spirits, dry wines.

Avoid ✗ — Avoid desserts, pasta, pizza, beer, cakes, biscuits, sweets, bread, rice, lentils, beans, fruit, starches such as corn and potatoes.

Based on KetoConnect Keto Food Pyramid https://www.ketoconnect.net/keto-food-pyramid/

The keto diet food pyramid.

carbohydrate or protein.[82] However, if both carbohydrates and fat are in short supply, as a last resort the body will use protein to generate energy.

The nature of the keto diet means that as much protein as possible is used to generate glucose through the process of gluconeogenesis. This can leave little excess for essential repair and maintenance of tissues.[83] And the breakdown of protein for energy increases levels of ammonia in the body, which can put pressure on both the liver and kidneys.[84]

Very low carbohydrate diets can also mean low intakes of fruit and vegetables, all of which contain not only carbohydrates, but also an abundance of vitamins, minerals, phytochemicals, and fibre. Individuals on keto diets can be at risk of insufficient intakes of vitamins A, E and K, thiamin, folate and B6 and the minerals calcium, magnesium, iron, and potassium.[83]

Fibre is also central to the health of the microbiome, and, given the importance of the microbiome, therefore to our own health. There is insufficient evidence to say what impact long-term adherence to a keto diet may have on the health of the microbiome. Studies on humans to date have been both small, and short term which makes studying the impact of anything on the microbiome difficult. The studies which have been carried out have found that low carbohydrate diets tend to reduce the numbers of bacteria which produce short-chain fatty acids, particularly butyrate, which is key to the health and integrity of the gut.[85] This shift in species has also been noted in a study which found that the altered microbial populations reduced the numbers of Th17 immune cells, which fight infectious diseases but which also promote inflammation.[86]

The keto diet does lead to weight loss, although that loss slows or even halts after about five months.[87] Keto diets are helpful in the management of type II diabetes and may reduce the risk of developing metabolic syndrome, a significant risk factor in cardiovascular disease, although here too, studies have been small and short term, which limits the value of the data generated.[88]

As with all restrictive diets, anyone considering following the keto diet should be advised to take a good quality multivitamin and mineral food supplement. Given the impact on the microbiome, it would also be advisable for them to consume fermented foods and a combination of fibre supplements which should include different forms of oligosaccharides.[89]

INTERMITTENT FASTING

Humanity has practiced intermittent fasting for thousands of years. It is part of religious observance in many different faiths, generally taking the form of abstaining from certain foods, or total fasting for specified periods of time. However, the modern idea of intermittent fasting is all about weight loss and/or weight control. It doesn't restrict the types of food that can be eaten, instead it controls the timing of eating.

Some patterns of fasting limit the hours during the day when food can be eaten, for example, the 16:8 diet limits eating to an eight-hour window; the other 16 hours of the day are fasting, although water, coffee, and zero-calorie drinks are permitted. Other intermittent fasts stipulate that calorie intake is restricted on two days out of a week. The recently revised 5:2 diet allows "normal" eating for five days, and then restricts intake to 800 calories on two non-consecutive days.

Intermittent fasting is not always appropriate for everyone. Many people may unconsciously "cheat", eating more calories than they would normally on non-fasting days, in which case the diet is unlikely to lead to weight loss.[90] Humanity's deep and complex relationship with food can make maintaining the diet difficult, particularly over any length of time.[91] There may also be some unpleasant side effects like headaches, constipation, bloating, irritability, and dehydration.[92,93]

The idea that some intermittent fasting regimes advocate the consumption of zero-calorie drinks is concerning. There have been concerns about the health impacts of low-calorie sweeteners for many years and long-term studies are bearing out some of those concerns, including "they give you cancer", the prevalent anxiety from a decade ago. A recent study found that aspartame and acesulfame-K, two of the most widely used sweeteners, do increase overall cancer risk.[94] However, the primary focus for artificial sweeteners and health risks are now focused on the impact on the microbiome and stimulation of inflammation. Some artificial sweeteners stimulate the production of pro-inflammatory chemicals by gut bacteria, while others increase immune reactivity in the gut wall which could trigger inappropriate autoimmune responses.[95] Some also influence glucose metabolism, increasing insulin resistance and impairing glucose homeostasis.[96]

There are some clear benefits to intermittent fasting, although it would probably be best done without the addition of artificial sweeteners. It stimulates weight loss, lowers blood pressure, and can improve insulin sensitivity and blood sugar control.[97,98] However, as is often the case, most studies have been conducted on animals; those run with humans have been relatively small and short term.[99] It can be difficult to maintain a long-term pattern of intermittent fasting and success is limited by compliance.[100] And, as with all weight loss diets, once the diet is no longer being followed, anecdotal evidence suggests that "bounce back" weight gain occurs.

It is also worth remembering that the decision to reduce calorie intake in a time-limited way will not necessarily impact on the quality or nature of the diet during "normal" eating pattern times. An individual could continue to eat a diet composed primarily of ultra-processed food, with limited fruit and vegetables. Low micronutrient intakes from this kind of diet would be compounded by the reduced intake of food during fast days, raising the risk of nutritional insufficiency, or even outright deficiency.[101]

Anyone considering intermittent fasting would be well advised to take a good quality multivitamin and mineral food supplement, along with a fish or algal oil omega-3 supplement.

THE PALAEOLITHIC (PALEO) DIET

The concept of the Palaeolithic diet was dreamed up in the 1970s by a gastro-enterologist. Although it did not really gain popularity until the early 2000s, it is now one of the most popular diets around.[102]

The idea behind the Paleo diet is to eat only what our Palaeolithic ancestors would have eaten, avoiding foods that would not have been available at the time. However, there is huge variability in the types of foods our ancestors would have eaten, depending on where they lived. Diets in coastal, mountain or savannah regions would all have been completely different, as would diets in tropical or northerly latitudes.[103] It is therefore impossible to definitively say exactly what Palaeolithic diets would have been, although they are likely to have included meat from large and small animals; seafood (in coastal and river areas); a wide range of plants including some grains, legumes, and tubers; and insects and their products, for example, honey.[104]

Of course, the foods we eat now bear little resemblance to the foods that our ancestors ate. The claim that Palaeolithic peoples did not eat grains has been debunked, but ancient grains were not the plump, carbohydrate-rich, domesticated grains we know now.[105,106,107] Thousands of years of selective breeding have changed the plant foods that we eat, making them larger, sweeter, and easier to cook and eat.[108] They generally require far less processing to make them edible and most have had toxic substances either reduced or eliminated entirely.[109]

Proponents of the Paleo diet claim that it will help with cholesterol balance, reduce blood pressure, improve glycaemic control, and lead to weight loss. There is some evidence that following the Paleo diet has a positive impact on weight, BMI and waist circumference and that it can lead to short-term improvements in factors linked to metabolic syndrome.[110,111] There is also evidence that the Paleo diet may reduce all-cause mortality, including mortality from cancer and cardiovascular disease, as well as reducing the risks of type II diabetes and high blood pressure.[112,113] But as with many of the diets discussed here, studies are generally neither large enough nor long enough to provide definitive evidence.

The human microbiome is not reacting well to the modern world, with our highly processed diet, wide use of antibiotics and overly sanitised lives.[114,115] This has led to the development of a theory that a Paleo diet could support a more beneficial microbiome with greater diversity, although there are concerns that the elimination of grains and legumes from the diet alters the profile of fibre, and therefore prebiotics, consumed. This could have a negative impact on the microbiome, particularly reducing species which are associated with better gut and heart health.[116]

One small study, conducted over a year did find high microbiome diversity, however within that were very high levels of some microorganisms that prosper in conditions that are not necessarily considered beneficial, particularly high fat and high bile acids.[117] The specific types of bacteria that thrive in a high-fat high bile environment have been linked with an increased risk of colorectal cancers.[118]

One key factor in the Paleo diet that can only be a good thing is the total elimination of modern processed food. Although it may be advisable, if following a Paleo diet, to ensure it includes rich sources of the varieties of fibre that are preferred by the microbiome. There is also the issue that eating fresh unprocessed food increases the cost of the food bill, and this may be a deterrent for many individuals.[119]

DETOX DIETS

Detoxification practices have a long history across many different cultures around the globe. Using a variety of methods they "cleanse" the body and mind by various forms of fasting, purging through the use of laxatives, emetics and enemas, and the consumption of specific "remedies".

Today, detox diets claim to eliminate toxins from the body, "clean" the blood, "rest" internal organs, enable weight loss, and improve overall health. They are generally short term with most lasting only a few days and are often viewed as a "quick fix."[120] Despite a lack of evidence for their effectiveness, and concerns about risks associated with them, celebrities and influencers promote the idea of detox diets, and advertising for them appears across social media.

Those at greatest risk of falling for the hype are young women between the ages of 15 and 29.[121] Although detox diets are not linked to eating disorders, they can trigger excessive use of laxative products, leading to diarrhoea which in turn causes dehydration and depletes electrolytes.[122] Laxatives also disrupt the microbiome because they alter the environment in the gut.[123] Among other things they speed up transit time, which prevents effective fermentation taking place, they change the fluid balance in the gut which impacts the diversity of the microbiome, and they disrupt the mucosal barrier in the gut.[124,125]

Because detox diets involve a drastic reduction in calorie intake, they can result in some short-term weight loss. They do not support weight loss over the long term.[126] And they lack sufficient macro and micronutrients to be sustained for any length of time.[120]

THE LIVER – KEY TO DETOXIFICATION

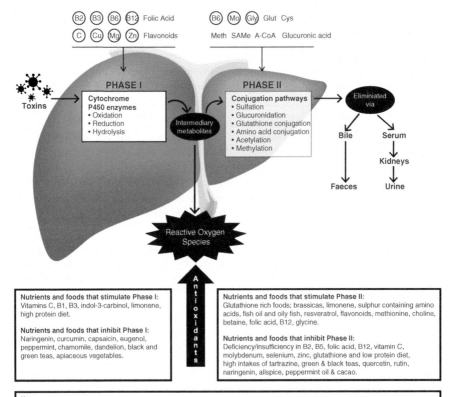

Nutrients needed for effective liver detoxification.

We don't need a special diet to stimulate detoxification because the body already has excellent in-built detoxification systems. One of the most important of these is the liver where blood is filtered, removing bacteria, debris from the breakdown of cells, and toxic substances. Bacteria and cellular debris are destroyed by macrophages whilst toxins are passed through sequences of enzymatic pathways known as Phase I and Phase II which act on ingested and metabolic toxins, changing them into other substances that can be excreted via urine, sweat and bile (and then faeces).[127] That excretion is sometimes referred to as Phase III.

Phase I is carried out by a group of enzymes, known collectively as the cytochrome P450 family. Through a series of reduction, oxidation, and hydrolysis reactions, toxic substances undergo biotransformation, changing their chemical structure. Some are immediately neutralised by making them water soluble for excretion via urine, but many cannot be made water soluble, so instead they are converted to intermediate forms for processing by Phase II.[128]

The intermediates are loaded with reactive oxygen species (ROS) and are often more cytotoxic than the original substances were.[129] It is therefore essential that they are picked up as rapidly as possible by the next stage of liver detoxification, Phase II.

In a process known as conjugation, Phase II liver enzymes combine the intermediate substances with other chemicals, making them suitable for excretion via urine, sweat, or bile.[130] There are six different conjugation pathways: glutathione conjugation; sulphation; glucuronidation; methylation; acetylation and amino acid conjugation.[130]

As with all biochemical reactions within the body, Phase I and Phase II require specific nutrients to function effectively with each Phase, and process requiring different nutrients, or metabolic chemicals to fund it. In addition, there are substances which can both speed up and inhibit both Phases. If Phase I is working more effectively, or faster than Phase II because the nutrients required for Phase II are in short supply, or substances which inhibit Phase II are present, then damaging intermediate metabolites can build up.[131]

Antioxidants can support and protect the liver against the oxidative damage that intermediates can cause. For example, the antioxidant curcumin, found in turmeric and often used as an anti-inflammatory, also has extremely broad antioxidant applications, inhibiting lipid peroxidation and neutralising ROS.[132] Resveratrol, a flavonoid found in the skin of dark purple fruits and vegetables (as well as chocolate and red wine) is a potent antioxidant that protects liver, kidney, and brain tissues, as well as having a positive impact on non-alcoholic fatty liver disease.[133] Quercetin, a flavonoid found in red wine, onions, apples, berries, and dark green vegetables, silymarin, found in the herb milk thistle, naringenin, a flavonoid found in grapefruit, as well as substances in coffee and green tea also have protective effects in the liver.[134]

There are concerns about UK intakes of many of the nutrients which are needed for liver function; vitamin C; riboflavin, folic acid, B12, choline, magnesium, selenium, and zinc all have low intakes in UK populations.[135] Probably, the best way to support the organs that detox us is to eat a varied and balanced diet that included a wide range of fruit and vegetables and a minimum of processed foods, get some exercise, get enough sleep, and drink enough water to stay hydrated (around 1.8 L/day).

RAW FOOD DIET

The idea that we should only eat raw food has been around for a while. Historically, it was practiced as an extreme form of religious observance, however, it is not something that occurs widely in traditional societies. The current version seems to be specific to industrialised societies with access to an abundance of every variety of food.

The raw food movement claims that it is more "natural" and "better" for you to eat only raw food because cooking destroys nutrients and enzymes that are present in food. There are variations which range from an entirely vegan diet, a raw vegetarian diet that includes raw milk and eggs, or something which also includes raw meat and fish. The foods eaten are largely unprocessed although juiced, blended, sprouted, pickled, or fermented foods still "count" as raw.

Cooking does destroy the enzymes that are naturally present in food. But the mouth, stomach, pancreas, gallbladder, and liver all produce enzymes that are specifically tailored to our digestive system. These, together with stomach acid, are more than adequate to digest the foods we eat, whether raw or cooked.[136]

Cooking can also reduce or destroy some nutrients, although the amount of loss depends on the type of cooking, and the types of foods being cooked.[137] Some nutrients may leach into cooking water, be destroyed by heat, or react to copper or iron in cooking vessels. But the benefits of cooking generally far outweigh the negatives.

Using fire for cooking was a significant turning point for our ancestors, indeed ancestral species that predate *Homo sapiens* appear to have been using fire for cooking for at least a million years.[138] There is evidence that about 2 million years ago, the gut of *Homo erectus* started shrinking whilst at the same time, their brain started growing and there is a theory this is linked to cooking.[139] Because cooking foods facilitates nutrient extraction. The application of heat alters cell structures in the food, making chewing and digestion easier, which in turn makes extracting energy and absorbing nutrients from food more straightforward.[140] This is particularly true of plant foods because the cell walls in plants are made from complex carbohydrates like cellulose and hemicellulose, which we cannot digest. Cooking softens and sometimes even breaks those cell walls, helping us to easily access the nutrients within the cells.[141]

Cooking also makes food safer, killing bacteria and parasites and removing or reducing naturally occurring toxins.[142,143] Many plant foods contain lectins, proteins which bind to carbohydrates which means we cannot digest them. Some lectins are also highly toxic. But cooking destroys lectins in foods.[144] Plant foods with high levels of toxic lectins include kidney and soya beans, lentils, peanuts, and plants in the Solanaceae family (potatoes, tomatoes, aubergine, peppers, chillies, paprika, and tobacco) many of which would make us very unwell if we were to eat them raw. In addition, some vegetables, particularly in the Brassica family, contain glucosinolates, chemicals that interfere with the uptake of iodine. Eating large quantities of raw glucosinolate containing vegetables can impact thyroid function, leading to the formation of a goitre, however, cooking destroys them.[145]

Raw food diets do lead to significant weight loss, probably because it is simply too difficult to extract sufficient energy from raw food. They can reduce LDL cholesterol and triglycerides, however, they can also increase homocysteine levels and reduce HDL cholesterol.[146] They can also result in nutrient deficiencies in vitamin B12, vitamin D and calcium, as well as being concerningly low in protein.[147]

As with so many of the "diets" that are currently in fashion, anyone following a raw food diet would be well advised to include some carefully considered micronutrient supplementation.

IS THERE A "BEST" DIET?

The "best" diet for any individual is the one that suits that individual the best. Weight loss diets tend not to work unless they are specifically intended to fundamentally change the way someone eats in the long term. As soon as the dieter stops following the diet and returns to "normal" eating, the weight begins to creep up again. Which then makes the dieter feel as if they have failed in their goals, potentially creating a repeating cycle of yo-yo dieting which in itself can have negative health consequences.[148] And to add to the problem, many diets can be difficult to maintain and, despite having some health benefits, may have hidden risks in micronutrient insufficiencies.

When it comes to diet, there are a few absolutes. Top of the list is the avoidance, as far as it possible of processed foods; applying the mantra "steer clear of ultra-processed foods" to all foodstuffs is probably a good place to start. Another is that a high intake of as wide a variety as possible of plant foods is good. The two most positive diets discussed here are the flexitarian and the Mediterranean diets. Both follow a "traditional" pattern, with high fruit and vegetable intakes, good quality protein in the form of limited amounts of meat, fish and dairy products, and low, or better yet, no modern processed food.

Where populations follow traditional diets, there is little heart disease, obesity or diabetes. However, those diseases rapidly appear in immigrant populations that shift their dietary patterns away from the traditional and towards the industrialised Western model.[149] Although some traditional dietary practices may be maintained, Western foods and patterns of eating start to creep in during the first generation and are widely consumed by the second generation.[150] As whole grains, traditional plant foods and saturated fats from animals are replaced with refined carbohydrates, highly processed vegetable oils, and increased sugar, chronic diseases linked to diets begin to appear.[151]

Equally, where populations within a country move away from their traditional diets and begin adopting Western eating habits, Western patterns of health deterioration arise. Japan is an excellent example. The traditional Japanese diet prevents obesity and reduces the risk of type II diabetes, heart disease, and some cancers.[152,153,154] But recent decades have seen an increasing Westernisation of diet in Japan, and this has been accompanied by a rise in the degenerative diseases common in the West.[155] The same holds true for many other countries.[156,157]

There are certain characteristics that all traditional diets share. They generally have high intake of plant foods, a low intake of sugars, and no intake of highly processed or refined foods. They often include some form of fermented food, and most include a range of animal foods.[157]

Instead of adopting the latest fad, or setting some unattainable "perfect diet", citizens in the UK should consider simply moving to a more traditional way of eating. But of course, the food industry wouldn't like that at all.

REFERENCES

1 Leite, F., Khandpur, N., Andrade, G.C., Anastasiou, K., Baker, P., Lawrence, M., & Monteiro, C.A. (2022). Ultra-processed foods should be central to global food systems dialogue and action on biodiversity. *BMJ Global Health*, *7*(3), e008269. https://doi.org/10.1136/bmjgh-2021-008269

2 Keys, A.B., & Keys, M. (1975). *How to Eat Well and Stay Well, the Mediterranean Way*. New York: Doubleday.

3 Smith, R. (2014). Are some diets "mass murder"?. *BMJ*, *349*, g7654. https://doi.org/10.1136/bmj.g7654

4 Altomare, R., Cacciabaudo, F., Damiano, G., Palumbo, V.D., Gioviale, M.C., Bellavia, M., Tomasello, G., & Lo Monte, A.I. (2013). The Mediterranean diet: A history of health. *Iranian Journal of Public Health*, *42*(5), 449–457. https://ijph.tums.ac.ir/index.php/ijph/article/view/4556

5 Franquesa, M., Pujol-Busquets, G., García-Fernández, E., Rico, L., Shamirian-Pulido, L., Aguilar-Martínez, A., Medina, F.X., Serra-Majem, L., & Bach-Faig, A. (2019). Mediterranean diet and cardiodiabesity: A systematic review through evidence-based answers to key clinical questions. *Nutrients*, *11*(3), 655. https://doi.org/10.3390/nu11030655

6 Guasch-Ferré, M., & Willett, W.C. (2021). The Mediterranean diet and health: A comprehensive overview. *Journal of Internal Medicine*, *290*(3), 549–566. https://doi.org/10.1111/joim.13333

7 Lăcătuşu, C.M., Grigorescu, E.D., Floria, M., Onofriescu, A., & Mihai, B.M. (2019). The Mediterranean diet: From an environment-driven food culture to an emerging medical prescription. *International Journal of Environmental Research and Public Health*, *16*(6), 942. https://doi.org/10.3390/ijerph16060942

8 Papadaki, A., Wood, L., Sebire, S.J., & Jago, R. (2015). Adherence to the Mediterranean diet among employees in South West England: Formative research to inform a web-based, work-place nutrition intervention. *Preventive Medicine Reports*, *2*, 223–228. https://doi.org/10.1016/j.pmedr.2015.03.009

9 Bonaccio, M., Di Castelnuovo, A., Pounis, G., Costanzo, S., Persichillo, M., Cerletti, C., Donati, M.B., de Gaetano, G., Iacoviello, L., & Moli-sani Study Investigators (2017). High adherence to the Mediterranean diet is associated with cardiovascular protection in higher but not in lower socioeconomic groups: Prospective findings from the Moli-sani study. *International Journal of Epidemiology*, *46*(5), 1478–1487. https://doi.org/10.1093/ije/dyx145

10 Dagevos, H., & Voordouw, J. (2013). Sustainability and meat consumption: Is reduction realistic? *Sustainability: Science, Practice and Policy*, *9*(2), 60–69. https://doi.org/10.1080/15487733.2013.11908115

11 Stewart, C., Piernas, C., Cook, B., & Jebb, S.A. (2021). Trends in UK meat consumption: Analysis of data from years 1–11 (2008–09 to 2018-19) of the National Diet and Nutrition Survey rolling programme. *The Lancet. Planetary Health*, *5*(10), e699–e708. https://doi.org/10.1016/S2542-5196(21)00228-X

12 Ellison K. (2021). The Attenborough effect: Brits want to be Greener. *3 Sided Cube.* https://3sidedcube.com/the-attenborough-effect-brits-want-to-be-greener/

13 Lai, A.E., Tirotto, F.A., Pagliaro, S., & Fornara, F. (2020). Two sides of the same coin: Environmental and health concern pathways toward meat consumption. *Frontiers in Psychology, 11,* 578582. https://doi.org/10.3389/fpsyg.2020.578582

14 YouGov (2021). What is making flexitarians in the US and UK shift towards a meatless diet? https://yougov.co.uk/topics/food/articles-reports/2021/05/31/what-making-flexitarians-us-and-uk-shift-towards-m

15 Clark, M.A., Springmann, M., Hill, J., & Tilman, D. (2019). Multiple health and environmental impacts of foods. *Proceedings of the National Academy of Sciences of the United States of America, 116*(46), 23357–23362. https://doi.org/10.1073/pnas.1906908116

16 Derbyshire, E.J. (2017). Flexitarian diets and health: A review of the evidence-based literature. *Frontiers in Nutrition, 3,* 55. https://doi.org/10.3389/fnut.2016.00055

17 Satija, A., Bhupathiraju, S.N., Rimm, E.B., Spiegelman, D., Chiuve, S.E., Borgi, L., Willett, W.C., Manson, J.E., Sun, Q., & Hu, F.B. (2016). Plant-based dietary patterns and incidence of type 2 diabetes in US men and women: Results from three prospective cohort studies. *PLoS Medicine, 13*(6), e1002039. https://doi.org/10.1371/journal.pmed.1002039

18 Wozniak, H., Larpin, C., de Mestral, C., Guessous, I., Reny, J. L., & Stringhini, S. (2020). Vegetarian, pescatarian and flexitarian diets: Sociodemographic determinants and association with cardiovascular risk factors in a Swiss urban population. *The British Journal of Nutrition, 124*(8), 844–852. https://doi.org/10.1017/S000711452 0001762

19 Orlich, M.J., Singh, P.N., Sabaté, J., Fan, J., Sveen, L., Bennett, H., Knutsen, S.F., Beeson, W.L., Jaceldo-Siegl, K., Butler, T.L., Herring, R.P., & Fraser, G.E. (2015). Vegetarian dietary patterns and the risk of colorectal cancers. *JAMA Internal Medicine, 175*(5), 767–776. https://doi.org/10.1001/jamainternmed.2015.59

20 Barrubés, L., Babio, N., Becerra-Tomás, N., Rosique-Esteban, N., & Salas-Salvadó, J. (2019). Association between dairy product consumption and colorectal cancer risk in adults: A systematic review and meta-analysis of epidemiologic studies. *Advances in Nutrition, 10*(suppl_2), S190–S211. https://doi.org/10.1093/advances/nmy114

21 Springmann, M., Wiebe, K., Mason-D'Croz, D., Sulser, T.B., Rayner, M., & Scarborough, P. (2018). Health and nutritional aspects of sustainable diet strategies and their association with environmental impacts: A global modelling analysis with country-level detail. *The Lancet. Planetary Health, 2*(10), e451–e461. https://doi.org/10.1016/S2542-5196(18)30206-7

22 Toribio-Mateas, M.A., Bester, A., & Klimenko, N. (2021). Impact of plant-based meat alternatives on the gut microbiota of consumers: A real-world study. *Foods, 10*(9), 2040. https://doi.org/10.3390/foods10092040

23 Cotillard, A., Cartier-Meheust, A., Litwin, N.S., Chaumont, S., Saccareau, M., Lejzerowicz, F., Tap, J., Koutnikova, H., Lopez, D.G., McDonald, D., Song, S. J., Knight, R., Derrien, M., & Veiga, P. (2022). A posteriori dietary patterns better explain variations of the gut microbiome than individual markers in the American Gut Project. *The American Journal of Clinical Nutrition, 115*(2), 432–443. https://doi.org/10.1093/ajcn/nqab332

24 Milton K. (2003). The critical role played by animal source foods in human (Homo) evolution. *The Journal of Nutrition, 133*(11 Suppl 2), 3886S–3892 S. https://doi.org/10.1093/jn/133.11.3886S

25 Pereira, P.M., & Vicente, A.F. (2013). Meat nutritional composition and nutritive role in the human diet. *Meat Science, 93*(3), 586–592. https://doi.org/10.1016/j.meatsci.2012.09.018

26 Hunter, P. (2018). The genetics of domestication: Research into the domestication of livestock and companion animals sheds light both on their "evolution" and human history. *EMBO Reports, 19*(2), 201–205. https://doi.org/10.15252/embr.201745664

27 Martínez, L.M., Estebaranz-Sánchez, F., Galbany, J., & Pérez-Pérez, A. (2016). Testing dietary hypotheses of East African hominines using buccal dental microwear data. *PloS One, 11*(11), e0165447. https://doi.org/10.1371/journal.pone.0165447

28 Ben-Dor, M., Sirtoli, R., & Barkai, R. (2021). The evolution of the human trophic level during the Pleistocene. *American Journal of Physical Anthropology, 175 Suppl 72,* 27–56. https://doi.org/10.1002/ajpa.24247

29 Mann, N.J. (2018). A brief history of meat in the human diet and current health implications. *Meat Science, 144,* 169–179. https://doi.org/10.1016/j.meatsci.2018.06.008

30 Furness, J.B., Cottrell, J.J., & Bravo, D.M. (2015). Comparative Gut Physiology Symposium: Comparative physiology of digestion. *Journal of Animal Science, 93*(2), 485–491. https://doi.org/10.2527/jas.2014-8481

31 Gehring, J., Touvier, M., Baudry, J., Julia, C., Buscail, C., Srour, B., Hercberg, S., Péneau, S., Kesse-Guyot, E., & Allès, B. (2021). Consumption of ultra-processed foods by pesco-vegetarians, vegetarians, and vegans: Associations with duration and age at diet initiation. *The Journal of Nutrition, 151*(1), 120–131. https://doi.org/10.1093/jn/nxaa196

32 van Vliet, S., Bain, J.R., Muehlbauer, M.J., Provenza, F.D., Kronberg, S.L., Pieper, C.F., & Huffman, K.M. (2021). A metabolomics comparison of plant-based meat and grass-fed meat indicates large nutritional differences despite comparable Nutrition Facts panels. *Scientific Reports, 11*(1), 13828. https://doi.org/10.1038/s41598-021-93100-3

33 Tso, R., & Forde, C.G. (2021). Unintended consequences: Nutritional impact and potential pitfalls of switching from animal- to plant-based foods. *Nutrients, 13*(8), 2527. https://doi.org/10.3390/nu13082527

34 Chen, D., Rocha-Mendoza, D., Shan, S., Smith, Z., García-Cano, I., Prost, J., Jimenez-Flores, R., & Campanella, O. (2022). Characterization and cellular uptake of peptides derived from in vitro digestion of meat analogues produced by a sustainable extrusion process. *Journal of Agricultural and Food Chemistry, 70*(26), 8124–8133. https://doi.org/10.1021/acs.jafc.2c01711

35 Bakaloudi, D.R., Halloran, A., Rippin, H.L., Oikonomidou, A.C., Dardavesis, T.I., Williams, J., Wickramasinghe, K., Breda, J., & Chourdakis, M. (2021). Intake and adequacy of the vegan diet. A systematic review of the evidence. *Clinical Nutrition, 40*(5), 3503–3521. https://doi.org/10.1016/j.clnu.2020.11.035

36 Tang, G. (2010). Bioconversion of dietary provitamin A carotenoids to vitamin A in humans. *The American Journal of Clinical Nutrition, 91*(5), 1468S–1473 S. https://doi.org/10.3945/ajcn.2010.28674G

37 Novotny, J.A., Harrison, D.J., Pawlosky, R., Flanagan, V.P., Harrison, E.H., & Kurilich, A.C. (2010). Beta-carotene conversion to vitamin A decreases as the dietary dose increases in humans. *The Journal of Nutrition, 140*(5), 915–918. https://doi.org/10.3945/jn.109.116947

38 Kristensen, N.B., Madsen, M.L., Hansen, T.H., Allin, K.H., Hoppe, C., Fagt, S., Lausten, M.S., Gøbel, R.J., Vestergaard, H., Hansen, T., & Pedersen, O. (2015). Intake of macro- and micronutrients in Danish vegans. *Nutrition Journal, 14,* 115. https://doi.org/10.1186/s12937-015-0103-3

39 Menzel, J., Abraham, K., Stangl, G.I., Ueland, P.M., Obeid, R., Schulze, M.B., Herter-Aeberli, I., Schwerdtle, T., & Weikert, C. (2021). Vegan diet and bone health-results from the cross-sectional rbvd study. *Nutrients, 13*(2), 685. https://doi.org/10.3390/nu13020685

40 Pawlak, R., Lester, S.E., & Babatunde, T. (2014). The prevalence of cobalamin deficiency among vegetarians assessed by serum vitamin B12: A review of literature.

European Journal of Clinical Nutrition, 68(5), 541–548. https://doi.org/10.1038/ejcn.2014.46

41 Majchrzak, D., Singer, I., Männer, M., Rust, P., Genser, D., Wagner, K.H., & Elmadfa, I. (2006). B-vitamin status and concentrations of homocysteine in Austrian omnivores, vegetarians and vegans. *Annals of Nutrition & Metabolism, 50*(6), 485–491. https://doi.org/10.1159/000095828

42 Schüpbach, R., Wegmüller, R., Berguerand, C., Bui, M., & Herter-Aeberli, I. (2017). Micronutrient status and intake in omnivores, vegetarians and vegans in Switzerland. *European Journal of Nutrition, 56*(1), 283–293. https://doi.org/10.1007/s00394-015-1079-7

43 Derbyshire, E. (2019). Could we be overlooking a potential choline crisis in the United Kingdom? *BMJ Nutrition, Prevention & Health, 2*(2), 86–89. https://doi.org/10.1136/bmjnph-2019-000037

44 Wallace, T.C., Blusztajn, J.K., Caudill, M.A., Klatt, K.C., Natker, E., Zeisel, S.H., & Zelman, K.M. (2018). Choline: The underconsumed and underappreciated essential nutrient. *Nutrition Today, 53*(6), 240–253. https://doi.org/10.1097/NT.0000000000000302

45 Martineau, A.R., Thummel, K.E., Wang, Z., Jolliffe, D.A., Boucher, B.J., Griffin, S.J., Forouhi, N.G., & Hitman, G. A. (2019). Differential effects of oral boluses of Vitamin D2 vs Vitamin D3 on Vitamin D metabolism: A randomized controlled trial. *The Journal of Clinical Endocrinology and Metabolism, 104*(12), 5831–5839. https://doi.org/10.1210/jc.2019-00207

46 Calame, W., Street, L., & Hulshof, T. (2020). Vitamin D serum levels in the uk population, including a mathematical approach to evaluate the impact of vitamin d fortified ready-to-eat breakfast cereals: Application of the NDNS database. *Nutrients, 12*(6), 1868. https://doi.org/10.3390/nu12061868

47 Sakkas, H., Bozidis, P., Touzios, C., Kolios, D., Athanasiou, G., Athanasopoulou, E., Gerou, I., & Gartzonika, C. (2020). Nutritional status and the influence of the vegan diet on the gut microbiota and human health. *Medicina, 56*(2), 88. https://doi.org/10.3390/medicina56020088

48 Rocha, C.P., Pacheco, D., Cotas, J., Marques, J.C., Pereira, L., & Gonçalves, A. (2021). Seaweeds as valuable sources of essential fatty acids for human nutrition. *International Journal of Environmental Research and Public Health, 18*(9), 4968. https://doi.org/10.3390/ijerph18094968

49 Burns-Whitmore, B., Froyen, E., Heskey, C., Parker, T., & San Pablo, G. (2019). Alpha-linolenic and linoleic fatty acids in the vegan diet: Do they require dietary reference intake/adequate intake special consideration?. *Nutrients, 11*(10), 2365. https://doi.org/10.3390/nu11102365

50 Greupner, T., Kutzner, L., Nolte, F., Strangmann, A., Kohrs, H., Hahn, A., Schebb, N.H., & Schuchardt, J.P. (2018). Effects of a 12-week high-α-linolenic acid intervention on EPA and DHA concentrations in red blood cells and plasma oxylipin pattern in subjects with a low EPA and DHA status. *Food & Function, 9*(3), 1587–1600. https://doi.org/10.1039/c7fo01809f

51 Derbyshire, E. (2019). Oily fish and omega-3s across the life stages: A focus on intakes and future directions. *Frontiers in Nutrition, 6*, 165. https://doi.org/10.3389/fnut.2019.00165

52 Craddock, J.C., Neale, E.P., Probst, Y.C., & Peoples, G.E. (2017). Algal supplementation of vegetarian eating patterns improves plasma and serum docosahexaenoic acid concentrations and omega-3 indices: A systematic literature review. *Journal of Human Nutrition and Dietetics, 30*(6), 693–699. https://doi.org/10.1111/jhn.12474

53 Gupta, S. (2016). Brain food: Clever eating. *Nature, 531*(7592), S12–S13. https://doi.org/10.1038/531S12a

54 Young, I., Parker, H.M., Rangan, A., Prvan, T., Cook, R.L., Donges, C.E., Steinbeck, K.S., O'Dwyer, N.J., Cheng, H. L., Franklin, J.L., & O'Connor, H.T. (2018). Association between haem and non-haem iron intake and serum ferritin in healthy young women. *Nutrients, 10*(1), 81. https://doi.org/10.3390/nu10010081

55 Gibson, R.S., Raboy, V., & King, J.C. (2018). Implications of phytate in plant-based foods for iron and zinc bioavailability, setting dietary requirements, and formulating programs and policies. *Nutrition Reviews, 76*(11), 793–804. https://doi.org/10.1093/nutrit/nuy028

56 Pawlak, R., Berger, J., & Hines, I. (2016). Iron status of vegetarian adults: A review of literature. *American Journal of Lifestyle Medicine, 12*(6), 486–498. https://doi.org/10.1177/1559827616682933

57 Agnoli, C., Baroni, L., Bertini, I., Ciappellano, S., Fabbri, A., Papa, M., Pellegrini, N., Sbarbati, R., Scarino, M.L., Siani, V., & Sieri, S. (2017). Position paper on vegetarian diets from the working group of the Italian Society of Human Nutrition. *Nutrition, Metabolism, and Cardiovascular Diseases, 27*(12), 1037–1052. https://doi.org/10.1016/j.numecd.2017.10.020

58 Iguacel, I., Miguel-Berges, M.L., Gómez-Bruton, A., Moreno, L.A., & Julián, C. (2019). Veganism, vegetarianism, bone mineral density, and fracture risk: A systematic review and meta-analysis. *Nutrition Reviews, 77*(1), 1–18. https://doi.org/10.1093/nutrit/nuy045

59 Neufingerl, N., & Eilander, A. (2021). Nutrient intake and status in adults consuming plant-based diets compared to meat-eaters: A systematic review. *Nutrients, 14*(1), 29. https://doi.org/10.3390/nu14010029

60 Aakre, I., Tveito Evensen, L., Kjellevold, M., Dahl, L., Henjum, S., Alexander, J., Madsen, L., & Markhus, M.W. (2020). Iodine status and thyroid function in a group of seaweed consumers in Norway. *Nutrients, 12*(11), 3483. https://doi.org/10.3390/nu12113483

61 Eveleigh, E.R., Coneyworth, L.J., Avery, A., & Welham, S. (2020). Vegans, vegetarians, and omnivores: How does dietary choice influence iodine intake? A systematic review. *Nutrients, 12*(6), 1606. https://doi.org/10.3390/nu12061606

62 Woodside, J.V., & Mullan, K.R. (2021). Iodine status in UK-An accidental public health triumph gone sour. *Clinical Endocrinology, 94*(4), 692–699. https://doi.org/10.1111/cen.14368

63 Eveleigh, E., Coneyworth, L., Zhou, M., Burdett, H., Malla, J., Nguyen, V.H., & Welham, S. (2022). Vegans and vegetarians living in Nottingham (UK) continue to be at risk of iodine deficiency. *The British Journal of Nutrition*, 1–46. https://doi.org/10.1017/S0007114522000113

64 Fallon, N., & Dillon, S.A. (2020). Low intakes of iodine and selenium amongst vegan and vegetarian women highlight a potential nutritional vulnerability. *Frontiers in Nutrition, 7*, 72. https://doi.org/10.3389/fnut.2020.00072

65 Stoffaneller, R., & Morse, N.L. (2015). A review of dietary selenium intake and selenium status in Europe and the Middle East. *Nutrients, 7*(3), 1494–1537. https://doi.org/10.3390/nu7031494

66 Gorini, F., Sabatino, L., Pingitore, A., & Vassalle, C. (2021). Selenium: An element of life essential for thyroid function. *Molecules, 26*(23), 7084. https://doi.org/10.3390/molecules26237084

67 Sobiecki, J.G. (2017). Vegetarianism and colorectal cancer risk in a low-selenium environment: Effect modification by selenium status? A possible factor contributing to the null results in British vegetarians. *European Journal of Nutrition, 56*(5), 1819–1832. https://doi.org/10.1007/s00394-016-1364-0

68 Hunt, J.R. (2003). Bioavailability of iron, zinc, and other trace minerals from vegetarian diets. *The American Journal of Clinical Nutrition, 78*(3), 633S–639S. https://doi.org/10.1093/ajcn/78.3.633 S

69 Maares, M., & Haase, H. (2020). A guide to human zinc absorption: General overview and recent advances of in vitro intestinal models. *Nutrients*, *12*(3), 762. https://doi.org/10.3390/nu12030762

70 Kondaiah, P., Yaduvanshi, P.S., Sharp, P.A., & Pullakhandam, R. (2019). Iron and zinc homeostasis and interactions: Does enteric zinc excretion cross-talk with intestinal iron absorption?. *Nutrients*, *11*(8), 1885. https://doi.org/10.3390/nu11081885

71 D'Andrea Meira, I., Romão, T.T., Pires do Prado, H.J., Krüger, L.T., Pires, M., & da Conceição, P.O. (2019). Ketogenic diet and epilepsy: What we know so far. *Frontiers in Neuroscience*, *13*, 5. https://doi.org/10.3389/fnins.2019.00005

72 Tanne, J.H. (2003). Low carbohydrate diet is vindicated. *BMJ: British Medical Journal*, *326*, 1133.

73 Spinelli, J.B., & Haigis, M.C. (2018). The multifaceted contributions of mitochondria to cellular metabolism. *Nature Cell Biology*, *20*(7), 745–754. https://doi.org/10.1038/s41556-018-0124-1

74 Dhillon, K.K., & Gupta, S. (2021). *Biochemistry, Ketogenesis*. In: *StatPearls* [Internet]. Treasure Island (FL): StatPearls Publishing. Available from: https://www.ncbi.nlm.nih.gov/books/NBK493179/

75 Yuan, X., Wang, J., Yang, S., Gao, M., Cao, L., Li, X., Hong, D., Tian, S., & Sun, C. (2020). Effect of the ketogenic diet on glycemic control, insulin resistance, and lipid metabolism in patients with T2DM: A systematic review and meta-analysis. *Nutrition & Diabetes*, *10*(1), 38. https://doi.org/10.1038/s41387-020-00142-z

76 Kolb, H., Kempf, K., Röhling, M., Lenzen-Schulte, M., Schloot, N.C., & Martin, S. (2021). Ketone bodies: From enemy to friend and guardian angel. *BMC Medicine*, *19*(1), 313. https://doi.org/10.1186/s12916-021-02185-0

77 Puchalska, P., & Crawford, P. A. (2017). Multi-dimensional roles of ketone bodies in fuel metabolism, signaling, and therapeutics. *Cell Metabolism*, *25*(2), 262–284. https://doi.org/10.1016/j.cmet.2016.12.022

78 von Geijer, L., & Ekelund, M. (2015). Ketoacidosis associated with low-carbohydrate diet in a non-diabetic lactating woman: A case report. *Journal of Medical Case Reports*, *9*, 224. https://doi.org/10.1186/s13256-015-0709-2

79 Blanco, J.C., Khatri, A., Kifayat, A., Cho, R., & Aronow, W.S. (2019). Starvation ketoacidosis due to the ketogenic diet and prolonged fasting – A possibly dangerous diet trend. *The American Journal of Case Reports*, *20*, 1728–1731. https://doi.org/10.12659/AJCR.917226

80 White-Cotsmire, A.J., & Healy, A.M. (2020). Ketogenic diet as a trigger for diabetic ketoacidosis in a misdiagnosis of diabetes: A case report. *Clinical Diabetes*, *38*(3), 318–321. https://doi.org/10.2337/cd20-0001

81 Charoensri, S., Sothornwit, J., Trirattanapikul, A., & Pongchaiyakul, C. (2021). Ketogenic diet-induced diabetic ketoacidosis in a young adult with unrecognized type 1 diabetes. *Case Reports in Endocrinology*, *2021*, 6620832. https://doi.org/10.1155/2021/6620832

82 National Agricultural Library. How many calories are in one gram of fat, carbohydrate, or protein? *U.S. Department of Agriculture*. https://www.nal.usda.gov/legacy/fnic/how-many-calories-are-one-gram-fat-carbohydrate-or-protein

83 Crosby, L., Davis, B., Joshi, S., Jardine, M., Paul, J., Neola, M., & Barnard, N.D. (2021). Ketogenic diets and chronic disease: Weighing the benefits against the risks. *Frontiers in Nutrition*, *8*, 702802. https://doi.org/10.3389/fnut.2021.702802

84 Holeček, M. (2020). Branched-chain amino acids and branched-chain keto acids in hyperammonemic states: Metabolism and as supplements. *Metabolites*, *10*(8), 324. https://doi.org/10.3390/metabo10080324

85 Rondanelli, M., Gasparri, C., Peroni, G., Faliva, M.A., Naso, M., Perna, S., Bazire, P., Sajuox, I., Maugeri, R., & Rigon, C. (2021). The potential roles of very low calorie,

very low calorie ketogenic diets and very low carbohydrate diets on the gut microbiota composition. *Frontiers in Endocrinology, 12,* 662591. https://doi.org/10.3389/fendo.2021.662591

86 Ang, Q.Y., Alexander, M., Newman, J.C., Tian, Y., Cai, J., Upadhyay, V., Turnbaugh, J.A., Verdin, E., Hall, K.D., Leibel, R.L., Ravussin, E., Rosenbaum, M., Patterson, A.D., & Turnbaugh, P.J. (2020). Ketogenic diets alter the gut microbiome resulting in decreased intestinal Th17 cells. *Cell, 181*(6), 1263–1275.e16. https://doi.org/10.1016/j.cell.2020.04.027

87 Ting, R., Dugré, N., Allan, G.M., & Lindblad, A.J. (2018). Ketogenic diet for weight loss. *Canadian Family Physician, 64*(12), 906. https://www.cfp.ca/content/64/12/906

88 Ludwig, D.S. (2020). The ketogenic diet: Evidence for optimism but high-quality research needed. *The Journal of Nutrition, 150*(6), 1354–1359. https://doi.org/10.1093/jn/nxz308

89 Paoli, A., Mancin, L., Bianco, A., Thomas, E., Mota, J.F., & Piccini, F. (2019). Ketogenic diet and microbiota: Friends or enemies? *Genes, 10*(7), 534. https://doi.org/10.3390/genes10070534

90 James, R., James, L.J., & Clayton, D.J. (2020). Anticipation of 24 h severe energy restriction increases energy intake and reduces physical activity energy expenditure in the prior 24 h, in healthy males. *Appetite, 152,* 104719. https://doi.org/10.1016/j.appet.2020.104719

91 Hajek, P., Przulj, D., Pesola, F., McRobbie, H., Peerbux, S., Phillips-Waller, A., Bisal, N., & Myers Smith, K. (2021). A randomised controlled trial of the 5:2 diet. *PLoS One, 16*(11), e0258853. https://doi.org/10.1371/journal.pone.0258853

92 Cui, Y., Cai, T., Zhou, Z., Mu, Y., Lu, Y., Gao, Z., Wu, J., & Zhang, Y. (2020). Health effects of alternate-day fasting in adults: A systematic review and meta-analysis. *Frontiers in Nutrition, 7,* 586036. https://doi.org/10.3389/fnut.2020.586036

93 Phillips M. (2019). Fasting as a therapy in neurological disease. *Nutrients, 11*(10), 2501. https://doi.org/10.3390/nu11102501

94 Debras, C., Chazelas, E., Srour, B., Druesne-Pecollo, N., Esseddik, Y., Szabo de Edelenyi, F., Agaësse, C., De Sa, A., Lutchia, R., Gigandet, S., Huybrechts, I., Julia, C., Kesse-Guyot, E., Allès, B., Andreeva, V. A., Galan, P., Hercberg, S., Deschasaux-Tanguy, M., & Touvier, M. (2022). Artificial sweeteners and cancer risk: Results from the NutriNet-Santé population-based cohort study. *PLoS Medicine, 19*(3), e1003950. https://doi.org/10.1371/journal.pmed.1003950

95 Basson, A.R., Rodriguez-Palacios, A., & Cominelli, F. (2021). Artificial sweeteners: History and new concepts on inflammation. *Frontiers in Nutrition, 8,* 746247. https://doi.org/10.3389/fnut.2021.746247

96 Pang, M.D., Goossens, G.H., & Blaak, E.E. (2021). The impact of artificial sweeteners on body weight control and glucose homeostasis. *Frontiers in Nutrition, 7,* 598340. https://doi.org/10.3389/fnut.2020.598340

97 Welton, S., Minty, R., O'Driscoll, T., Willms, H., Poirier, D., Madden, S., & Kelly, L. (2020). Intermittent fasting and weight loss: Systematic review. *Canadian Family Physician, 66*(2), 117–125. https://www.cfp.ca/content/66/2/117

98 Sutton, E.F., Beyl, R., Early, K.S., Cefalu, W.T., Ravussin, E., & Peterson, C.M. (2018). Early time-restricted feeding improves insulin sensitivity, blood pressure, and oxidative stress even without weight loss in men with prediabetes. *Cell Metabolism, 27*(6), 1212–1221.e3. https://doi.org/10.1016/j.cmet.2018.04.010

99 Stockman, M.C., Thomas, D., Burke, J., & Apovian, C.M. (2018). Intermittent fasting: Is the wait worth the weight?. *Current Obesity Reports, 7*(2), 172–185. https://doi.org/10.1007/s13679-018-0308-9

100 Patterson, R.E., Laughlin, G.A., LaCroix, A.Z., Hartman, S.J., Natarajan, L., Senger, C.M., Martínez, M.E., Villaseñor, A., Sears, D.D., Marinac, C.R., & Gallo, L.C. (2015).

Intermittent fasting and human metabolic health. *Journal of the Academy of Nutrition and Dietetics*, *115*(8), 1203–1212. https://doi.org/10.1016/j.jand.2015.02.018

101 Grajower, M.M., & Horne, B.D. (2019). Clinical management of intermittent fasting in patients with diabetes mellitus. *Nutrients*, *11*(4), 873. https://doi.org/10.3390/nu11040873

102 Passos, J.A., Vasconcellos-Silva, P.R., & Santos, L. (2020). Cycles of attention to fad diets and internet search trends by Google trends. *Ciencia & saude coletiva*, *25*(7), 2615–2631. https://www.scielo.br/j/csc/a/nqtgQMFf3CFhkdRVKscqfSK/?lang=en

103 Garn, S.M., & Leonard, W.R. (1989). What did our ancestors eat?. *Nutrition Reviews*, *47*(11), 337–345. https://doi.org/10.1111/j.1753-4887.1989.tb02765.x

104 Challa, H.J., Bandlamudi, M., & Uppaluri, K.R. (2021). *Paleolithic Diet*. In: *StatPearls* [Internet]. Treasure Island (FL): StatPearls Publishing. Available from: https://www.ncbi.nlm.nih.gov/books/NBK482457/

105 Henry, A.G., Brooks, A.S., & Piperno, D.R. (2014). Plant foods and the dietary ecology of Neanderthals and early modern humans. *Journal of Human Evolution*, *69*, 44–54. https://doi.org/10.1016/j.jhevol.2013.12.014

106 Mariotti Lippi, M., Foggi, B., Aranguren, B., Ronchitelli, A., & Revedin, A. (2015). Multistep food plant processing at Grotta Paglicci (Southern Italy) around 32,600 cal B.P. *Proceedings of the National Academy of Sciences of the United States of America*, *112*(39), 12075–12080. https://doi.org/10.1073/pnas.1505213112

107 Revedin, A., Aranguren, B., Becattini, R., Longo, L., Marconi, E., Lippi, M.M., Skakun, N., Sinitsyn, A., Spiridonova, E., & Svoboda, J. (2010). Thirty thousand-year-old evidence of plant food processing. *Proceedings of the National Academy of Sciences of the United States of America*, *107*(44), 18815–18819. https://doi.org/10.1073/pnas.1006993107

108 Wieczorek, A.M. & Wright, M.G. (2012) History of agricultural biotechnology: How crop development has evolved. *Nature Education Knowledge*, *3*(10), 9. https://www.nature.com/scitable/knowledge/library/history-of-agricultural-biotechnology-how-crop-development-25885295/

109 Rupp R. (2014). Prehistoric dining: The real paleo diet. *National Geographic*. https://www.nationalgeographic.com/culture/article/prehistoric-dining-the-real-paleo-diet

110 de Menezes, E., Sampaio, H., Carioca, A., Parente, N.A., Brito, F.O., Moreira, T., de Souza, A., & Arruda, S. (2019). Influence of Paleolithic diet on anthropometric markers in chronic diseases: Systematic review and meta-analysis. *Nutrition Journal*, *18*(1), 41. https://doi.org/10.1186/s12937-019-0457-z

111 Manheimer, E.W., van Zuuren, E.J., Fedorowicz, Z., & Pijl, H. (2015). Paleolithic nutrition for metabolic syndrome: Systematic review and meta-analysis. *The American Journal of Clinical Nutrition*, *102*(4), 922–932. https://doi.org/10.3945/ajcn.115.113613

112 Whalen, K.A., Judd, S., McCullough, M.L., Flanders, W.D., Hartman, T.J., & Bostick, R.M. (2017). Paleolithic and Mediterranean diet pattern scores are inversely associated with all-cause and cause-specific mortality in adults. *The Journal of Nutrition*, *147*(4), 612–620. https://doi.org/10.3945/jn.116.241919

113 Shah, S., MacDonald, C.J., El Fatouhi, D., Mahamat-Saleh, Y., Mancini, F.R., Fagherazzi, G., Severi, G., Boutron-Ruault, M.C., & Laouali, N. (2021). The associations of the Palaeolithic diet alone and in combination with lifestyle factors with type 2 diabetes and hypertension risks in women in the E3N prospective cohort. *European Journal of Nutrition*, *60*(7), 3935–3945. https://doi.org/10.1007/s00394-021-02565-5

114 Sonnenburg, E.D., & Sonnenburg, J.L. (2014). Starving our microbial self: The deleterious consequences of a diet deficient in microbiota-accessible carbohydrates. *Cell Metabolism*, *20*(5), 779–786. https://doi.org/10.1016/j.cmet.2014.07.003

115 Blaser, M.J. (2017). The theory of disappearing microbiota and the epidemics of chronic diseases. *Nature Reviews. Immunology*, *17*(8), 461–463. https://doi.org/10.1038/nri. 2017.77

116 Genoni, A., Christophersen, C.T., Lo, J., Coghlan, M., Boyce, M.C., Bird, A.R., Lyons-Wall, P., & Devine, A. (2020). Long-term Paleolithic diet is associated with lower resistant starch intake, different gut microbiota composition and increased serum TMAO concentrations. *European Journal of Nutrition*, *59*(5), 1845–1858. https://doi.org/10.1007/s00394-019-02036-y

117 Barone, M., Turroni, S., Rampelli, S., Soverini, M., D'Amico, F., Biagi, E., Brigidi, P., Troiani, E., & Candela, M. (2019). Gut microbiome response to a modern Paleolithic diet in a Western lifestyle context. *PloS One*, *14*(8), e0220619. https://doi.org/10.1371/ journal.pone.0220619

118 Wirbel, J., Pyl, P.T., Kartal, E., Zych, K., Kashani, A., Milanese, A., Fleck, J.S., Voigt, A.Y., Palleja, A., Ponnudurai, R., Sunagawa, S., Coelho, L.P., Schrotz-King, P., Vogtmann, E., Habermann, N., Niméus, E., Thomas, A.M., Manghi, P., Gandini, S., Serrano, D., Zeller, G. (2019). Meta-analysis of fecal metagenomes reveals global microbial signatures that are specific for colorectal cancer. *Nature Medicine*, *25*(4), 679–689. https://doi.org/10.1038/s41591-019-0406-6

119 Genoni, A., Lo, J., Lyons-Wall, P., & Devine, A. (2016). Compliance, palatability and feasibility of PALEOLITHIC and Australian guide to healthy eating diets in healthy women: A 4-week dietary intervention. *Nutrients*, *8*(8), 481. https://doi.org/10.3390/ nu8080481

120 Klein, A.V., & Kiat, H. (2015). Detox diets for toxin elimination and weight management: A critical review of the evidence. *Journal of Human Nutrition and Dietetics*, *28*(6), 675–686. https://doi.org/10.1111/jhn.12286

121 Carrotte, E.R., Vella, A.M., & Lim, M.S. (2015). Predictors of "Liking" three types of health and fitness-related content on social media: A cross-sectional study. *Journal of Medical Internet Research*, *17*(8), e205. https://doi.org/10.2196/jmir.4803

122 National Institute for Clinical Excellence (2021). Constipation: Adverse effects of laxatives. https://cks.nice.org.uk/topics/constipation/prescribing-information/adverse-effects-of-laxatives/

123 Weersma, R.K., Zhernakova, A., & Fu, J. (2020). Interaction between drugs and the gut microbiome. *Gut*, *69*(8), 1510–1519. https://doi.org/10.1136/gutjnl-2019-320204

124 Vich Vila, A., Collij, V., Sanna, S., Sinha, T., Imhann, F., Bourgonje, A.R., Mujagic, Z., Jonkers, D., Masclee, A., Fu, J., Kurilshikov, A., Wijmenga, C., Zhernakova, A., & Weersma, R.K. (2020). Impact of commonly used drugs on the composition and metabolic function of the gut microbiota. *Nature Communications*, *11*(1), 362. https://doi.org/10.1038/s41467-019-14177-z

125 Tropini, C., Moss, E.L., Merrill, B.D., Ng, K.M., Higginbottom, S.K., Casavant, E.P., Gonzalez, C.G., Fremin, B., Bouley, D.M., Elias, J.E., Bhatt, A.S., Huang, K.C., & Sonnenburg, J.L. (2018). Transient osmotic perturbation causes long-term alteration to the gut microbiota. *Cell*, *173*(7), 1742–1754.e17. https://doi.org/10.1016/j.cell. 2018.05.008

126 Obert, J., Pearlman, M., Obert, L., & Chapin, S. (2017). Popular weight loss strategies: A review of four weight loss techniques. *Current Gastroenterology Reports*, *19*(12), 61. https://doi.org/10.1007/s11894-017-0603-8

127 Kalra, A., Yetiskul, E., Wehrle, C.J., & Tuma, F. (2021). *Physiology, Liver*. In: *StatPearls* [Internet]. Treasure Island (FL): StatPearls Publishing. Available from: https://www.ncbi.nlm.nih.gov/books/NBK535438/

128 Phang-Lyn, S., & Llerena, V.A. (2021). *Biochemistry, Biotransformation*. In: *StatPearls* [Internet]. Treasure Island (FL): StatPearls Publishing. Available from: https://www. ncbi.nlm.nih.gov/books/NBK544353/

129 Esteves, F., Rueff, J., & Kranendonk, M. (2021). The central role of Cytochrome P450 in xenobiotic metabolism – A brief review on a fascinating enzyme family. *Journal of Xenobiotics*, *11*(3), 94–114. https://doi.org/10.3390/jox11030007

130 Pizzorno, J. (1996). *Total Wellness*. Rocklin CA: Prima Health.

131 Hodges, R.E., & Minich, D.M. (2015). Modulation of metabolic detoxification pathways using foods and food-derived components: A scientific review with clinical application. *Journal of Nutrition and Metabolism*, *2015*, 760689. https://doi.org/10.1155/2015/760689

132 Farzaei, M.H., Zobeiri, M., Parvizi, F., El-Senduny, F.F., Marmouzi, I., Coy-Barrera, E., Naseri, R., Nabavi, S.M., Rahimi, R., & Abdollahi, M. (2018). Curcumin in liver diseases: A systematic review of the cellular mechanisms of oxidative stress and clinical perspective. *Nutrients*, *10*(7), 855. https://doi.org/10.3390/nu10070855

133 Izzo, C., Annunziata, M., Melara, G., Sciorio, R., Dallio, M., Masarone, M., Federico, A., & Persico, M. (2021). The role of resveratrol in liver disease: A comprehensive review from in vitro to clinical trials. *Nutrients*, *13*(3), 933. https://doi.org/10.3390/nu13030933

134 Casas-Grajales, S., & Muriel, P. (2015). Antioxidants in liver health. *World Journal of Gastrointestinal Pharmacology and Therapeutics*, *6*(3), 59–72. https://doi.org/10.4292/wjgpt.v6.i3.59

135 Derbyshire, E. (2018). Micronutrient intakes of British adults across mid-life: A secondary analysis of the UK National Diet and Nutrition Survey. *Frontiers in Nutrition*,*5*, 55. https://doi.org/10.3389/fnut.2018.00055

136 Goodman, B.E. (2010). Insights into digestion and absorption of major nutrients in humans. *Advances in Physiology Education*, *34*(2), 44–53. https://doi.org/10.1152/advan.00094.2009

137 Lee, S., Choi, Y., Jeong, H.S., Lee, J., & Sung, J. (2017). Effect of different cooking methods on the content of vitamins and true retention in selected vegetables. *Food Science and Biotechnology*, *27*(2), 333–342. https://doi.org/10.1007/s10068-017-0281-1

138 Berna, F., Goldberg, P., Horwitz, L.K., Brink, J., Holt, S., Bamford, M., & Chazan, M. (2012). Microstratigraphic evidence of in situ fire in the Acheulean strata of Wonderwerk Cave, Northern Cape province, South Africa. *Proceedings of the National Academy of Sciences of the United States of America*, *109*(20), E1215–E1220. https://doi.org/10.1073/pnas.1117620109

139 Gowlett, J.A. (2016). The discovery of fire by humans: A long and convoluted process. *Philosophical Transactions of the Royal Society of London. Series B, Biological Sciences*, *371*(1696), 20150164. https://doi.org/10.1098/rstb.2015.0164

140 Carmody, R.N., Weintraub, G.S., & Wrangham, R.W. (2011). Energetic consequences of thermal and nonthermal food processing. *Proceedings of the National Academy of Sciences of the United States of America*, *108*(48), 19199–19203. https://doi.org/10.1073/pnas.1112128108

141 Fabbri A.D.T., & Crosby G.A., (2016). A review of the impact of preparation and cooking on the nutritional quality of vegetables and legumes. *International Journal of Gastronomy and Food Science*, *3*, 2–11. https://doi.org/10.1016/j.ijgfs.2015.11.001

142 Food Standards Agency (2018). Cooking your food. https://www.food.gov.uk/safety-hygiene/cooking-your-food

143 Franssen, F., Gerard, C., Cozma-Petruț, A., Vieira-Pinto, M., Jambrak, A.R., Rowan, N., Paulsen, P., Rozycki, M., Tysnes, K., Rodriguez-Lazaro, D., & Robertson, L. (2019). Inactivation of parasite transmission stages: Efficacy of treatments on food of animal origin. *Trends in Food Science & Technology*, *83*, 114–128 https://doi.org/10.1016/j.tifs.2018.11.009

144 Dolan, L.C., Matulka, R.A., & Burdock, G.A. (2010). Naturally occurring food toxins. *Toxins*, *2*(9), 2289–2332. https://doi.org/10.3390/toxins2092289

145 Felker, P., Bunch, R., & Leung, A.M. (2016). Concentrations of thiocyanate and goitrin in human plasma, their precursor concentrations in brassica vegetables, and associated potential risk for hypothyroidism. *Nutrition Reviews*, *74*(4), 248–258. https://doi.org/10.1093/nutrit/nuv110

146 Koebnick, C., Garcia, A.L., Dagnelie, P.C., Strassner, C., Lindemans, J., Katz, N., Leitzmann, C., & Hoffmann, I. (2005). Long-term consumption of a raw food diet is associated with favorable serum LDL cholesterol and triglycerides but also with elevated plasma homocysteine and low serum HDL cholesterol in humans. *The Journal of Nutrition*, *135*(10), 2372–2378. https://doi.org/10.1093/jn/135.10.2372

147 Fontana, L., Shew, J.L., Holloszy, J.O., & Villareal, D.T. (2005). Low bone mass in subjects on a long-term raw vegetarian diet. *Archives of Internal Medicine*, *165*(6), 684–689. https://doi.org/10.1001/archinte.165.6.684

148 Strohacker, K., Carpenter, K.C., & McFarlin, B.K. (2009). Consequences of weight cycling: An increase in disease risk?. *International Journal of Exercise Science*, *2*(3), 191–201. https://www.ncbi.nlm.nih.gov/pmc/articles/PMC4241770/

149 Jones, R., Haardoerfer, R., Riosmena, F., & Cunningham, S. (2021). Does place matter? Dietary change among immigrants to the US. *Current Developments in Nutrition*, *5*(S2), 1045. https://doi.org/10.1093/cdn/nzab053_038

150 Calandre, N., & Ribert, E. (2019). Sharing norms and adapting habits. The eating practices of immigrants and immigrants' children from Malian and Moroccan origins in France. *Social Science Information*, *58*(1), 141–192. https://doi.org/10.1177/053901 8419843408

151 Pressler, M., Devinsky, J., Duster, M., Lee, J.H., Glick, C.S., Wiener, S., Laze, J., Friedman, D., Roberts, T., & Devinsky, O. (2022). Dietary transitions and health outcomes in four populations – Systematic review. *Frontiers in Nutrition*, *9*, 748305. https://doi.org/10.3389/fnut.2022.748305

152 Imai, T., Miyamoto, K., Sezaki, A., Kawase, F., Shirai, Y., Abe, C., Fukaya, A., Kato, T., Sanada, M., & Shimokata, H. (2019). Traditional Japanese Diet Score – Association with obesity, incidence of ischemic heart disease, and healthy life expectancy in a global comparative study. *The Journal of Nutrition, Health & Aging*, *23*(8), 717–724. https://doi.org/10.1007/s12603-019-1219-5

153 Maruyama, C., Nakano, R., Shima, M., Mae, A., Shijo, Y., Nakamura, E., Okabe, Y., Park, S., Kameyama, N., Hirai, S., Nakanishi, M., Uchida, K., & Nishiyama, H. (2017). Effects of a Japan Diet Intake Program on metabolic parameters in middle-aged men. *Journal of Atherosclerosis and Thrombosis*, *24*(4), 393–401. https://doi.org/10.5551/jat.36780

154 Abe, C., Imai, T., Sezaki, A., Miyamoto, K., Kawase, F., Shirai, Y., Inden, A., Kato, T., Sanada, M., & Shimokata, H. (2021). 64 Traditional Japanese Diet Score and cancer incidence and mortality – A 23-year longitudinal global study. *International Journal of Epidemiology*, *50*(S1), September 2021, dyab168.004. https://doi.org/10.1093/ije/dyab168.004

155 Gabriel, A.S., Ninomiya, K., & Uneyama, H. (2018). The role of the Japanese traditional diet in healthy and sustainable dietary patterns around the world. *Nutrients*, *10*(2), 173. https://doi.org/10.3390/nu10020173

156 Popkin, B.M., Adair, L.S., & Ng, S.W. (2012). Global nutrition transition and the pandemic of obesity in developing countries. *Nutrition Reviews*, *70*(1), 3–21. https://doi.org/10.1111/j.1753-4887.2011.00456.x

157 Sproesser, G., Ruby, M.B., Arbit, N., Akotia, C.S., Alvarenga, M., Bhangaokar, R., Furumitsu, I., Hu, X., Imada, S., Kaptan, G., Kaufer-Horwitz, M., Menon, U., Fischler, C., Rozin, P., Schupp, H.T., & Renner, B. (2019). Understanding traditional and modern eating: The TEP10 framework. *BMC Public Health*, *19*(1), 1606. https://doi.org/10.1186/s12889-019-7844-4

Conclusion

To the reader who made it this far, hopefully this book has aroused interest, kindled excitement, and motivated you, the reader, to go and find out more. It was always intended to be a narrative, a starter book to engage the reader rather than a textbook. Any book that tried to cover every nutrient, body system, and disease in intricate detail would be unreadable – and unmanageably huge. Although nutrition is not the answer to all ills, it certainly underpins all health, from before the cells of an oocyte start dividing, all the way through to the last breath a body takes.

For the last century, modern medicine has tried to strip back diagnosis and treatment to a simplified one-size-fits-all model of mechanistic materialism that looks through a narrow window of symptom and disease, rather than the holistic approach of looking at a whole individual. Although this does seem to be changing, it is happening very slowly. But at least there are some elements within medicine that are looking beyond the route of big pharma to see what else could be helpful to patients. This book will hopefully give some indication to practitioners about how digestive health might make a difference to immunity. How the microbiome might impact mental health. How inflammation is systemic and one inflammatory condition could trigger a whole cascade of inflammation. And how what a patient eats can influence the health and wellbeing of the next generation.

The subject matter for chapters was carefully chosen deep dives into selected areas that are relevant to primary care practitioners. For example, vitamin D has a dedicated chapter because research over the last decade has made it increasingly apparent that $1\alpha,25(OH)_2$ is central to almost every aspect of our health and wellbeing. Of course all of the other micronutrients are important, but the relevance of vitamin D has really come to the fore recently. So other nutrients are discussed, in context, in multiple chapters without the same depth as vitamin D. Hopefully the quick reference "nutrient cheat sheets" at the back of the book on 14 vitamins, 17 minerals, the essential fatty acids, as well as a number of other substances will prove useful to practitioners.

Most systems do not have dedicated chapters and those which have been selected (the digestive system, the immune system, and reproduction) were chosen because nutrition is so fundamental to their function, and their functions are so essential to the health and wellbeing of every one of us.

The digestive system is generally not particularly well understood by primary care practitioners, other than in the context of pathology. It is often thought of as being rather simple and straightforward, food and energy in, waste out. But the reality is that the gastrointestinal tract is one of the most complex of our body systems. Without a well-functioning digestive system, all sorts of other things in other systems start to falter; body systems are not neatly boxed up in separate parcels, everything is interconnected.

DOI: 10.1201/b22900-11

Likewise, the relevance of nutrition to the functioning of the immune system is not something most primary care practitioners are likely to think about. But without an effective supply of appropriate micronutrients, the immune system falters and lets us down. And as for the systems of reproduction, their importance to the health of future generations is entirely based on good nutrition. Which, once again, is something that too many healthcare practitioners in the UK simply do not think about.

Heart disease, cancer, and neurodegenerative diseases are extraordinarily complex in both their development and their subsequent management. It would take an entire book to fully explore the aetiology and depths of nutritional understanding relating to each, and even that would probably be insufficient because new research is stimulating new ideas all the time. So these and other diseases are referenced in relation to specific nutrients which are discussed throughout the book.

Life expectancy in parts of the UK is falling, with an increasing disparity between areas of deprivation and areas of wealth.[1] Health inequalities are rising, so too is food insecurity.[2,3] Health inequalities and life expectancy are closely linked to diet; individuals in lower socioeconomic groups have lower intakes of fruit and vegetables of any kind as well as low intakes of whole grains, nuts and seeds, and legumes.[4] And greater levels of food insecurity increases the intake of ultra-processed foods.[5] Poor diet is one of the leading causes of avoidable harm to our health and better access to, and knowledge of, healthy affordable food would make a huge difference to the lives of many millions of UK citizens.

And while quality of life declines, the rate of autoimmune conditions in the UK is rising at an alarming rate. The incidence of rheumatic disease is increasing by around 7% a year, type I diabetes is not far behind at 6.3% a year whilst multiple sclerosis is increasing by 3.7% a year.[6] In 2018 these three diseases alone were collectively estimated to cost the UK more than £13 billion a year.[6] Yet they can all be modified, and in some cases reversed or even prevented entirely, with diet and lifestyle changes. An understanding of how what we eat influences our health, our biochemistry, and our immune responses could help healthcare practitioners support their patients, whilst potentially reducing their reliance on an overburdened and under resourced health service.

No book on nutrition can ever be absolutely up to date. As soon as the writing process is finished, before it is even published, thousands of new peer review papers highlighting extraordinary research and, in some cases, revolutionary ideas will have come out. The majority of the peer review research used as the evidence base in this book is open access. This was a deliberate choice, because if a reader wants to pursue an issue, yet cannot access the full reference, then that could close down the interest this book is intended to stimulate.

When doing some research about nutrition and diet, for a patient, or for yourself, it may not necessarily be wise to swallow the UK government or NHS line whole. Some of it needs to be taken with a substantial pinch of salt because it is not necessarily based on the most recent thinking. There are ideas out in the nutrition world that are considered to be deeply controversial. For example, the consumption of saturated fat. The NHS is sticking doggedly to the party line, that saturated fat is "bad" and that polyunsaturated fat is "good", despite much of the nutrition world changing its thinking on this one and issuing a call to rethink national dietary guidelines on fat intake.[7] It takes time for new ideas to filter through. Think about how long it took for the world to accept that stomach ulcers are caused by *Helicobacter pylori* (23 years for anyone who was wondering).

There are no easy answers in health or nutrition. Perhaps the biggest lie that modern healthcare has promoted is the "easy" option of the pharmaceutical magic bullet. The trouble is, everyone's biochemistry is as unique at the individual themselves. Whilst clearly there are broad similarities, tiny details are likely to be different in everyone, for example how well or badly β-carotene is converted to retinoid; or how well or badly any individual will respond to a medication. Genetic factors, environmental impacts, the health (or otherwise) of the micro-biome, social influences, personal likes and dislikes will all shape our health, just as much as how we eat and what we eat. But there is one basic principle that is unlikely to change, regardless of any new and exciting research, or shiny new products on the shelves. Real food is the foundation of good health. Real food that involves peeling and chopping and cooking and flavour and chewing and socialising and family and love.

REFERENCES

1 Wise J. (2022). Life expectancy: Parts of England and Wales see "shocking" fall. *BMJ*, *377*, o1056. https://doi.org/10.1136/bmj.o1056

2 Ralston, R., Smith, K., O'Connor, C. H., & Brown, A. (2022). Levelling up the UK: is the government serious about reducing regional inequalities in health?. *BMJ*, *377*, e070589. https://doi.org/10.1136/bmj-2022-070589

3 The Food Foundation (2022). New data shows food insecurity major challenge to levelling up agenda. https://foodfoundation.org.uk/press-release/new-data-shows-food-insecurity-major-challenge-levelling-agenda

4 Patel, L., Alicandro, G., & La Vecchia, C. (2020). Dietary Approaches to Stop Hypertension (DASH) diet and associated socio-economic inequalities in the UK. *The British Journal of Nutrition*, *124*(10), 1076–1085. https://doi.org/10.1017/S0007114520001087

5 Leung, C. W., Fulay, A. P., Parnarouskis, L., Martinez-Steele, E., Gearhardt, A. N., & Wolfson, J. A. (2022). Food insecurity and ultra-processed food consumption: the modifying role of participation in the Supplemental Nutrition Assistance Program (SNAP). *The American Journal of Clinical Nutrition*, *116*(1), 197–205. https://doi.org/10.1093/ajcn/nqac049

6 Connect Immune Research (2018). Are you AutoimmuneAware? *British Society for Immunology* https://www.immunology.org/sites/default/files/connect-immune-research-are-you-autoimmune-report.pdf

7 Astrup, A., Magkos, F., Bier, D. M., Brenna, J. T., de Oliveira Otto, M. C., Hill, J. O., King, J. C., Mente, A., Ordovas, J. M., Volek, J. S., Yusuf, S., & Krauss, R. M. (2020). Saturated Fats and Health: A Reassessment and Proposal for Food-Based Recommendations: JACC State-of-the-Art Review. *Journal of the American College of Cardiology*, *76*(7), 844–857. https://doi.org/10.1016/j.jacc.2020.05.077

Nutrient "Cheat Sheets"

Fat soluble vitamins:

- A
- D
- E
- K

Water soluble vitamins

- C
- B1 (Thiamin)
- B2 (Riboflavin)
- B3 (Niacin)
- B5 (Pantothenic Acid)
- B6 (Pyridoxine)
- Folic acid
- B12 (Cyanocobalamin)
- Biotin
- Choline

Minerals

- Potassium
- Chloride
- Calcium
- Phosphorus
- Magnesium
- Sodium

Trace elements

- Iron
- Zinc
- Copper
- Manganese
- Fluoride
- Selenium
- Chromium
- Molybdenum
- Iodine

- Boron
- Silicon

Other substances

- Alpha Linolenic Acid
- Eicosapentaenoic Acid & Docosahexaenoic Acid
- Omega-6 fatty acids
- Co-enzyme Q10
- Flavonoids

The acronyms used in this section are explained in the chapter on Nutrition Basics, however for quick reference:

- RNI Reference Nutrient Intake
- LRNI Lower Reference Nutrient Intake
- SUL Safe Upper intake Level
- EU DRV Dietary Reference Values set by the European Food Safety Authority who have evaluated all of the micronutrients much more recently than the UK authorities.

Levels given for RNI, LRNI, SUL and EU DRV are all those for an average adult male.

RNI, LRNI, SUL and DRV can vary across age ranges and genders and therefore in some instances, additional intake levels are provided.

In some instances SULs provided refer to additional nutrients provided by supplementation, in which case this is noted as "supplemental rather than total intake".

Food sources are listed with the richest sources first, descending to adequate sources.

The UK government tracks nutrient intakes through the National Diet and Nutrition Survey (NDNS) which has been running for three decades.

Vitamin A (retinol & β-carotene); fat soluble

Daily intakes[1,2,3]	• RNI 700 μg • LRNI 300 μg • SUL 1500 μg • EU DRV 750 μg	Vitamin A is measured in micrograms (μg) in food supplements and International Units (IU) in medicines. 1 IU = 0.3 μg of vitamin A.
Nutrient of concern?[4,5]	• **Yes.** • 17% of adults aged 18–79 and 21% of children aged 11–18 have intakes below the LRNI putting them at risk of deficiency.	
Functions[6,7,8]	• Normal growth and function of the retina. • Structure, integrity, and function of all epithelial tissues. • Immune function (growth and distribution of T-cells). • Cellular differentiation and proliferation including red blood cell production and bone growth. • Foetal and child growth and development.	

Risks from insufficiency[4,9]	• Insufficiency during pregnancy and lactation negatively impacts:
	  • Maternal vision and foetal ocular development.
	  • Foetal development (heart, central nervous system, skeletal, circulatory, urogenital, and respiratory systems).
	• Night blindness and xeropthalmia.
	• Increased risk of infections, particularly respiratory and urinary tract.	

Risks from excess[2,4,10]	• Risks ONLY relate to excess consumption of retinol form. • Teratogenic effects at intakes >3000 μg supplemental **retinol.** • Dry, itchy, flaking skin. • Bone and joint pain. • Reduced bone density, possible increased fracture risk. • With chronic over consumption, potential hepatotoxicity.	
Food sources[11]	**Retinol:** Liver and other organ meats, cod liver oil, eggs, full fat dairy products.	**β-carotene:** Brightly coloured fruit and vegetables, particularly sweet potato, pumpkin and squash, carrot, leafy greens (spinach and kale).
Additional notes[12]	The UK has a precautionary stance on supplementary vitamin A. There is NO RISK from high consumption of natural β-carotene. Possible risk to smokers: high consumption of synthetic β-carotene may increase cancer risk in some individuals.	

Vitamin D (cholecalciferol, ergocalciferol) (fat soluble)

Daily intakes[3, 13, 14]	• RNI (>age 5) 10 μg (400 IU) • LRNI none set • SUL 25 μg (1,000 IU) • EU DRV (>12 months) 15 μg (600 IU)	Vitamin D is measured in micrograms (μg) in food supplements and International Units (IU) in medicines. 1 IU = 0.025 μg of vitamin D.
Nutrient of concern?[4, 15, 16, 17]	• **Yes.** • All UK populations have intakes below what is considered optimum. • Increase in rickets and osteoporosis in recent decades.	
Functions[18, 19]	• Facilitates calcium and phosphorus absorption and utilisation to ensure bone health. • Positive impact on mental health. • Essential for immune function. • Modulates inflammation. • Essential in reproduction.	
Risks from insufficiency[18, 20, 21]	• Increased incidence of rickets, osteomalacia and osteoporosis. • Muscle weakness and pain. • Increased risk of some cancers, autoimmune diseases, hypertension and infectious diseases. • Poor mental health, increased depression, increased risk of suicidal thoughts and behaviours.	
Risks from excess[6, 22]	• Hypercalcaemia can cause constipation, diarrhoea, dehydration, nausea and vomiting, headache. • Vitamin D toxicity is extremely rare; long term daily intake of more than 500 μg (20,000 IU) in adults found no evidence of toxicity.	
Food sources[11]	Oily fish and cod liver oil, eggs, mushrooms exposed to UV light and some fortified foods.	
Additional notes	As a fat-soluble substance, vitamin D food supplements must be taken with food or drink which contains fat, otherwise it cannot be absorbed. The UK government recommends that everyone should consider taking a vitamin D food supplement of 10 μg during the autumn and winter. This is completely inadequate; everyone should be taking at least 25 μg/d from early September to early April.	

Vitamin E (tocopherols) (fat soluble)

Daily intakes[2,3]	• RNI Not set • LRNI Not set • SUL 560 mg α-tocopherol equivalents • EU DRV 12 mg
Nutrient of concern?	• No RNI for vitamin E is set in the UK and intakes are not tracked in the NDNS.
Functions[6,23,24]	• Potent antioxidant particularly active in cell membranes, red blood cells and plasma. • Facilitates greater stability in cell membranes. • Enhances immune function. • Regulates platelet aggregation, reducing the risk of blood clots.
Risks from insufficiency[25]	• Rare; related to malabsorption and metabolic issues. • Increased risk of respiratory complaints. • Increased risk of blood clots. • Nerve and muscle damage leading to loss of sensation and reduced movement, muscle weakness, and vision problems.
Risks from excess[6]	• Relatively non-toxic, chronic intake over 1,000 mg/d can increase bleeding and lead to nausea, headache, fatigue, weakness and altered endocrine function (thyroid, adrenal and pituitary).
Food sources[11]	Wheatgerm, sunflower seeds & sunflower oil, hazelnuts, almonds, peanuts, avocado, leafy green vegetables.
Additional notes	As with all fat-soluble vitamins, low fat diets may impact on vitamin E status as it requires sufficient dietary fat to be absorbed and utilised.

Vitamin K (phylloquinone (K1), menaquinone (K2)) (fat soluble)

Daily intakes[2,3]	• RNI Not set • LRNI Not set • SUL 1 mg (supplemental rather than total intake) • EU DRV 75 µg
Nutrient of concern?	• No RNI for vitamin K is set in the UK and intakes are not tracked in the NDNS.

Functions[26,27]	• Synthesis of vitamin K-dependent proteins used in:
	  • Proper coagulation; prevention of inappropriate coagulation including prevention of blood clots.
	  • Prevention of vascular calcification, protecting against cardiovascular disease.
	  • Formation and maintenance of bones and teeth, improving bone quality, protection against fractures and degeneration.
	  • Regulation of cell differentiation and proliferation, inhibition of metastasis in a range of cancers.
	• Modulation of immune cell synthesis.
	• Anti-inflammatory.

Risks from insufficiency[26,27,28]	• Increased risk of bleeding. • Increased risk of cardiovascular disease. • Increased risk of osteo and rheumatoid arthritis. • Increased risk of bone fracture and reduced mobility.
Risks from excess[6]	• Oral vitamin K is not toxic. • There have been rare hypersensitivity reactions to phytomenadione (injectable vitamin K).

Food sources[11]	**Phylloquinone:** Green vegetables (kale, spinach, broccoli, cabbage, Brussels sprouts), soya beans, carrots, and grapes.	**Menaquinone:** Small quantities in fermented foods like natto (Japanese fermented soyabeans), sauerkraut, and hard cheeses, as well as organ meats.

Additional notes	Menaquinone is found in limited foods but is primarily produced by the gut microbiome. Vitamin K deficiency in adults may be the result of malabsorption issue, the use of anticoagulated medication, or prolonged antibiotic use.

Vitamin C (ascorbic acid) (water soluble)

Daily intakes[1,2,3]	• RNI 40 mg • LRNI 10 mg • SUL 1000 mg (supplemental rather than total intake) • EU DRV 80 mg
Nutrient of concern?[29,30,31,32]	• **Yes.** • Optimum intake 200 mg/day; UK RNI is inadequate. • 86% of the population eat <3.5 portions of fruit and vegetables a day. • Poor vitamin C status is common in low-income families. • The 2019 UK NDNS found many women have plasma vitamin C levels that puts them at risk of deficiency.
Functions[6,8,33]	• Potent electron donor in reduction reactions; primary antioxidant in aqueous mediums. • Regenerates vitamin E's antioxidant capability. • Cofactor in synthesis of hormones, neurotransmitters, and collagen. • Essential in production and function of many immune cells. • Facilitation of non-heme iron absorption.
Risks from insufficiency[29,34,35]	• In extreme cases, scurvy. • Reduced collagen synthesis = weak blood vessels, connective tissue, and bone = easy bruising, poor wound healing, bone and join pain, hair, and tooth loss. • Reduced immune function. • Increased risk of respiratory infections. • Increased risk of coronary heart disease, stroke, and cancer. • Increased risk of metabolic disorders.
Risks from excess[6]	• Relatively non-toxic. • Excessively high intakes (over 10 grams/d) may cause diarrhoea and gastrointestinal distress in some individuals.
Food sources[11]	All fresh fruit and vegetables, particularly high in guavas, Kiwi fruit, red and green peppers, blackcurrants, cantaloupe melon, strawberries, kale, Brussels sprouts, and cabbage.
Additional notes	The reason more of the UK population are not deemed at risk of deficiency is probably due to the extremely low bar set by the British government.

Vitamin B1 (thiamin)

Daily intakes[1,2,3]	• RNI 0.9 mg • LRNI 0.23 mg • SUL 100 mg (supplemental rather than total intake) • EU DRV 1.1 mg
Nutrient of concern?	• UK intakes of thiamine have not been measured by the NDNS for over a decade. It is not possible to say if current UK intakes are adequate or not.
Functions[6,36,37]	• An enzyme cofactor in energy production (Krebs cycle, protein metabolism and β-oxidation of fatty acids). • Direct antioxidant protection of nerves. • Protects nerve tissues from hyperglycaemia and increases nerve conduction. • Facilitates process of nerve regeneration.
Risks from insufficiency[38,39]	• In extreme cases, beriberi. • Tiredness, fatigue, and apathy. • Loss of appetite, nausea, abdominal pain, and anorexia. • Poor tendon reflexes and progressive muscle weakness. • Water retention, swelling of legs, body, and face. • Loss of muscle coordination, confusion, and memory loss. • Neurological issues including depression, cognitive deficits, and dementia.
Risks from excess	• No established toxic level.
Food sources[11]	Brewer's yeast, nutritional yeast, wheatgerm, pork, Brazil nuts, green peas, fortified breakfast cereals.
Additional notes	Industrial food processing depletes thiamine, and the high calorie content of ultra-processed food increases requirement for thiamine. This could be creating a significant problem that is not being looked at.

Vitamin B2 (riboflavin)

Daily intakes[1,2,3]	• RNI 1.3 mg • LRNI 0.8 mg • SUL 43 mg • EU DRV 1.4 mg
Nutrient of concern?[4,5,40]	• **Yes.** • 95% of adolescent girls & 41% of elderly free-living people are riboflavin insufficient. • UK intakes have fallen 11% over the last 20 years.
Functions[6,41]	• Component of coenzymes flavin adenine dinucleotide (FAD) and flavin mononucleotide (FMN), both central to energy metabolism. • Required for redox reactions in the glutathione, superoxide dismutase, and xanthine oxidase antioxidant systems. • Essential in the absorption, utilisation and metabolism of iron, folate, B6, and B12.
Risks from insufficiency[42]	• In extreme cases, ariboflavinosis. • Tiredness and fatigue. • Sore throat, swollen tongue, cracked, inflamed lips. • Increased oxidative stress. • Reduced iron absorption and potential anaemia. • Increased risk of cataracts.
Risks from excess	• No known toxicity.
Food sources[11]	Organ meats, dairy products, eggs, meat, chicken, and fish, fortified breakfast cereals.
Additional notes	Low intakes of riboflavin increase the risk of cognitive impairment in later life.

Vitamin B3 (niacin; nicotinic acid, niacinamide, nicotinamide)

Daily intakes[1,2,3]	<ul><li>RNI 17 mg</li><li>LRNI 4.4 mg</li><li>SUL 560 mg</li><li>EU DRV 16 mg</li></ul>
Nutrient of concern?	<ul><li>UK intakes of niacin have not been measured in the NDNS since 2012. It is not possible to say if current UK intakes are adequate or not.</li></ul>
Functions[6,43,44]	<ul><li>Component of nicotinamide adenine dinucleotide (NAD) and nicotinamide adenine dinucleotide phosphate (NADP) which provide electron transfers in over 400 redox reactions.</li><li>NAD is used in the energy metabolism of carbohydrates, fats and proteins.</li><li>NADP is used in the biosynthesis of cholesterol, steroid hormones and fatty acids, and in oxidant defence.</li><li>NAD is also used as a substrate by other enzymes involved in alcohol detoxification, immunity, DNA repair, cell signalling, and calcium mobilisation.</li></ul>
Risks from insufficiency[43,45,46]	<ul><li>In extreme cases, pellagra.</li><li>Tiredness and fatigue.</li><li>Headache, depression, and memory loss.</li><li>Increased risk of cardiovascular disease and some cancers.</li><li>Increased risk of age-related cognitive decline.</li></ul>
Risks from excess[2]	<ul><li>Varies depending on the form.</li><li>≥50 mg/d nicotinic acid can cause skin flushing, itching, nausea, and GI disturbance.</li><li>≥3000 mg/d nicotinamide may cause liver dysfunction.</li><li>Symptoms are reversible.</li></ul>
Food sources[11]	Organ meats, red meat, chicken, fish, peanuts, brown rice, fortified breakfast cereals.
Additional notes[47,48]	Niacin can be synthesised from the amino acid tryptophan; this requires riboflavin (B2) and pyridoxine (B6) for several of the reactions and low levels of these vitamins can lead to niacin deficiency. Niacin in plant foods it is often bound to sugars that reduce its bioavailability, preventing it from being absorbed.

Vitamin B5 (pantothenic acid)

Daily intakes[2,3]	• RNI Not set • LRNI Not set • SUL 210 mg • EU DRV6 mg
Nutrient of concern?	• No RNI for pantothenic acid is set in the UK and intakes are not tracked in the NDNS.

Functions[49,50,51]	• A component of co-enzyme A which is essential for:
	  • Energy metabolism.
	  • Synthesis of cholesterol, steroid hormones and neurotransmitters.
	  • Metabolism and detoxification pathways within the liver.
	• May reduce C-reactive protein and low grade inflammation; C-reactive protein and inflammation are associated with increased risk of heart disease.
	• May alter the balance of cholesterol, shifting the ratio to lower LDL, higher HDL and increase CoQ10 levels, thereby improving cardiovascular risk markers.

Risks from insufficiency[49,52]	• Numbness and burning of the hands and feet. • Headaches. • Fatigue & disturbed sleep. • Irritability & restlessness. • Gastrointestinal disturbances.
Risks from excess[2]	• No known toxicity.
Food sources[11]	Organ meats, shiitake mushrooms, fish and shellfish, chicken, eggs, avocados, peanuts, dairy products, legumes and pulses, fortified breakfast cereal.
Additional notes	Deficiency is extremely rare except in severe malnutrition and is often accompanied by multiple micronutrient deficiencies, particularly other B vitamins. It has only been noted in humans who are prisoners of war, particularly during World War II.

Vitamin B6 (pyridoxin)

Daily intakes[1,2,3]	• RNI 1.4 mg • LRNI 11 µg • SUL 10 mg (supplemental rather than total intake) • EU DRV1.4 mg
Nutrient of concern?	• No.
Functions[8,53]	• A cofactor for more than 60 enzymes involved in over 100 biochemical reactions in protein, lipid, and carbohydrate metabolism. • Essential for RNA & DNA synthesis, the synthesis of neurotransmitters, the production of red blood cells. • Acts with B12 and folic acid in the conversion of homocysteine to the less toxic methionine.
Risks from insufficiency[6]	• Dermatitis, glossitis, cheilosis, angular stomatitis. • Tiredness and fatigue. • Irritability and depression.
Risks from excess[6]	• Toxicity is rare; supplemental intakes above 117 mg/d can cause neurological symptoms (numbness & tingling), unsteady gait, impaired tendon reflexes. • Symptoms are reversible when dose is reduced.
Food sources[11]	Fish, organ meats, poultry, grains, legumes, fortified breakfast cereals, potatoes, avocadoes, dairy products.
Additional notes[54]	Deficiency is rare, usually associated with other B vitamin deficiencies; may be linked to alcoholism, extreme obesity, malnutrition, and inflammatory GI diseases that cause absorptive issues.

Vitamin B12 (cyanocobalamin)

Daily intakes[1,2,3]	• RNI 1.5 µg • LRNI 1 µg • SUL 2000 µg (supplemental rather than total intake) • EU DRV 2.5 µg
Nutrient of concern?	• **Yes** in vegetarians, vegans, and individuals with absorptive issues.
Functions[8,53]	• Essential in the development and function of the central nervous system. • Required for the synthesis of fatty acids in the myelin sheath of nerves. • Involved in red blood cell formation and RNA & DNA synthesis. • Acts with B6 and folic acid in the conversion of homocysteine to the less toxic methionine.
Risks from insufficiency[6,55]	• Anaemia (both pernicious and megaloblastic); palpitations. • Fatigue. • Glossitis. • Dementia. • Weight loss. • Numbness and tingling in hands and feet.
Risks from excess[6]	• None known.
Food sources[11]	Organ meats, shellfish, oily fish, white fish, meat, dairy products, fortified breakfast cereal, fortified vegetarian yeast flakes.
Additional notes[56]	Low maternal B12 increases the risk of neural tube defects; it is also linked with developmental delay, failure to thrive and anaemia in offspring.

Folic Acid

Daily intakes[1,2,3]	• RNI 200 μg • LRNI 100 μg • SUL 1.5 mg • EU DRV 200 μg	• For women, 400 μg for three months prior to pregnancy and for the first three months of pregnancy.
Nutrient of concern?	• **Yes**, particularly in women of childbearing age.	
Functions[8,53,57]	• Co-factor in cell division and synthesis of RNA, DNA, and proteins. • Key nutrient in the prevention of neural tube defects. • Acts with B6 and B12 in the conversion of homocysteine to the less toxic methionine. • Required for red blood cell formation. • Has a role in supporting cognitive function.	
Risks from insufficiency[6,58]	• Increased risk of neural tube defects. • Increased tiredness and fatigue. • Increased risk of megaloblastic anaemia. • Increased risk of cardiovascular events.	
Risks from excess[6,58,]	• Debate is ongoing about possible masking of B12 deficiency; however concerns are largely historical, dating from before there were B12 blood assays. These days a simple blood test will determine any issues. • Extremely high doses may cause GI disturbances which cease once dose is reduced.	
Food sources[11]	Leafy green vegetables, beans and pulses, potatoes whole grains, liver, brewer's yeast, and fortified foods.	
Additional notes[4]	90% of UK women of childbearing age have red blood cell folate levels below the level that protects against neural tube defects.	

Biotin

Daily intakes[2,3]	• RNI Not set • LRNI Not set • SUL 900 µg (supplemental rather than total intake) • EU DRV 50 µg
Nutrient of concern?	• No RNI for biotin is set in the UK and intakes are not tracked in the NDNS.
Functions[59,60,61]	• Key co-factor in enzymes involved in metabolism of fats and proteins, in gluconeogenesis, and the formation of oxaloacetate, the starter molecule of the Kreb's cycle. • Modulates gene expression, including in DNA replication and transcription. • Improves pancreatic function, increases insulin secretion, and reduces diabetic complications by supporting glucose homeostasis.
Risks from insufficiency[62,63]	• Insufficiency during pregnancy may increase the risk of foetal growth restriction, birth defects, and preterm delivery. • Thinning hair and alopecia, dermatitis, brittle nails.
Risks from excess[64]	• No known risks to health. • High levels of biotin may skew test results for troponin (used to diagnose heart attacks); hormone tests for TSH, T4, T3, PHT, FSH, LH and cortisol; and vitamin D levels.
Food sources[6]	Organ meats, eggs, fish, red meat, soya beans, peanuts, dairy products, whole grains.
Additional notes[65]	Biotin requirements increase in pregnancy and lactation.

Choline

Daily intakes[66,67]	• RNI Not set • LRNI Not set • SUL Not set; Institute of Medicine (USA) set 3.5 g/d • EU AI (adequate intake) 400 mg, increased in pregnancy to 480 mg, and lactation to 520 mg
Nutrient of concern?[68]	• **Yes** • No RNI for choline is set in the UK and intakes are not tracked in the NDNS.
Functions[66,69]	• Essential in foetal brain and spinal cord development and foetal and infant cognitive development. • Synthesis of neurotransmitters. • Component of phospholipids in cell membranes. • Key constituent of very-low-density lipoprotein. • Facilitates the methylation of homocysteine to methionine.
Risks from insufficiency[66,70,71]	• Increased risk of neural tube defects. • Liver damage and non-alcoholic fatty liver disease. • Muscle damage that resolves if adequate choline is consumed. • Poor cognitive function and potential neurological disorders.
Risks from excess[67]	• Intakes over 3.5 g/d in adults can result in fishy body odour, vomiting, excessive sweating, hypotension, and liver toxicity.
Food sources[72]	Eggs, beef and beef liver, fish, pork, chicken, almonds, full fat milk; soya beans, quinoa, wheat germ.
Additional notes[68]	Requirements increase in pregnancy and lactation. Plasma choline levels in pregnant women are significantly higher than in non-pregnant women while choline concentrations in amniotic fluid are 10× higher than those circulating in maternal blood.

Potassium

Daily intakes[1,2,3]	• RNI 3500 mg • LRNI 2000 mg • SUL 3700 mg (supplemental rather than total intake) • EU DRV 2000 mg
Nutrient of concern?[5]	• **Yes.** • A significant proportion of children aged 11–18 and adults across all age ranges have intakes below the LRNI.
Functions[6]	• Works with sodium and chloride to maintain intercellular and extracellular fluid balance. • Regulates acid-base balance. • Regulates blood pressure. • Essential for transmission of nerve impulses and control of skeletal muscle contractions.
Risks from insufficiency[73]	• Increased blood pressure and greater likelihood that changes in sodium intake will affect blood pressure. • Increased risk of kidney stones. • Increased bone turnover. • Hypokalaemia which causes constipation, fatigue, muscle weakness and cardiac arrhythmias.
Risks from excess[6,73]	• Nausea, vomiting, diarrhoea, and abdominal cramps may occur if taken on an empty stomach. • Excess can be an indicator of kidney disease, type I diabetes, congestive heart failure, adrenal insufficiency or liver disease.
Food sources[11]	Potatoes, baked beans, green vegetables, peas, beans and pulses, dried apricots, prunes, raisins, bananas.
Additional notes[74]	The more potassium that is consumed, the more sodium is excreted in urine. Excess plasma potassium may be an indicator of impaired elimination.

Chloride

Daily intakes[3]	<ul><li>RNI Not set</li><li>LRNI Not set</li><li>SUL Not set</li><li>EU DRV 800 mg</li></ul>
Nutrient of concern?	<ul><li>No RNI for chloride is set in the UK and intakes are not tracked in the NDNS.</li></ul>
Functions[75, 76]	<ul><li>Works with sodium and potassium to maintain intercellular and extracellular fluid balance.</li><li>Maintains acid-base and salt balance.</li><li>Enables transport across cell membranes through specific chloride channels.</li><li>Needed for muscle contraction, particularly in smooth muscle in the heart and GI tract.</li><li>Transmission of nerve signals.</li><li>Essential in the formation of hydrochloric acid in the stomach.</li></ul>
Risks from insufficiency[77]	<ul><li>Rare; chloride loss mirrors sodium loss.</li><li>Metabolic alkalosis (pH>7.45).</li><li>Weakness and fatigue.</li><li>Dehydration, linked to vomiting and diarrhoea.</li></ul>
Risks from excess[77]	<ul><li>Metabolic acidosis (pH<7.35).</li><li>Fatigue and muscle weakness.</li><li>High blood pressure.</li></ul>
Food sources[6]	Found in very small amounts in most foods, found in higher amounts in any food that contains salt.
Additional notes[77]	Individuals who have a particularly low salt intake, or breastfed infants of mother's who have a very low salt intake may be at risk of insufficiency. Vomiting, diarrhoea, excessive sweating, and excessive loss through urine may result in insufficiency.

Calcium

Daily intakes[1,2,3]	• RNI 700 mg • LRNI 400 mg • SUL 1500 mg (supplemental rather than total intake) • EU DRV 800 mg
Nutrient of concern?[4]	• **Yes** • 22% of teenage girls have low intakes that put them at risk of deficiency.
Functions[8,78]	• Structural mineral needed for bone density, tooth enamel, and cellular structures. • Regulates the flow of nutrients (and other substances) in and out of cells. • Calcium concentration maintains blood pH. • Intercellular messenger mediates muscle contraction and the transmission of nerve impulses. • Essential in insulin synthesis.
Risks from insufficiency[78,79]	• Poor bone density and osteoporosis. • High blood pressure and cardiovascular disease. • Increased risk of inflammatory bowel disease and colorectal cancers. • Increased risk of Type I and Type II diabetes.
Risks from excess[80]	• Headaches and fatigue. • Extreme thirst and excessive urination. • Kidney stones. • Bloating and constipation. • Increased risk of vascular calcification and cardiovascular disease.
Food sources[11]	Dairy products, green leafy vegetables, tinned fish, nuts and seeds, beans and pulses and white bread (fortified with calcium in the UK).
Additional notes	Calcium cannot be absorbed and utilised unless sufficient vitamin D is present. As the UK is suffering population wide deficiency in vitamin D, it is likely that calcium is also a nutrient of far wider concern than suggested by NDNS data which only evaluates intakes, not absorption and utilisation.

Phosphorus

Daily intakes[2,3]	• RNI Not set • LRNI Not set • SUL 2400 mg • EU DRV 700 mg
Nutrient of concern?	• No RNI for phosphorus is set in the UK and intakes are not tracked in the NDNS.
Functions[8,81,82]	• Structural component in cell membranes. • Essential in the formation and function of nucleic acids DNA and RNA. • Central to energy production because of its function within ADP & ATP. • Acts with calcium in forming hydroxyapatite, the mineral that provides strength in bone.
Risks from insufficiency[81,83]	• Rare. Seen in near starvation (particularly anorexia); inbuilt error of phosphate metabolism; alcoholics; diabetics recovering from diabetic ketoacidosis. • Loss of appetite, anaemia, muscle weakness, rickets and osteomalacia, increased susceptibility to infection.
Risks from excess[84]	• Disrupts hormonal regulation of mineral absorption and utilisation. • Increased risk of cardiovascular disease. • Increased risk of tissue calcification in blood vessels and kidneys. • Loss of bone mineralisation.
Food sources[81,85]	Meat, chicken, fish, milk, cheese, eggs, lentils, nuts, potatoes. Ultra-processed foods, which make up over 57% of the calories consumed in the UK, contain very high levels of inorganic phosphates which presents a risk of anyone with kidney issues.
Additional notes	Impaired kidney function and low levels of parathyroid hormone both reduce excretion of phosphorus which can lead to elevated serum phosphorus concentrations.

Magnesium

Daily intakes[1,2,3]	• RNI 300 mg • LRNI 190 mg • SUL 400 mg (supplemental rather than total intake) • EU DRV 375 mg
Nutrient of concern?[5]	• **Yes** • 100% of the UK population have intakes below the RNI and nearly 13% of adults have intakes below the LRNI.

Functions[86,87]	• Co-factor in hundreds of enzymes involved in multiple processes including:
	  • Vitamin D absorption and utilisation.
	  • Energy metabolism.
	  • RNA synthesis and DNA replication.
	  • Neuromuscular impulse transmission (including to the heart).
	  • Supporting vascular tone.
	• Preserves bone by stimulating calcitonin production.

Risks from insufficiency[86,87]	• Loss of appetite, nausea, vomiting, fatigue, and muscle weakness. • Numbness, tingling, muscle contractions, and cramps. • Abnormal heart rhythms and heart spasms. • Disrupted mineral homeostasis, particularly low calcium and or potassium.
Risks from excess[88]	• Unlikely to occur from food alone, excess is the result of supplementation, medication, or under-excretion by kidneys. • Diarrhoea, nausea, and vomiting. • Muscle weakness. • Low blood pressure. • Extreme excess can lead to respiratory paralysis and heart failure.
Food sources[11]	Nuts (particularly Brazil nuts, peanuts, hazelnuts, and almonds), seeds (particularly pumpkin and chia seeds), green leafy vegetables, whole grains, meat, fish and shellfish, peas, beans and other pulses, and dark chocolate.
Additional notes	60% of total magnesium is found in bone. 39% is stored intracellularly and only 1% is found in plasma.

Sodium

Daily intakes[89]	• RNI not set • LRNI Not set • SUL Not set • EU DRV Not set	• UK government advises maximum intake of 2.4 g of sodium per day
Nutrient of concern?[90]	• **Yes** • Unique among micronutrients, excess rather than insufficiency is the concern.	
Functions[91]	• Regulates fluid, electrolyte and acid-base balance in blood and tissues. • Action in fluid balance also regulates blood pressure. • Essential in transport of chemicals across cell membranes. • Combines with chloride in the formation of hydrochloric acid in the stomach. • Works with potassium to enable nerve function and muscle contraction and expansion.	
Risks from insufficiency[92]	• Rare, linked to sodium depleting kidney diseases, extensive burns, chronic diarrhoea or vomiting, extreme sweating, or excessive water intake. • Nausea, vomiting, headache, muscle cramps, fatigue, disorientation, fainting.	

Risks from excess[8,91]	• Thirst, dehydration, reduced urination, vomiting, diarrhoea.
	• Increased extracellular fluid volume.
	  • Leading to increased blood pressure.
	• Reduced elasticity in blood vessels.
	  • Leading to increased blood pressure.
	• Increased blood pressure increases risk of cardiovascular disease and stroke as well as kidney disease.
	• Increased risk of gastric cancer and osteoporosis.	

Food sources	Widely available in all processed foods.	
Additional notes[93]	A UK government programme to reduce salt intake, which ran from 2003 to 2018 only managed to reduce daily salt intake by an average of one gram.	

Iron

Daily intakes[1,2,3]	• RNI 8.7 mg • LRNI 4.7 mg • SUL 17 mg (supplemental rather than total intake) • EU DRV 14 mg	
Nutrient of concern?[5]	• **Yes.** • 54% of teenage girls and more than 25% of all women are at risk of iron deficiency.	
Functions[8,94,95,96]	• Essential in the formation and function of proteins that transport and store oxygen. • Used in energy metabolism. • Co-factor in the synthesis and repair of DNA. • Needed for the proliferation and maturation of immune cells. • Essential for cognitive development and function.	
Risks from insufficiency[6,8]	• Breathlessness, tiredness, and fatigue. • Pallor. • Palpitations. • Reduced immune function. • Negative impact on foetal brain development and lifelong cognition.	
Risks from excess[8]	• GI upset, nausea, constipation. • Tissue damage to heart, pancreas and liver. • Chronic excess leads to fibrosis and ultimately cirrhosis of the liver.	
Food sources[11]	**Haem iron:** Meat, organ meats, fish, and shellfish.	**Non-haem iron:** Beans, pulses, dried fruit (particularly figs, prunes, and apricots), green vegetables, wholemeal flour, and fortified foods.
Additional notes	There is no mechanism to eliminate iron from the body, iron loss only occurs through blood loss, or the shedding of epithelial cells. Therefore it is one of the more high-risk micronutrients to supplement with; children, men and post-menopausal women should be monitored if taking supplemental iron.	

Zinc

Daily intakes[1,2,3]	• RNI 9.5 mg • LRNI 5.5 mg • SUL 42 mg • EU DRV 10 mg
Nutrient of concern?[4]	• **Yes.** • 10% of males and 14% of females have intakes below LRNI.

Functions[97,98]	• Thousands of zinc dependent proteins and over 300 enzymes with wide ranging functions:
	    • Storage and transportation of nutrients.
	    • Maintaining the structure and integrity of cell membranes & facilitating wound healing.
	    • RNA and DNA synthesis, repair, and translation.
	    • Cell communication, proliferation and differentiation.
	    • Regulation of inflammatory and immune responses.
	    • Energy metabolism and insulin synthesis.
	    • Absorption and utilisation of folic acid & vitamin A.
	    • Senses of smell and taste.
	    • Fertility and foetal development.

Risks from insufficiency[99]	• Loss of appetite. • Loss of sense of taste and smell. • Poor wound healing and skin lesions. • Fatigue. • Reduced fertility. • Reduced immunity. • Increased maternal morbidity.
Risks from excess[6]	• Nausea, vomiting, diarrhoea. • Chronic excess may result in copper deficiency as the two minerals compete for the same absorption pathways.
Food sources[11]	Shellfish, red meat, organ meat, chickpeas, pumpkin and sunflower seeds, wheatgerm, dark chocolate, nuts and dairy products.
Additional notes	Virtually no-one in the UK achieves 100% of the RNI. Chronic low-grade insufficiency will impact on the health and wellbeing of the nation as a whole.

Copper

Daily intakes[1,2,3]	<ul><li>RNI 1.2 mg</li><li>LRNI Not set</li><li>SUL 10 mg</li><li>EU DRV 1 mg</li></ul>
Nutrient of concern?	<ul><li>NDNS years 1–4 found nearly 90% of respondents had intakes below the RNI. UK intakes of copper have not been measured since. It is not possible to say if current UK intakes are adequate or not.</li></ul>
Functions[100,101]	<ul><li>Needed for iron absorption, metabolism, and transport.</li><li>Critical role in energy metabolism.</li><li>Involved in the formation of haemoglobin and red blood cells.</li><li>Essential in the formation and maintenance of strong, flexible connective tissue.</li><li>Used in the formation of the myelin sheath, and in the synthesis of some neurotransmitters.</li><li>A component of the antioxidant enzyme superoxide dismutase.</li><li>Utilised in the metabolism of both cholesterol and glucose.</li></ul>
Risks from insufficiency[6,8]	<ul><li>Feeling cold and tired all the time.</li><li>Pallor.</li><li>Low immunity.</li><li>Impaired glucose tolerance.</li><li>Poor growth and bone fragility in children.</li></ul>
Risks from excess[100]	<ul><li>Abdominal pain, cramps, nausea, diarrhoea and vomiting.</li><li>Chronic excess may cause liver and kidney damage.</li></ul>
Food sources[11]	Liver (calf and lamb) and liver products, shellfish, nuts and seeds, dark chocolate, and cocoa powder.
Additional notes	Copper accumulates in the foetal liver prior to birth to ensure sufficiency in early life; therefore lamb and calf liver have higher levels of copper than beef or sheep liver.

Manganese

Daily intakes[2,3]	• RNI Not set • LRNI Not set • SUL 12.2 mg • EU DRV 2 mg
Nutrient of concern?	• No RNI for manganese is set in the UK and intakes are not tracked in the NDNS.
Functions[102, 103]	• A constituent of multiple enzymes involved in: • Gluconeogenesis. • Ammonia detoxification in amino acid metabolism. • Cholesterol metabolism. • The formation of healthy cartilage and bone. • Wound healing through the formation of collagen. • An activator in the antioxidant enzyme superoxide dismutase (the key antioxidant enzyme in the mitochondria).
Risks from insufficiency[102, 103]	• Possible bone demineralisation and poor growth in children. • Skin rashes. • Hair depigmentation. • Reduced serum cholesterol. • Abnormal glucose regulation.
Risks from excess[102, 103]	• Where toxicity occurs it is primarily from inhalation in mines and industrial plants. • Toxicity from ingestion is rare and is generally the result of high levels in drinking water.
Food sources[6]	Shellfish, brown rice, lentils, kidney beans and other pulses, pineapple, blackberries, hazelnuts.
Additional notes	Both deficiency and excess are rare in humans.

Fluoride

Daily intakes[3]	• RNI Not set • LRNI Not set • SUL Not set • EU DRV 3.5 mg
Nutrient of concern?	• No RNI for fluoride is set in the UK and intakes are not tracked in the NDNS.
Functions[104]	• Fluoride ions form part of oral plaque. • If the oral environment is too acidic, fluoride actively pulls minerals from saliva to remineralise tooth enamel and slow decay.
Risks from insufficiency[105, 106]	• Insufficiency has not been established. • Low levels of fluoride have been linked with increased levels of tooth decay, particularly in deprived areas. • Poor diet, health inequalities, and poor dental hygiene are as much of an influence on dental health as fluoridated water.

Risks from excess[107, 108, 109]	• As little as 2 parts per million (1.99 mg/L) of fluoride in water consumed by pregnant women shows significant reduction in cognitive function and IQ in offspring.
	• Dental fluorosis.
	   • Changes to tooth enamel colour and texture due to excess exposure during the first eight years of life.
	• Skeletal fluorosis.
	   • Chronic intake of water containing more than 1.5 parts per million (1.5 mg/L), particularly in women, leads to weakened and painful bones and joints.

Food sources[110]	Water. May be naturally occurring or artificially added, levels are variable. Any plants grown in areas with high levels of fluoride in the water (tea, coffee, grapes, raisins, green vegetables, fruit etc).
Additional notes[111]	Fluoride does not need to be ingested to be effective; topical application through toothpaste, gels or mouthwashes are equally effective.

Selenium

Daily intakes[1,2,3]	• RNI 75 μg • LRNI 40 μg • SUL 450 μg • EU DRV 55 μg
Nutrient of concern?[5]	• **Yes** • More than half of all women and over a quarter of all men have intakes below the LRNI.
Functions[6,8]	• Essential in multiple antioxidant systems. • Regulates cell proliferation and growth. • Regulates thyroid function and thyroid hormone production. • Regulation and modulation of immunity and inflammation. • Essential in reproductive health for both sexes.
Risks from insufficiency[112,113,114,115]	• Increased inflammation; reduced immune function. • Increased risk of developing certain cancers. • Increased risk of impaired cardiovascular function. • Increased rate of cognitive decline in older populations. • Increased risk of cataracts. • Reduced fertility. • Impaired thyroid function.
Risks from excess[116,117]	• Smell of garlic on the breath and metallic taste in the mouth. • Brittleness and loss of hair and nails and skin rashes. • Irritability and fatigue. • GI disturbances. • Neurological symptoms including tremors.
Food sources[11]	Liver and kidneys (pig, ox and sheep are the richest sources), Brazil nuts, fish and shellfish, eggs from hens eating a selenium enriched diet, lentils, cashew nuts, mushrooms.
Additional notes[118]	As with all minerals, the selenium content of food is dependent on how much is present in the soil, and soil levels of selenium in Europe are low.

Chromium

Daily intakes[2,3]	• RNI Not set • LRNI Not set • SUL 10 mg • EU DRV 40 µg
Nutrient of concern?	• No RNI for chromium is set in the UK and intakes are not tracked in the NDNS.
Functions[119]	• Acts as a co-factor to insulin, activating insulin receptors and increasing insulin efficiency. • Improves insulin sensitivity and facilitates glucose use in insulin target tissues.
Risks from insufficiency[120]	• No deficiency symptoms have been established.
Risks from excess[121]	• Limited data; may have a negative impact on individuals with renal or liver function issues. • Possibly linked to excessive weight loss, anaemia, thrombocytopenia, and dermatitis.
Food sources[121]	Grape juice, processed ham, whole grain wheat and wheat germ, brewer's yeast, orange juice.
Additional notes	The mechanism of exactly how chromium influences carbohydrate, lipid and protein metabolism by enhancing insulin activity remains unclear.

Molybdenum

Daily intakes[3]	<ul><li>RNI Not set</li><li>LRNI Not set</li><li>SUL Not set</li><li>EU DRV 50 μg</li></ul>
Nutrient of concern?	<ul><li>No RNI for chromium is set in the UK and intakes are not tracked in the NDNS.</li></ul>
Functions[122]	<ul><li>Co-factor in sulfite oxidase which transforms sulfite to sulphate in amino acid metabolism, and nitrate to nitric oxide.</li><li>Co-factor in xanthine oxidase, needed in the production of uric acid.</li><li>Co-factor in aldehyde oxidase which plays a role in the metabolism of toxins.</li><li>Co-factor in mitochondrial amidoxime reducing component (mARC) which plays a role in drug metabolism.</li></ul>
Risks from insufficiency[123]	<ul><li>Unknown in healthy individuals.</li><li>Only seen in individuals with rare genetic mutations which prevent the formation of molybdenum dependent enzymes.</li></ul>
Risks from excess[6]	<ul><li>Rarely seen.</li><li>Intakes above 10 mg daily can lead to elevated uric acid concentrations and an increased incidence of gout.</li></ul>
Food sources[123]	Legumes (peas, beans, lentils), whole grains, nuts and seeds, beef liver, milk and dairy products.
Additional notes[124]	Soil in some areas of Armenia has very high level of molybdenum, leading to intakes of 10–15 mg/d. The population there have very high serum levels of uric acid and suffer gout like symptoms which has been linked to extremely high intakes of molybdenum.

Iodine

Daily intakes[1,2,3]	• RNI 140 µg • LRNI 70 µg • SUL 940 µg • EU DRV 150 µg
Nutrient of concern?[125,126]	• **Yes**, particularly among women of childbearing age. • The UK ranks seventh amongst the ten most iodine deficient nations in the world. • Despite this, the UK government claims that iodine deficiency is rare in this country.
Functions[127,128,129]	• Key component of the T4 and T3 thyroid hormones. • Essential in regulating energy metabolism. • Central to the growth and development of the foetal and infant brain and central nervous system. • Antioxidant and immune modulator.
Risks from insufficiency[127,130]	• Hypothyroidism and goiter. • Maternal insufficiency increases risk of impaired growth and development in babies and children. • Increased risk of brain damage and reduced cognitive ability throughout life. • Reduced immune response.
Risks from excess[131]	• Iodine induced hyperthyroidism and thyroiditis. • Weight loss, rapid heartbeat, muscle weakness. • Abdominal pain, nausea, vomiting, diarrhoea.
Food sources[132]	Iodised salt (not widely available in the UK), white fish and shellfish, milk and dairy products; a limited amount in eggs and meat; very little iodine in plant foods other than seaweed.
Additional notes[133,134]	Although seaweed contains iodine, the content is variable depending on species. Seaweed should not be used as an iodine source unless it is presented in a product which has been titrated to ensure consistency of dose. Plant based milk alternatives do not contain iodine which may put vegan and vegetarian children at risk of severe deficiency.

Boron

Daily intakes[2]	• RNI Not set • LRNI Not set • SUL 9.6 mg • EU DRV Not set
Nutrient of concern?	• No RNI for boron is set in the UK and intakes are not tracked in the NDNS.
Functions[135, 136]	• Bone development and turnover, stabilising and extending the half-life of vitamin D and oestrogen. • Facilitates improved wound healing. • Production and metabolism of sex hormones. • Facilitates the absorption and deposit in bone of calcium and magnesium. • Reduces inflammatory chemicals.
Risks from insufficiency[137, 138]	• Poor bone development and reduced regeneration. • Slower wound healing. • Impaired growth. • Impaired reproductive ability.

Risks from excess[139]	• None known from intakes from food and water.
	• Accidental consumption of boric acid or borax results in:
	  • Nausea, GI discomfort, vomiting and diarrhoea.
	  • Skin flushing, dermatitis, and rash.
	  • Headache, restlessness, and possible renal injury.

Food sources[139]	Prunes, avocado, raisins, peaches, apples, pears, peanuts, pulses. Content will be dependent on boron content of the soil in which plants are grown.
Additional notes[140, 141]	Boron deficiency is widespread in plants; it negatively impacts growth and reproductive capabilities and increases deformity in growing plants. There is little research on boron deficiency in humans but if it is low in plants, it is likely to be low in human diets.

Silicon

Daily intakes[2]	• RNI Not set • LRNI Not set • SUL 760 mg • EU DRV Not set
Nutrient of concern?	• No RNI for silicon is set in the UK and intakes are not tracked in the NDNS.
Functions[142, 143]	• Essential in the formation of all connective tissues. • Structural component of collagen, supporting strong hair, skin, nails, ligaments, tendons, and bone. • Improves strength and integrity of the bone matrix. • Blocks the uptake of aluminium from the gut, reducing the risk of neurodegenerative disease.
Risks from insufficiency[144, 145]	• Reduced bone mass. • Increased risk of osteoporosis. • Increased risk of hip fracture. • Increased fragility of skin, hair and nails. • Increased susceptibility to neurodegenerative disease.
Risks from excess[142]	• Toxicity depends on both the chemical form and route of entry to the human body of silicone. • High oral intakes of ground silicates (including in medications) may lead to kidney inflammation and kidney stones. • Chronic inhalation of crystalline fibres results in lung scarring, reduce lung capacity, increased risk of lung cancer and tuberculosis.
Food sources[145]	Water, particularly mineral waters, brown rice, whole grain wheat, barley and rye products, whole oats, beer (silicon content of barley and hops is high), green beans, beetroot, corn, carrots, bananas, pineapple, antacid, and anti-diarrhoeal medications.
Additional notes[145]	Silicon in soil reduces the bioavailability of toxic metals such as aluminium, arsenic and cadmium, preventing uptake by plants.

Omega 3 fatty acids: Alpha-linolenic acid (ALA)

Daily intakes	• RNI Not set • LRNI Not set • SUL Not set • EU DRV Not set
Nutrient of concern?	• Unknown.
Functions[146, 147]	• Reduces pro-inflammatory cytokines through production of anti-inflammatory prostaglandins. • Protective against cardiovascular disease and stroke. • Neuroprotective, supports neuronal maintenance, learning and memory, neuronal survival, and neurogenesis. • May have a role in gene expression during foetal development that programmes health throughout life.
Risks from insufficiency[146, 148, 149]	• Increased risk of cardiovascular disease and stroke. • Reduced synthesis of DHA and EPA. • Dermatitis and folliculitis.
Risks from excess	No known toxicity.
Food sources[150]	Nuts and seeds (flax, chia, hemp, pumpkin, walnuts); soyabeans, seed oils from of the above and rape seed oil, cruciferous vegetables, algal oil.
Additional notes[151]	ALA can be converted to EPA and DHA in humans, however this conversion is extremely inefficient.

Omega 3 fatty acids: Eicosapentaenoic Acid (EPA) & Docosahexaenoic acid (DHA)

Daily intakes	• RNI Not set • LRNI Not set • SUL Not set • EU DRV Not set
Nutrient of concern?[152]	• **Yes.** • Oily fish intake in the UK is extremely low.
Functions[153,154,155]	• Formation of phospholipids in cell membranes, enabling fluidity, flexibility, and permeability. • DHA supports the normal development and function of the retina and in the formation and function of rhodopsin. • EPA is essential in healthy vascular function. • Both are essential in the formation, development, and lifelong function of the central nervous system, including neuronal growth and synapse formation. • Needed for the synthesis of prostaglandins which control inflammation, maintain normal blood pressure, regulate blood triglyceride levels, support heart function, and inhibit platelet stickiness. • Facilitation of cell signalling pathways.
Risks from insufficiency[150,155]	• Rough scaly skin and dermatitis. • Increased risk of coronary heart disease and more general cardiovascular disease. • Poor foetal cognitive and visual development. • Increased risk of cognitive decline.
Risks from excess[156]	• No safety issues known at intakes up to 5 g/d. • Potential for excessive bleeding at intakes >6.5 g/d.
Food sources[11]	Oily fish (mackerel, salmon, herring, sardines, fresh tuna); marine algae; eggs from hens fed omega-3 fortified diets.
Additional notes[157,158]	The UK has one of the lowest intakes of EPA and DHA in the world. Supplementing with omega-3 increases the chances of becoming pregnant during IVF treatment.

Omega 6 fatty acids: Linoleic Acid (LA) and Arachidonic Acid (AA)

Daily intakes	• RNI Not set • LRNI Not set • SUL Not set • EU DRV Not set
Nutrient of concern?	• No.
Functions[159, 160]	• LA and AA provide structure within phospholipids in cell membranes. • LA is essential in maintaining the transdermal water barrier of the epidermis. • Both facilitate cell signalling. • Precursors to pro-inflammatory prostaglandins which contribute to inflammatory processes, mediate inflammation, and facilitate wound healing. • Modulation of gene expression, particularly in fatty acid metabolism.
Risks from insufficiency[159, 161]	• Potential increased risk of major cardiovascular events. • Growth retardation and scaly skin in infants consuming formula or breastmilk containing insufficient LA.
Risks from excess[162]	• Increased risk of chronic inflammatory disease including cardiovascular disease, obesity, inflammatory bowel disease, arthritic conditions, and dementias.
Food sources[162]	Soyabean, corn and sunflower oils, soya products, nuts and seeds, meat, fish, shellfish poultry, eggs.
Additional notes[163, 164]	The ideal ratio between omega 3 and omega 6 is 1:1; the ratio in the modern western diet is more like 20:1 and this may be a factor in driving chronic inflammatory diseases.

Co-enzyme Q10 (CoQ10)

Daily intakes	• RNI not set • LRNI Not set • SUL Not set • EU DRV Not set
Nutrient of concern?[165]	• Unknown. • CoQ10 is synthesised within the body, however synthesis declines with age, and is further reduced by the use of statin medications.
Functions[166, 167]	• Central to energy metabolism as an electron carrier in the manufacture of ATP within the electron transport chain. • Potent antioxidant that is present in all cell membranes where it protects against lipid peroxidation. • Reactivates the antioxidant capacity of vitamins C and E.
Risks from insufficiency[168, 169, 170]	• Tiredness and fatigue. • Increased risk of heart failure. • Increased risk of metabolic disease and reduced insulin sensitivity. • Increased risk of any condition related to high oxidative stress (cancer, diabetes, cardiovascular disease, neurogenerative disease).
Risks from excess[171]	• None noted at doses below 3,000 mg.
Food sources[172]	Organ meats, oily fish, whole grains, cold pressed seed oils.
Additional notes[173]	CoQ10 synthesis peaks at around age 25 and then declines, falling increasingly rapidly from age 50. Supplementation with 100mg of CoQ10 3×/d reduces the risk of mortality from cardiovascular disease. Supplementation with 500 mg/d of CoQ10 reduces inflammation and inflammatory markers. Supplementing with CoQ10 may also slow the growth of some cancer tumour cells.

Flavonoids (polyphenols, alkaloids, terpenoids, flavones etc)

Daily intakes	• RNI Not set • LRNI Not set • SUL Not set • EU DRV Not set
Nutrient of concern?	• Unknown.
Functions [174, 175, 176, 177, 178, 179, 180]	• Regulation of inflammatory mechanisms. • Potent antioxidants. • Boosts antioxidant activity of antioxidant enzyme systems. • Modulates scavenging activity of reactive oxygen species and triggers apoptosis in cancer cells. • Disrupts pathogen membrane function and permeability, blocks pathogen energy metabolism, suppresses nucleic acid synthesis. • Disrupts fungal cell wall formation and cell division, inhibits fungal RNA, DNA and protein synthesis, suppresses fungal mitochondrial functions. • Inhibits gut wall inflammation and nourishes the microbiome. • Improves vascular health and reduces arterial stiffness.
Risks from insufficiency	• Unknown, but benefits noted above will not occur.
Risks from excess [181]	• Limited data, toxicity depends on flavonoid variety and the amount consumed, average consumption is unlikely to cause adverse events.
Food sources [182]	All plant foods, particularly brightly coloured fruit and vegetables, berries, soyabeans, citrus fruit, whole grains, legumes, nuts and seeds, tea, coffee, red wine, chocolate.
Additional notes	Coffee, tea, wine, and chocolate are widely consumed in the UK, fruit and vegetables less so. Therefore some flavonoids are likely to be of concern in the UK diet.

REFERENCES

1 Department of Health (1991). *Dietary Reference Values, A Guide*. London Her Majesty's Stationery Office. https://assets.publishing.service.gov.uk/government/uploads/system/uploads/attachment_data/file/743790/Dietary_Reference_Values_-_A_Guide__1991_.pdf

2 Expert Group on Vitamins and Minerals (2003). Safe Upper Levels for Vitamins and Minerals. https://cot.food.gov.uk/sites/default/files/vitmin2003.pdf

3 European Food Safety Authority (2017). Dietary Reference Values for nutrients Summary Report EFSA supporting publication *EFSA Journal;* 2017:e15121. 98 pp. doi:10.2903/sp.efsa.2017.e15121

4 Derbyshire E. (2019). UK Dietary Changes Over the Last Two Decades: A Focus on Vitamin & Mineral Intakes. *Journal of Vitamins and Minerals* 2: 104. https://www.gavinpublishers.com/assets/articles_pdf/1562406424article_pdf1056672662.pdf

5 Derbyshire E. (2018). Micronutrient Intakes of British Adults Across Mid-Life: A Secondary Analysis of the UK National Diet and Nutrition Survey. *Frontiers in Nutrition, 5*, 55. https://doi.org/10.3389/fnut.2018.00055

6 Mason P. (2001). *Dietary Supplements*, Second Edition, London: Pharmaceutical Press.

7 Linus Pauling Institute (2021). Vitamin A. *Micronutrient Information Center, Oregon State University*. https://lpi.oregonstate.edu/mic/vitamins/vitamin-A

8 Eastwood M. (2003). *Principles of Human Nutrition*, Second Edition. Wiley-Blackwell; Hoboken, New Jersey.

9 Bastos Maia, S., Rolland Souza, A. S., Costa Caminha, M. F., Lins da Silva, S., Callou Cruz, R., Carvalho Dos Santos, C., & Batista Filho, M. (2019). Vitamin A and Pregnancy: A Narrative Review. *Nutrients, 11*(3), 681. https://doi.org/10.3390/nu11030681

10 National Institutes of Health (2021). Fact Sheet for Health Professionals; Vitamin A. *Office of Dietary Supplements* https://ods.od.nih.gov/factsheets/VitaminA-HealthProfessional/

11 Public Health England (2021). McCance and Widdowson's Composition of Foods Integrated Dataset (CoFID). https://www.gov.uk/government/publications/composition-of-foods-integrated-dataset-cofid

12 Hemilä H. (2020). The effect of β-carotene on the mortality of male smokers is modified by smoking and by vitamins C and E: evidence against a uniform effect of nutrient. *Journal of Nutritional Science*, 9, e11. https://doi.org/10.1017/jns.2020.3

13 Public Health England (2016). Government Dietary Recommendations for energy and nutrients for males and females aged 1-18 years and 19+ years. https://assets.publishing.service.gov.uk/government/uploads/system/uploads/attachment_data/file/618167/government_dietary_recommendations.pdf

14 Rizzoli R. (2021). Vitamin D supplementation: upper limit for safety revisited? *Aging Clinical and Experimental Research, 33*(1), 19–24. https://doi.org/10.1007/s40520-020-01678-x

15 Calame, W., Street, L., & Hulshof, T. (2020). Vitamin D Serum Levels in the UK Population, including a Mathematical Approach to Evaluate the Impact of Vitamin D Fortified Ready-to-Eat Breakfast Cereals: Application of the NDNS Database. *Nutrients, 12*(6), 1868. https://doi.org/10.3390/nu12061868

16 AL Callaghan, RJD Moy, IW Booth, G Debelle & NJ Shaw (2006). Incidence of symptomatic vitamin D deficiency. *Archives of Disease in Childhood*; 91:606-607. http://adc.bmj.com/content/91/7/606.full

17 Royal Osteoporosis Society Annual Impact Report 2017. https://strwebstgmedia.blob.core.windows.net/media/dqab05ky/impact-report-2017.pdf

18 Föcker M., Antel J., Ring S., Hahn D., Özlem K., Öztürk D., Hebebrand J., Libuda L., (2017). Vitamin D and mental health in children and adolescents *European Child & Adolescent Psychiatry* Feb 26:1043-1066. https://doi.org/10.1007/s00787-017-0949-3

19 Cannell J.J., Grant W.B., Holick M.F. (2015). Vitamin D and inflammation. *Dermato-Endocrinology* 6:1. https://doi.org/10.4161/19381980.2014.983401

20 Holick, M. F., & Chen, T. C. (2008). Vitamin D deficiency: a worldwide problem with health consequences. *The American Journal of Clinical Nutrition*, *87*(4), 1080S–6S. https://doi.org/10.1093/ajcn/87.4.1080S

21 Kim, S. Y., Jeon, S. W., Lim, W. J., Oh, K. S., Shin, D. W., Cho, S. J., Park, J. H., Kim, Y. H., & Shin, Y. C. (2020). Vitamin D deficiency and suicidal ideation: A cross-sectional study of 157,211 healthy adults. *Journal of Psychosomatic Research*, *134*, 110125. https://doi.org/10.1016/j.jpsychores.2020.110125

22 Marcinowska-Suchowierska, E., Kupisz-Urbańska, M., Łukaszkiewicz, J., Płudowski, P., & Jones, G. (2018). Vitamin D Toxicity-A Clinical Perspective. *Frontiers in Endocrinology*, *9*, 550. https://doi.org/10.3389/fendo.2018.00550

23 Almoosawi, S., & Palla, L. (2020). Association between vitamin intake and respiratory complaints in adults from the UK National Diet and Nutrition Survey years 1-8. *BMJ Nutrition, Prevention & Health*, *3*(2), 403–408. https://doi.org/10.1136/bmjnph-2020-000150

24 Rizvi, S., Raza, S. T., Ahmed, F., Ahmad, A., Abbas, S., & Mahdi, F. (2014). The role of vitamin e in human health and some diseases. *Sultan Qaboos University Medical Journal*, *14*(2), e157–e165. https://www.ncbi.nlm.nih.gov/pmc/articles/PMC3997530/

25 Kemnic T.R., Coleman M., (2021). Vitamin E Deficiency. In: StatPearls [Internet]. Treasure Island (FL): StatPearls Publishing. Available from: https://www.ncbi.nlm.nih.gov/books/NBK519051/

26 Simes, D. C., Viegas, C., Araújo, N., & Marreiros, C. (2020). Vitamin K as a Diet Supplement with Impact in Human Health: Current Evidence in Age-Related Diseases. *Nutrients*, *12*(1), 138. https://doi.org/10.3390/nu12010138

27 Halder, M., Petsophonsakul, P., Akbulut, A. C., Pavlic, A., Bohan, F., Anderson, E., Maresz, K., Kramann, R., & Schurgers, L. (2019). Vitamin K: Double Bonds beyond Coagulation Insights into Differences between Vitamin K1 and K2 in Health and Disease. *International Journal of Molecular Sciences*, *20*(4), 896. https://doi.org/10.3390/ijms20040896

28 Simes, D. C., Viegas, C., Araújo, N., & Marreiros, C. (2019). Vitamin K as a Powerful Micronutrient in Aging and Age-Related Diseases: Pros and Cons from Clinical Studies. *International Journal of Molecular Sciences*, *20*(17), 4150. https://doi.org/10.3390/ijms20174150

29 Frei, B., Birlouez-Aragon, I., & Lykkesfeldt, J. (2012). Authors' perspective: What is the optimum intake of vitamin C in humans?. *Critical Reviews in Food Science and Nutrition*, *52*(9), 815–829. https://doi.org/10.1080/10408398.2011.649149

30 Veg Facts 2021 (2021). The Food Foundation. https://foodfoundation.org.uk/publication/veg-facts-2021/

31 Mosdøl, A., Erens, B., & Brunner, E. J. (2008). Estimated prevalence and predictors of vitamin C deficiency within UK's low-income population. *Journal of Public Health*, *30*(4), 456–460. https://doi.org/10.1093/pubmed/fdn076

32 Public Health England (2019). NDNS: time trend and income analyses for Years 1 to 9: report. https://assets.publishing.service.gov.uk/government/uploads/system/uploads/attachment_data/file/772434/NDNS_UK_Y1-9_report.pdf

33 Linus Pauling Institute (2018). Vitamin C. *Micronutrient Information Center, Oregon State University*. https://lpi.oregonstate.edu/mic/vitamins/vitamin-C

34 Hemilä H. (2017). Vitamin C and Infections. *Nutrients*, *9*(4), 339. https://doi.org/10.3390/nu9040339

35 Wilson, R., Willis, J., Gearry, R., Skidmore, P., Fleming, E., Frampton, C., & Carr, A. (2017). Inadequate Vitamin C Status in Prediabetes and Type 2 Diabetes Mellitus: Associations with Glycaemic Control, Obesity, and Smoking. *Nutrients*, *9*(9), 997. https://doi.org/10.3390/nu9090997

36 Calderón-Ospina, C. A., & Nava-Mesa, M. O. (2020). B Vitamins in the nervous system: Current knowledge of the biochemical modes of action and synergies of thiamine, pyridoxine, and cobalamin. *CNS Neuroscience & Therapeutics*, *26*(1), 5–13. https://doi.org/10.1111/cns.13207

37 Baltrusch S. (2021). The Role of Neurotropic B Vitamins in Nerve Regeneration. *BioMed Research International*, Article ID 9968228; 9 pages. https://doi.org/10.1155/2021/9968228

38 Dhir, S., Tarasenko, M., Napoli, E., & Giulivi, C. (2019). Neurological, Psychiatric, and Biochemical Aspects of Thiamine Deficiency in Children and Adults. *Frontiers in Psychiatry*, *10*, 207. https://doi.org/10.3389/fpsyt.2019.00207

39 Gibson, G. E., Hirsch, J. A., Fonzetti, P., Jordan, B. D., Cirio, R. T., & Elder, J. (2016). Vitamin B1 (thiamine) and dementia. *Annals of the New York Academy of Sciences*, *1367*(1), 21–30. https://doi.org/10.1111/nyas.13031

40 Powers, H. J., Hill, M. H., Mushtaq, S., Dainty, J. R., Majsak-Newman, G., & Williams, E. A. (2011). Correcting a marginal riboflavin deficiency improves hematologic status in young women in the United Kingdom (RIBOFEM). *The American Journal of Clinical Nutrition*, *93*(6), 1274–1284. https://doi.org/10.3945/ajcn.110.008409

41 Powers H. J. (2003). Riboflavin (vitamin B-2) and health. *The American Journal of Clinical Nutrition*, *77*(6), 1352–1360. https://doi.org/10.1093/ajcn/77.6.1352

42 Suwannasom, N., Kao, I., Pruß, A., Georgieva, R., & Bäumler, H. (2020). Riboflavin: The Health Benefits of a Forgotten Natural Vitamin. *International Journal of Molecular Sciences*, *21*(3), 950. https://doi.org/10.3390/ijms21030950

43 Linus Pauling Institute (2018). Niacin. *Micronutrient Information Center, Oregon State University* https://lpi.oregonstate.edu/mic/vitamins/niacin

44 National Institutes of Health (2021). Fact Sheet for Health Professionals. Niacin. *Office of Dietary Supplements.* https://ods.od.nih.gov/factsheets/Niacin-HealthProfessional/

45 Meyer-Ficca, M., & Kirkland, J. B. (2016). Niacin. *Advances in Nutrition*, *7*(3), 556–558. https://doi.org/10.3945/an.115.011239

46 Morris, M. C., Evans, D. A., Bienias, J. L., Scherr, P. A., Tangney, C. C., Hebert, L. E., Bennett, D. A., Wilson, R. S., & Aggarwal, N. (2004). Dietary niacin and the risk of incident Alzheimer's disease and of cognitive decline. *Journal of Neurology, Neurosurgery and Psychiatry*, *75*(8), 1093–1099. https://doi.org/10.1136/jnnp.2003.025858

47 Fukuwatari, T., & Shibata, K. (2013). Nutritional aspect of tryptophan metabolism. *International Journal of Tryptophan Research*, *6*(Suppl 1), 3–8. https://doi.org/10.4137/IJTR.S11588

48 Wall J. S., Carpenter K. J., (1988). Variation in Availability of Niacin in Grain Products; Changes in chemical composition during grain development and processing affect the nutritional availability of niacin. *Food Technology;* October 198-204. https://pubag.nal.usda.gov/download/23799/pdf

49 Linus Pauling Institute (2015). Pantothenic Acid. *Micronutrient Information Center, Oregon State University.* https://lpi.oregonstate.edu/mic/vitamins/pantothenic-acid

50 Jung, S., Kim, M. K., & Choi, B. Y. (2017). The long-term relationship between dietary pantothenic acid (vitamin B_5) intake and C-reactive protein concentration in adults aged 40 years and older. *Nutrition, Metabolism, and Cardiovascular Diseases*, *27*(9), 806–816. https://doi.org/10.1016/j.numecd.2017.05.008

51 Evans, M., Rumberger, J. A., Azumano, I., Napolitano, J. J., Citrolo, D., & Kamiya, T. (2014). Pantethine, a derivative of vitamin B5, favorably alters total, LDL and non-HDL cholesterol in low to moderate cardiovascular risk subjects eligible for statin therapy: a triple-blinded placebo and diet-controlled investigation. *Vascular Health and Risk Management*, *10*, 89–100. https://doi.org/10.2147/VHRM.S57116

52 National Institutes of Health (2021). Fact Sheet for Health Professionals. Pantothenic Acid. *Office of Dietary Supplements.* https://ods.od.nih.gov/factsheets/PantothenicAcid-HealthProfessional/

53 Yuan, S., Mason, A. M., Carter, P., Burgess, S., & Larsson, S. C. (2021). Homocysteine, B vitamins, and cardiovascular disease: a Mendelian randomization study. *BMC Medicine, 19*(1), 97. https://doi.org/10.1186/s12916-021-01977-8

54 Brown M.J., Ameer M.A., Beier K., (2021). Vitamin B6 Deficiency. In: StatPearls [Internet]. Treasure Island (FL): StatPearls Publishing. Available from: https://www.ncbi.nlm.nih.gov/books/NBK470579/

55 Linus Pauling Institute (2015). Vitamin B12. *Micronutrient Information Center, Oregon State University.* https://lpi.oregonstate.edu/mic/vitamins/vitamin-B12

56 Molloy A.M., (2018). Should vitamin B12 status be considered in assessing risk of neural tube defects? *Annals of the New York Academy of Sciences* 1414(1): 109-125. https://doi.org/10.1111/nyas.13574

57 Ma, F., Wu, T., Zhao, J., Song, A., Liu, H., Xu, W., & Huang, G. (2016). Folic acid supplementation improves cognitive function by reducing the levels of peripheral inflammatory cytokines in elderly Chinese subjects with MCI. *Scientific Reports, 6,* 37486. https://doi.org/10.1038/srep37486

58 Linus Pauling Institute (2014). Folate. *Micronutrient Information Center, Oregon State University.* https://lpi.oregonstate.edu/mic/vitamins/folate

59 Pacheco-Alvarez, D., Solórzano-Vargas, R. S., & Del Río, A. L. (2002). Biotin in metabolism and its relationship to human disease. *Archives of Medical Research, 33*(5), 439–447. https://doi.org/10.1016/s0188-4409(02)00399-5

60 Rodriguez-Melendez, R., & Zempleni, J. (2009). Nitric oxide signaling depends on biotin in Jurkat human lymphoma cells. *The Journal of Nutrition, 139*(3), 429–433. https://doi.org/10.3945/jn.108.101840

61 Lazo de la Vega-Monroy, M. L., Larrieta, E., German, M. S., Baez-Saldana, A., & Fernandez-Mejia, C. (2013). Effects of biotin supplementation in the diet on insulin secretion, islet gene expression, glucose homeostasis and beta-cell proportion. *The Journal of Nutritional Biochemistry, 24*(1), 169–177. https://doi.org/10.1016/j.jnutbio.2012.03.020

62 Ichihara, Y., Suga, K., Fukui, M., Yonetani, N., Shono, M., Nakagawa, R., & Kagami, S. (2020). Serum biotin level during pregnancy is associated with fetal growth and preterm delivery. *The Journal of Medical Investigation, 67*(1.2), 170–173. https://doi.org/10.2152/jmi.67.170

63 Mock D. M. (2017). Biotin: From Nutrition to Therapeutics. *The Journal of Nutrition, 147*(8), 1487–1492. https://doi.org/10.3945/jn.116.238956

64 Testing.com (2017). Biotin Affects Some Blood Test Results. https://www.testing.com/articles/biotin-affects-some-blood-test-results/

65 Perry, C. A., West, A. A., Gayle, A., Lucas, L. K., Yan, J., Jiang, X., Malysheva, O., & Caudill, M. A. (2014). Pregnancy and lactation alter biomarkers of biotin metabolism in women consuming a controlled diet. *The Journal of Nutrition, 144*(12), 1977–1984. https://doi.org/10.3945/jn.114.194472

66 Panel on Dietetic Products, Nutrition and Allergies (2016). Dietary reference values for choline. *EFSA Journal:* 14(8):4484. https://efsa.onlinelibrary.wiley.com/doi/epdf/10.2903/j.efsa.2016.4484

67 Institute of Medicine, National Academy of Sciences USA (1998). Dietary reference intakes for folate, thiamin, riboflavin, niacin, vitamin B12, pantothenic acid, biotin, and choline. *National Academy Press* 390-422. Washington D.C. https://www.ncbi.nlm.nih.gov/books/NBK114310/

68 Derbyshire E (2019). Could we be overlooking a potential choline crisis in the United Kingdom? *BMJ Nutrition, Prevention & Health* 2(2), 86–89. https://doi.org/10.1136/bmjnph-2019-000037

69 da Costa, K. A., Gaffney, C. E., Fischer, L. M., & Zeisel, S. H. (2005). Choline deficiency in mice and humans is associated with increased plasma homocysteine concentration after a methionine load. *The American Journal of Clinical Nutrition, 81*(2), 440–444. https://doi.org/10.1093/ajcn.81.2.440

70 National Institutes of Health (2021). Fact Sheet for Health Professionals. Choline. *Office of Dietary Supplements.* https://ods.od.nih.gov/factsheets/Choline-HealthProfessional/

71 Zeisel, S. H., & da Costa, K. A. (2009). Choline: an essential nutrient for public health. *Nutrition Reviews, 67*(11), 615–623. https://doi.org/10.1111/j.1753-4887.2009.00246.x

72 Wiedeman, A. M., Barr, S. I., Green, T. J., Xu, Z., Innis, S. M., & Kitts, D. D. (2018). Dietary Choline Intake: Current State of Knowledge Across the Life Cycle. *Nutrients, 10*(10), 1513. https://doi.org/10.3390/nu10101513

73 National Institutes of Health (2021). Fact Sheet for Health Professionals. Potassium. *Office of Dietary Supplements.* https://ods.od.nih.gov/factsheets/Potassium-HealthProfessional/

74 Morris, R. C., Jr., Schmidlin, O., Frassetto, L. A., & Sebastian, A. (2006). Relationship and interaction between sodium and potassium. *Journal of the American College of Nutrition, 25*(3 Suppl), 262S–270S. https://doi.org/10.1080/07315724.2006.10719576

75 Berend, K., van Hulsteijn, L. H., & Gans, R. O. (2012). Chloride: the queen of electrolytes?. *European Journal of Internal Medicine, 23*(3), 203–211. https://doi.org/10.1016/j.ejim.2011.11.013

76 Chipperfield, A. R., & Harper, A. A. (2000). Chloride in smooth muscle. *Progress in Biophysics and Molecular Biology, 74*(3-5), 175–221. https://doi.org/10.1016/s0079-6107(00)00024-9

77 Signorelli, G. C., Bianchetti, M. G., Jermini, L., Agostoni, C., Milani, G. P., Simonetti, G. D., & Lava, S. (2020). Dietary Chloride Deficiency Syndrome: Pathophysiology, History, and Systematic Literature Review. *Nutrients, 12*(11), 3436. https://doi.org/10.3390/nu12113436

78 Linus Pauling Institute (2017). Calcium. *Micronutrient Information Center, Oregon State University.* https://lpi.oregonstate.edu/mic/minerals/calcium

79 Peterlik, M., Cross, H. Vitamin D and calcium insufficiency-related chronic diseases: molecular and cellular pathophysiology. *European Journal of Clinical Nutrition* **63,** 1377–1386 (2009). https://doi.org/10.1038/ejcn.2009.105

80 Daly, R. M., & Ebeling, P. R. (2010). Is excess calcium harmful to health?. *Nutrients, 2*(5), 505–522. https://doi.org/10.3390/nu2050505

81 Linus Pauling Institute (2014). Phosphorus. *Micronutrient Information Center, Oregon State University.* https://lpi.oregonstate.edu/mic/minerals/phosphorus

82 Bonjour J. P. (2011). Calcium and phosphate: a duet of ions playing for bone health. *Journal of the American College of Nutrition, 30*(5 Suppl 1), 438S–48S. https://doi.org/10.1080/07315724.2011.10719988

83 National Institutes of Health (2021). Fact Sheet for Health Professionals. Phosphorus. *Office of Dietary Supplements.* https://ods.od.nih.gov/factsheets/Phosphorus-HealthProfessional/

84 Uribarri, J., & Calvo, M. S. (2013). Dietary phosphorus excess: a risk factor in chronic bone, kidney, and cardiovascular disease?. *Advances in Nutrition, 4*(5), 542–544. https://doi.org/10.3945/an.113.004234

85 Rey-García, J., Donat-Vargas, C., Sandoval-Insausti, H., Bayan-Bravo, A., Moreno-Franco, B., Banegas, J. R., Rodríguez-Artalejo, F., & Guallar-Castillón, P. (2021). Ultra-Processed Food Consumption is Associated with Renal Function Decline in Older Adults: A Prospective Cohort Study. *Nutrients, 13*(2), 428. https://doi.org/10.3390/nu13020428

86 Linus Pauling Institute (2019). Magnesium. *Micronutrient Information Center, Oregon State University.* https://lpi.oregonstate.edu/mic/minerals/magnesium

87 National Institutes of Health (2022). Fact Sheet for Health Professionals. Magnesium. *Office of Dietary Supplements.* https://ods.od.nih.gov/factsheets/Magnesium-HealthProfessional/

88 Ajib F. A., Childress J. M. (2021). Magnesium Toxicity. In: StatPearls [Internet]. Treasure Island (FL): StatPearls Publishing; Available from: https://www.ncbi.nlm.nih. gov/books/NBK554593/

89 NHS (2021). Salt: the facts. https://www.nhs.uk/live-well/eat-well/food-types/salt-nutrition/

90 UK Salt Reduction Strategy. *Action on Salt.* https://www.actiononsalt.org.uk/media/ action-on-salt/about/FINAL-Action-on-Salt-Policy-Brief.pdf

91 Strazzullo, P., & Leclercq, C. (2014). Sodium. *Advances in Nutrition, 5*(2), 188–190. https://doi.org/10.3945/an.113.005215

92 Linus Pauling Institute (2016). Sodium. *Micronutrient Information Center, Oregon State University.* https://lpi.oregonstate.edu/mic/minerals/sodium

93 Alonso, S., Tan, M., Wang, C., Kent, S., Cobiac, L., MacGregor, G. A., He, F. J., & Mihaylova, B. (2021). Impact of the 2003 to 2018 Population Salt Intake Reduction Program in England: A Modeling Study. *Hypertension 77*(4), 1086–1094. https:// doi.org/10.1161/HYPERTENSIONAHA.120.16649

94 Puig, S., Ramos-Alonso, L., Romero, A. M., & Martínez-Pastor, M. T. (2017). The elemental role of iron in DNA synthesis and repair. *Metallomics: Integrated Biometal Science, 9*(11), 1483–1500. https://doi.org/10.1039/c7mt00116a

95 Dev, S., & Babitt, J. L. (2017). Overview of iron metabolism in health and disease. *Hemodialysis international. International Symposium on Home Hemodialysis, 21* (Suppl 1), S6–S20. https://doi.org/10.1111/hdi.12542

96 Ferreira, A., Neves, P., & Gozzelino, R. (2019). Multilevel Impacts of Iron in the Brain: The Cross Talk between Neurophysiological Mechanisms, Cognition, and Social Behavior. *Pharmaceuticals, 12*(3), 126. https://doi.org/10.3390/ph12030126

97 Linus Pauling Institute (2019). Zinc. *Micronutrient Information Center, Oregon State University.* https://lpi.oregonstate.edu/mic/minerals/zinc

98 Maret W. (2013). Zinc biochemistry: from a single zinc enzyme to a key element of life. *Advances in Nutrition, 4*(1), 82–91. https://doi.org/10.3945/an.112.003038

99 Prasad A. S. (2013). Discovery of human zinc deficiency: its impact on human health and disease. *Advances in Nutrition, 4*(2), 176–190. https://doi.org/10.3945/an.112. 003210

100 National Institutes of Health (2021). Fact Sheet for Health Professionals. Copper. *Office of Dietary Supplements.* https://ods.od.nih.gov/factsheets/Copper-HealthProfessional/

101 Linus Pauling Institute (2014). Copper. *Micronutrient Information Center, Oregon State University.* https://lpi.oregonstate.edu/mic/minerals/copper

102 Linus Pauling Institute (2021). Manganese. *Micronutrient Information Center, Oregon State University.* https://lpi.oregonstate.edu/mic/minerals/manganese

103 National Institutes of Health (2021). Fact Sheet for Health Professionals. Manganese. *Office of Dietary Supplements.* https://ods.od.nih.gov/factsheets/Manganese-HealthProfessional/

104 Guntermann, L., Rohrbach, A., Schäfer, E., & Dammaschke, T. (2022). Remineralization and protection from demineralization: effects of a hydroxyapatite-containing, a fluoride-containing and a fluoride- and hydroxyapatite-free toothpaste on human enamel in vitro. *Head & Face Medicine, 18*(1), 26. https://doi.org/10.1186/s13005-022-00330-5

105 Marques, R. B., Lima, C., de Abreu Costa, M., de Deus Moura de Lima, M., de Fátima Almeida de Deus Moura, L., Tabchoury, C., & de Moura, M. S. (2021). Fluoridated water impact on tooth decay and fluorosis in 17-20-year-olds exposed to fluoride toothpaste. *Journal of Public Health Dentistry*, 10.1111/jphd.12472. Advance online publication. https://doi.org/10.1111/jphd.12472

106 Peckham, S., & Awofeso, N. (2014). Water fluoridation: a critical review of the physiological effects of ingested fluoride as a public health intervention. *The Scientific World Journal, 2014*, 293019. https://doi.org/10.1155/2014/293019

107 Grandjean, P., Hu, H., Till, C., Green, R., Bashash, M., Flora, D., Tellez-Rojo, M. M., Song, P., Lanphear, B., & Budtz-Jørgensen, E. (2021). A Benchmark Dose Analysis for Maternal Pregnancy Urine-Fluoride and IQ in Children. *Risk Analysis 42*(3): 439–449. https://doi.org/10.1111/risa.13767

108 DenBesten, P., & Li, W. (2011). Chronic fluoride toxicity: dental fluorosis. *Monographs in Oral Science, 22,* 81–96. https://doi.org/10.1159/000327028

109 Mohammadi, A. A., Yousefi, M., Yaseri, M., Jalilzadeh, M., & Mahvi, A. H. (2017). Skeletal fluorosis in relation to drinking water in rural areas of West Azerbaijan, Iran. *Scientific Reports, 7*(1), 17300. https://doi.org/10.1038/s41598-017-17328-8

110 National Institutes of Health (2022). Fact Sheet for Health Professionals. Fluoride. *Office of Dietary Supplements.* https://ods.od.nih.gov/factsheets/Fluoride-HealthProfessional/

111 Hellwig, E., & Lennon, A. M. (2004). Systemic versus topical fluoride. *Caries Research, 38*(3), 258–262. https://doi.org/10.1159/000077764

112 Kieliszek M. (2019). Selenium-Fascinating Microelement, Properties and Sources in Food. *Molecules, 24*(7), 1298. https://doi.org/10.3390/molecules24071298

113 Shimada, B. K., Alfulaij, N., & Seale, L. A. (2021). The Impact of Selenium Deficiency on Cardiovascular Function. *International Journal of Molecular Sciences, 22*(19), 10713. https://doi.org/10.3390/ijms221910713

114 Steinbrenner, H., & Sies, H. (2013). Selenium homeostasis and antioxidant selenoproteins in brain: implications for disorders in the central nervous system. *Archives of Biochemistry and Biophysics, 536*(2), 152–157. https://doi.org/10.1016/j.abb.2013.02.021

115 Mojadadi, A., Au, A., Salah, W., Witting, P., & Ahmad, G. (2021). Role for Selenium in Metabolic Homeostasis and Human Reproduction. *Nutrients, 13*(9), 3256. https://doi.org/10.3390/nu13093256

116 Linus Pauling Institute (2015). Selenium. *Micronutrient Information Center, Oregon State University.* https://lpi.oregonstate.edu/mic/minerals/selenium

117 National Institutes of Health (2021). Fact Sheet for Health Professionals. Selenium. *Office of Dietary Supplements..* https://ods.od.nih.gov/factsheets/Selenium-HealthProfessional/

118 Stoffaneller, R., & Morse, N. L. (2015). A review of dietary selenium intake and selenium status in Europe and the Middle East. *Nutrients, 7*(3), 1494–1537. https://doi.org/10.3390/nu7031494

119 Kooshki, F., Tutunchi, H., Vajdi, M., Karimi, A., Niazkar, H. R., Shoorei, H., & Pourghassem Gargari, B. (2021). A Comprehensive insight into the effect of chromium supplementation on oxidative stress indices in diabetes mellitus: A systematic review. *Clinical and Experimental Pharmacology and Physiology, 48*(3), 291–309. https://doi.org/10.1111/1440-1681.13462

120 Vincent, J. B., & Lukaski, H. C. (2018). Chromium. *Advances in Nutrition, 9*(4), 505–506. https://doi.org/10.1093/advances/nmx021

121 National Institutes of Health (2022). Fact Sheet for Health Professionals. Chromium. *Office of Dietary Supplements.* https://ods.od.nih.gov/factsheets/Chromium-HealthProfessional/

122 Linus Pauling Institute (2021). Molybdenum. *Micronutrient Information Center, Oregon State University.* https://lpi.oregonstate.edu/mic/minerals/molybdenum

123 National Institutes of Health (2021). Fact Sheet for Health Professionals. Molybdenum. *Office of Dietary Supplements.* https://ods.od.nih.gov/factsheets/Molybdenum-HealthProfessional/

124 Novotny J.A. (2011). Molybdenum Nutriture in Humans. *Journal of Evidence-Based Integrative Medicine* 6(3): 164-168. https://doi.org/10.1177/2156587211406732

125 Patience S. (2018). Iodine deficiency: Britain's hidden nutrition crisis. *Independent Nurse.* https://www.independentnurse.co.uk/clinical-article/iodine-deficiency-britains-hidden-nutrition-crisis/174833/

126 Editorial (2016). Iodine deficiency in the UK: grabbing the low-hanging fruit. *The Lancet. Diabetes & Endocrinology, 4*(6), 469. https://doi.org/10.1016/S2213-8587(16)30055-9

127 Linus Pauling Institute (2015). Iodine. *Micronutrient Information Center, Oregon State University*. https://lpi.oregonstate.edu/mic/minerals/iodine

128 L. Harder S. Dudazy-Gralla H. Müller-Fielitz J. Hjerling Leffler B. Vennström H. Heuer J. Mittag (2018). Maternal thyroid hormone is required for parvalbumin neurone development in the anterior hypothalamic area, *Journal of Neuroendocrinology*, 30(3), pp. https://doi.org/10.1111/jne.12573

129 Aceves, C., Mendieta, I., Anguiano, B., & Delgado-González, E. (2021). Molecular Iodine Has Extrathyroidal Effects as an Antioxidant, Differentiator, and Immunomodulator. *International Journal of Molecular Sciences*, 22(3), 1228. https://doi.org/10.3390/ijms22031228

130 Bilal, M. Y., Dambaeva, S., Kwak-Kim, J., Gilman-Sachs, A., & Beaman, K. D. (2017). A Role for Iodide and Thyroglobulin in Modulating the Function of Human Immune Cells. *Frontiers in Immunology*, 8, 1573. https://doi.org/10.3389/fimmu.2017.01573

131 National Institutes of Health (2022). Fact Sheet for Health Professionals. Iodine. *Office of Dietary Supplements*. https://ods.od.nih.gov/factsheets/Iodine-HealthProfessional/

132 Eveleigh, E. R., Coneyworth, L. J., Avery, A., & Welham, S. (2020). Vegans, Vegetarians, and Omnivores: How Does Dietary Choice Influence Iodine Intake? A Systematic Review. *Nutrients*, 12(6), 1606. https://doi.org/10.3390/nu12061606

133 Tai S.Y, Hung N.H., Lin T.C., (2014). Analysis of iodine content in seaweed by GC.ECD and estimation of iodine intake. *Journal of Food and Drug Analysis* 22(2): 189-196. https://doi.org/10.1016/j.jfda.2014.01.014

134 Woodside, J. V., & Mullan, K. R. (2021). Iodine status in UK-An accidental public health triumph gone sour. *Clinical Endocrinology*, 94(4), 692–699. https://doi.org/10.1111/cen.14368

135 Price, C. T., Langford, J. R., & Liporace, F. A. (2012). Essential Nutrients for Bone Health and a Review of their Availability in the Average North American Diet. *The Open Orthopaedics Journal*, 6, 143–149. https://doi.org/10.2174/1874325001206010143

136 Pizzorno L. (2015). Nothing Boring About Boron. *Integrative Medicine*, 14(4), 35–48. https://www.ncbi.nlm.nih.gov/pmc/articles/PMC4712861/

137 Nielsen F. H. (2008). Is boron nutritionally relevant? *Nutrition Reviews*, 66(4), 183–191. https://doi.org/10.1111/j.1753-4887.2008.00023.x

138 Nielsen F.H., Meacham S.L., (2011). Growing Evidence for Human Health Benefits of Boron. *Journal of Evidence-Based Integrative Medicine* 16(3):169-180. https://doi.org/10.1177/2156587211407638

139 National Institutes of Health (2022). Fact Sheet for Health Professionals. Boron. *Office of Dietary Supplements*. https://ods.od.nih.gov/factsheets/Boron-HealthProfessional/

140 Koshiba, T., Kobayashi, M., & Matoh, T. (2009). Boron deficiency: how does the defect in cell wall damage the cells?. *Plant Signaling & Behavior*, 4(6), 557–558. https://doi.org/10.1093/pcp/pcn184

141 Wang, N., Yang, C., Pan, Z., Liu, Y., & Peng, S. (2015). Boron deficiency in woody plants: various responses and tolerance mechanisms. *Frontiers in Plant Science*, 6, 916. https://doi.org/10.3389/fpls.2015.00916

142 Jugdaohsingh R. (2007). Silicon and bone health. *The Journal of Nutrition, Health & Aging*, 11(2), 99–110. https://www.ncbi.nlm.nih.gov/pmc/articles/PMC2658806/

143 Domingo, J. L., Gómez, M., & Colomina, M. T. (2011). Oral silicon supplementation: an effective therapy for preventing oral aluminum absorption and retention in mammals. *Nutrition Reviews*, 69(1), 41–51. https://doi.org/10.1111/j.1753-4887.2010.00360.x

144 Price C. T., Koval K. J., Langford J. R., (2012). Silicon: A Review of Its Potential Role in the Prevention and Treatment of Postmenopausal Osteoporosis. *International Journal of Endocrinology*, 2013, 316783. https://doi.org/10.1155/2013/316783

145 Farooq, M. A., & Dietz, K. J. (2015). Silicon as Versatile Player in Plant and Human Biology: Overlooked and Poorly Understood. *Frontiers in Plant Science*, *6*, 994. https://doi.org/10.3389/fpls.2015.00994

146 Blondeau, N., Lipsky, R. H., Bourourou, M., Duncan, M. W., Gorelick, P. B., & Marini, A. M. (2015). Alpha-linolenic acid: an omega-3 fatty acid with neuroprotective properties-ready for use in the stroke clinic? *BioMed Research International*, *2015*, 519830. https://doi.org/10.1155/2015/519830

147 Leikin-Frenkel A. I. (2016). Is there A Role for Alpha-Linolenic Acid in the Fetal Programming of Health? *Journal of Clinical Medicine*, *5*(4), 40. https://doi.org/10.3390/jcm5040040

148 Connor W. E. (1999). Alpha-linolenic acid in health and disease. *The American Journal of Clinical Nutrition*, *69*(5), 827–828. https://doi.org/10.1093/ajcn/69.5.827

149 Bjerve, K. S., Fischer, S., Wammer, F., & Egeland, T. (1989). alpha-Linolenic acid and long-chain omega-3 fatty acid supplementation in three patients with omega-3 fatty acid deficiency: effect on lymphocyte function, plasma and red cell lipids, and prostanoid formation. *The American Journal of Clinical Nutrition*, *49*(2), 290–300. https://doi.org/10.1093/ajcn/49.2.290

150 National Institutes of Health (2022). Fact Sheet for Health Professionals. Omega-3 fatty acids. *Office of Dietary Supplements*. https://ods.od.nih.gov/factsheets/Omega3FattyAcids-HealthProfessional/

151 Brenna, J. T., Salem, N., Jr, Sinclair, A. J., Cunnane, S. C., & International Society for the Study of Fatty Acids and Lipids, ISSFAL (2009). alpha-Linolenic acid supplementation and conversion to n-3 long-chain polyunsaturated fatty acids in humans. *Prostaglandins, Leukotrienes, and Essential Fatty Acids*, *80*(2-3), 85–91. https://doi.org/10.1016/j.plefa.2009.01.004

152 Derbyshire E. (2019). Oily Fish and Omega-3s Across the Life Stages: A Focus on Intakes and Future Directions. *Frontiers in Nutrition*, *6*, 165. https://doi.org/10.3389/fnut.2019.00165

153 Cholewski, M., Tomczykowa, M., & Tomczyk, M. (2018). A Comprehensive Review of Chemistry, Sources and Bioavailability of Omega-3 Fatty Acids. *Nutrients*, *10*(11), 1662. https://doi.org/10.3390/nu10111662

154 Yagi, S., Hara, T., Ueno, R., Aihara, K., Fukuda, D., Takashima, A., Hotchi, J., Ise, T., Yamaguchi, K., Tobiume, T., Iwase, T., Yamada, H., Soeki, T., Wakatsuki, T., Shimabukuro, M., Akaike, M., & Sata, M. (2014). Serum concentration of eicosapentaenoic acid is associated with cognitive function in patients with coronary artery disease. *Nutrition Journal*, *13*(1), 112. https://doi.org/10.1186/1475-2891-13-112

155 Linus Pauling Institute (2019). Essential Fatty Acids. Micronutrient Information Center, *Oregon State University*. https://lpi.oregonstate.edu/mic/other-nutrients/essential-fatty-acids

156 Panel on Dietetic Products, Nutrition and Allergies (2012). Scientific Opinion on the Tolerable Upper Intake Level of eicosapentaenoic acid (EPA), docosahexaenoic acid (DHA) and docosapentaenoic acid (DPA). *EFSA Journal 10*(7). https://doi.org/10.2903/j.efsa.2012.2815

157 Stark, K. D., Van Elswyk, M. E., Higgins, M. R., Weatherford, C. A., & Salem, N., Jr (2016). Global survey of the omega-3 fatty acids, docosahexaenoic acid and eicosapentaenoic acid in the blood stream of healthy adults. *Progress in Lipid Research*, *63*, 132–152. https://doi.org/10.1016/j.plipres.2016.05.001

158 Stanhiser, J., Jukic, A., McConnaughey, D. R., & Steiner, A. Z. (2022). Omega-3 fatty acid supplementation and fecundability. *Human Reproduction*, *37*(5), 1037–1046. https://doi.org/10.1093/humrep/deac027

159 Whelan, J., & Fritsche, K. (2013). Linoleic acid. *Advances in Nutrition*, *4*(3), 311–312. https://doi.org/10.3945/an.113.003772

160 Tallima, H., & El Ridi, R. (2017). Arachidonic acid: Physiological roles and potential health benefits - A review. *Journal of Advanced Research, 11*, 33–41. https://doi.org/10.1016/j.jare.2017.11.004

161 Marklund, M., Wu, J., Imamura, F., Del Gobbo, L. C., Fretts, A., de Goede, J., Shi, P., Tintle, N., Wennberg, M., Aslibekyan, S., Chen, T. A., de Oliveira Otto, M. C., Hirakawa, Y., Eriksen, H. H., Kröger, J., Laguzzi, F., Lankinen, M., Murphy, R. A., Prem, K., Samieri, C., (2019) Cohorts for Heart and Aging Research in Genomic Epidemiology (CHARGE) Fatty Acids and Outcomes Research Consortium (FORCE). Biomarkers of Dietary Omega-6 Fatty Acids and Incident Cardiovascular Disease and Mortality. *Circulation, 139*(21), 2422–2436. https://doi.org/10.1161/CIRCULATIONAHA.118.038908

162 Patterson, E., Wall, R., Fitzgerald, G. F., Ross, R. P., & Stanton, C. (2012). Health implications of high dietary omega-6 polyunsaturated Fatty acids. *Journal of Nutrition and Metabolism, 2012*, 539426. https://doi.org/10.1155/2012/539426

163 Simopoulos A. P. (2011). Importance of the omega-6/omega-3 balance in health and disease: evolutionary aspects of diet. *World Review of Nutrition and Dietetics, 102*, 10–21. https://doi.org/10.1159/000327785

164 DiNicolantonio, J. J., & O'Keefe, J. H. (2018). Importance of maintaining a low omega-6/omega-3 ratio for reducing inflammation. *BMJ Open Heart, 5*(2), e000946. https://doi.org/10.1136/openhrt-2018-000946

165 Qu, H., Guo, M., Chai, H., Wang, W. T., Gao, Z. Y., & Shi, D. Z. (2018). Effects of Coenzyme Q10 on Statin-Induced Myopathy: An Updated Meta-Analysis of Randomized Controlled Trials. *Journal of the American Heart Association, 7*(19), e009835. https://doi.org/10.1161/JAHA.118.009835

166 Linus Pauling Institute (2018). Coenzyme Q10. *Micronutrient Information Center, Oregon State University*. https://lpi.oregonstate.edu/mic/dietary-factors/coenzyme-Q10

167 Hargreaves, I., Heaton, R. A., & Mantle, D. (2020). Disorders of Human Coenzyme Q10 Metabolism: An Overview. *International Journal of Molecular Sciences, 21*(18), 6695. https://doi.org/10.3390/ijms21186695

168 Zozina, V. I., Covantev, S., Goroshko, O. A., Krasnykh, L. M., & Kukes, V. G. (2018). Coenzyme Q10 in Cardiovascular and Metabolic Diseases: Current State of the Problem. *Current Cardiology Reviews, 14*(3), 164–174. https://doi.org/10.2174/1573403X14666180416115428

169 Zhang, S. Y., Yang, K. L., Zeng, L. T., Wu, X. H., & Huang, H. Y. (2018). Effectiveness of Coenzyme Q10 Supplementation for Type 2 Diabetes Mellitus: A Systematic Review and Meta-Analysis. *International Journal of Endocrinology, 2018*, 6484839. https://doi.org/10.1155/2018/6484839

170 Dhanasekaran, M., & Ren, J. (2005). The emerging role of coenzyme Q-10 in aging, neurodegeneration, cardiovascular disease, cancer and diabetes mellitus. *Current Neurovascular Research, 2*(5), 447–459. https://doi.org/10.2174/156720205774962656

171 Yeung, C. K., Billings, F. T., 4th, Claessens, A. J., Roshanravan, B., Linke, L., Sundell, M. B., Ahmad, S., Shao, B., Shen, D. D., Ikizler, T. A., & Himmelfarb, J. (2015). Coenzyme Q10 dose-escalation study in hemodialysis patients: safety, tolerability, and effect on oxidative stress. *BMC Nephrology, 16*, 183. https://doi.org/10.1186/s12882-015-0178-2

172 Saini R. (2011). Coenzyme Q10: The essential nutrient. *Journal of Pharmacy & Bioallied Sciences, 3*(3), 466–467. https://doi.org/10.4103/0975-7406.84471

173 Barcelos, I. P., & Haas, R. H. (2019). CoQ10 and Aging. *Biology, 8*(2), 28. https://doi.org/10.3390/biology8020028

174 Kim, H. P., Son, K. H., Chang, H. W., & Kang, S. S. (2004). Anti-inflammatory plant flavonoids and cellular action mechanisms. *Journal of Pharmacological Sciences, 96*(3), 229–245. https://doi.org/10.1254/jphs.crj04003x

175 Zeng, Y., Song, J., Zhang, M., Wang, H., Zhang, Y., & Suo, H. (2020). Comparison of In Vitro and In Vivo Antioxidant Activities of Six Flavonoids with Similar Structures. *Antioxidants*, *9*(8), 732. https://doi.org/10.3390/antiox9080732

176 Kopustinskiene, D. M., Jakstas, V., Savickas, A., & Bernatoniene, J. (2020). Flavonoids as Anticancer Agents. *Nutrients*, *12*(2), 457. https://doi.org/10.3390/nu12020457

177 Shamsudin, N. F., Ahmed, Q. U., Mahmood, S., Ali Shah, S. A., Khatib, A., Mukhtar, S., Alsharif, M. A., Parveen, H., & Zakaria, Z. A. (2022). Antibacterial Effects of Flavonoids and Their Structure-Activity Relationship Study: A Comparative Interpretation. *Molecules*, *27*(4), 1149. https://doi.org/10.3390/molecules27041149

178 Aboody, M., & Mickymaray, S. (2020). Anti-Fungal Efficacy and Mechanisms of Flavonoids. *Antibiotics*, *9*(2), 45. https://doi.org/10.3390/antibiotics9020045

179 Pei R., Lui X., Bolling B., (2020). Flavonoids and gut health. *Current Opinion in Biotechnology 61*:153-159. https://doi.org/10.1016/j.copbio.2019.12.018

180 Ullah, A., Munir, S., Badshah, S. L., Khan, N., Ghani, L., Poulson, B. G., Emwas, A. H., & Jaremko, M. (2020). Important Flavonoids and Their Role as a Therapeutic Agent. *Molecules*, *25*(22), 5243. https://doi.org/10.3390/molecules25225243

181 Vogiatzoglou, A., Mulligan, A. A., Lentjes, M. A., Luben, R. N., Spencer, J. P., Schroeter, H., Khaw, K. T., & Kuhnle, G. G. (2015). Flavonoid intake in European adults (18 to 64 years). *PloS One*, *10*(5), e0128132. https://doi.org/10.1371/journal.pone.0128132

182 Waheed Janabi, A. H., Kamboh, A. A., Saeed, M., Xiaoyu, L., BiBi, J., Majeed, F., Naveed, M., Mughal, M. J., Korejo, N. A., Kamboh, R., Alagawany, M., & Lv, H. (2020). Flavonoid-rich foods (FRF): A promising nutraceutical approach against lifespan-shortening diseases. *Iranian Journal of Basic Medical Sciences*, *23*(2), 140–153. https://doi.org/10.22038/IJBMS.2019.35125.8353

Index

Note: Page locators followed by *f* and *t* indicate figures and tables, respectively.